Renal
Physiology

Renal
Physiology

Second Edition

Bruce M. Koeppen, MD, PhD

Professor of Medicine & Physiology
Dean, Academic Affairs and Education
University of Connecticut Health Center
Farmington, Connecticut

Bruce A. Stanton, PhD

Professor of Physiology
Department of Physiology
Dartmouth Medical School
Hanover, New Hampshire

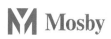 Mosby

St. Louis Baltimore Boston Carlsbad Chicago Naples New York Philadelphia Portland
London Madrid Mexico City Singapore Sydney Tokyo Toronto Wiesbaden

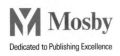

Mosby
Dedicated to Publishing Excellence

A Times Mirror Company

Vice President and Publisher: Anne S. Patterson
Editor: Emma D. Underdown
Developmental Editor: Christy Wells
Project Manager: Linda McKinley
Production Editor: René Spencer
Designer: Elizabeth Fett
Manufacturing Supervisor: Linda Ierardi

SECOND EDITION

Copyright © 1997 by Mosby–Year Book, Inc.

Previous edition copyrighted 1992

Printed in the United States of America
Composition by Top Graphics
Lithography/color film by Top Graphics
Printing/binding by R.R. Donnelley & Sons Co.

Mosby–Year Book, Inc.
11830 Westline Industrial Drive
St. Louis, Missouri 63146

Library of Congress Cataloging in Publication Data
Koeppen, Bruce M.
    Renal physiology / Bruce M. Koeppen, Bruce A. Stanton. — 2nd ed.
      p. cm.
    Includes bibliographical references and index.
    ISBN 0-8151-5202-7
    1. Kidneys—Physiology.   2. Water-electrolyte balance (Physiology)
  I. Stanton, Bruce A. II. Title.
    [DNLM: 1. Kidney—physiology. WJ 301 K78r 1996]
  QP249.K64 1996
  612.4'63—dc20
  DNLM/DLC
  for Library of Congress   96-16798
                                                 CIP

97 98 99 00 01 / 9 8 7 6 5 4 3 2 1

This book is dedicated to our students.
They have challenged and inspired us to be better teachers,
and for this we are indebted to them, because in the process of being their teachers
we too have learned much. Thank you.

Preface

In this, the second edition, we have maintained our original goal to write a textbook that provides the basics of renal physiology for the health professions student studying the kidney for the first time. In addition to updating all chapters, we have added new emphasis to several topics, including renal blood flow, calcium and phosphate homeostasis, and the renal adaptation to progressive nephron loss. As a study aid, an additional appendix summarizes the function of each nephron segment. In addition to a multiple-choice examination, clinical cases were included to assist the student in integrating the material. Answers are provided for student self-evaluation. Finally, we have emphasized the clinical relevance of important physiologic principles in boxes throughout the text. For every addition that we made, we deleted material where appropriate. Thus, the second edition is similar to the first in length.

To the instructor: This book is intended to provide students in the biomedical and health sciences with a basic understanding of the workings of the kidneys. We feel it is better for the student at this stage to master a few central concepts and ideas rather than assimilate a large array of facts. Consequently, this book is designed to teach the important aspects and fundamental concepts of normal renal function. We have em-

phasized clarity and conciseness in presenting the material. To accomplish this goal, we have been selective in the material included. The broader field of nephrology, with its current and future frontiers, is better learned at a later time and only after the "big picture" has been well established. For clarity and simplicity, we have made statements as assertions of fact, even though we recognize that not all aspects of a particular problem have been resolved.

To the student: As an aid to learning this material, each chapter includes a listing of objectives that reflect the fundamental concepts to be mastered. At the end of each chapter, we have provided a summary and a listing of key words and concepts that should serve as a checklist while working through the chapter. We have also provided a series of self-study questions. These questions review the central principles to be mastered. Because these questions are learning tools, answers and explanations are provided in an appendix. A multiple-choice exam and comprehensive clinical cases are included in another appendix. We recommend working through these tests and clinical cases only after completing the book. In this way they can serve to indicate where additional work or review is required.

We have provided an updated annotated bibliography of selected books, monographs, and papers. This highly selective bibliography is intended to provide the next step in the study of the kidney; it is a place to begin to add details to the subjects presented here and a resource for exploring other aspects of the kidney not treated in this book.

We encourage all who use this book to send us your comments and suggestions. Please let us know what we've done right, as well as what needs improvement.

Acknowledgments: We thank our students at the University of Connecticut Medical School and Dartmouth Medical School and our colleagues, who made helpful comments and suggestions on the first edition of this book. Most of their suggestions and comments have been incorporated into this edition. We thank Drs. Nancy Adams, William Arendhorst, Peter Friedman, Andre Kaplan, John Mills, David Pollack, Brian Remillard, and Cynthia Short, who read early versions of the second edition and provided excellent criticism and suggestions. We also thank Emma Underdown and Christy Wells at Mosby for their support and commitment to quality and Karen Majeski for her help in preparing the manuscript.

Bruce M. Koeppen
Bruce A. Stanton

Contents

Introduction to the Kidney

"The kidney presents in the highest degree the phenomenon of sensibility, the power of reacting to various stimuli in a direction which is appropriate for the survival of the organism; a power of adaptation which almost gives one the idea that its component parts must be endowed with intelligence."

E. Starling - 1909

As Starling recognized, the kidneys are viewed more appropriately as regulatory, rather than excretory, organs. However, it is clear that the excretory function of the kidneys is central to their ability to regulate the composition and volume of the body fluids.

In this book, various aspects of renal physiology are explored. Emphasis is placed on providing insight and understanding into the major functions of the kidneys, which are as follows:

- Regulation of body fluid osmolality and volume
- Regulation of electrolyte balance
- Regulation of acid-base balance
- Excretion of metabolic products and foreign substances
- Production and secretion of hormones

In the chapters that follow, these aspects of renal function are considered in detail. However, in order to provide a broad perspective and overview, they are briefly described here.

Regulation of body fluid osmolality and volume (Chapters 1, 5, and 6): The kidneys are critical components of the system involved in the control of both the osmolality and volume of the body fluids. The control of body fluid osmolality is important for the maintenance of normal cell volume in virtually all tissues of the body, and control of the volume of body fluids is necessary for normal function of the cardiovascular system. The kidneys, working in an integrated fashion with components of the cardiovascular and central nervous systems, accomplish these tasks by regulating the excretion of water and NaCl.

Regulation of electrolyte balance (Chapters 4, 5, 6, 7, 8, and 9): The kidneys play an essential role in regulating the amount of several important inorganic ions in the body, including sodium (Na^+), potassium (K^+), chloride (Cl^-), bicarbonate (HCO_3^-), hydrogen ion (H^+), calcium (Ca^{++}), and phosphate (Pi). The kidneys also contribute to the maintenance of organic ion balance. For example, the excretion of many of the intermediates of the Krebs cycle (e.g., citrate, succinate) is controlled by the kidneys. In order to maintain appropriate balance the excretion of any one of these electrolytes must be balanced to the daily intake. If intake exceeds excretion, the amount of a particular electrolyte in the body increases. Conversely, if excretion exceeds intake, the amount decreases. For many of these electrolytes the kidney is the sole or primary route for excretion from the body. Thus, electrolyte balance is achieved by carefully matching daily excretion by the kidneys with daily intake.

Regulation of acid-base balance (Chapter 8): Many of the metabolic functions of the body are exquisitely sensitive to pH. Thus, the pH of the body fluids must be maintained within very narrow limits. This is accomplished by buffers within the body fluids and the coordinated action of the lungs and kidneys. The importance of the kidneys in acid-base balance is underscored by the fact that acid accumulates in the body fluids of individuals with reduced renal function.

Excretion of metabolic products and foreign substances (Chapters 3 and 4): The kidneys excrete a number of end products of metabolism that are no longer needed by the body. These so-called waste products include urea (from amino acids), uric acid (from nucleic acids), creatinine (from muscle creatine), end products of hemoglobin metabolism, and metabolites of hormones. These substances are eliminated from the body by the kidneys at a rate that matches their production. Thus, their concentrations within the body fluids are maintained at a constant level. The kidneys also represent an important route for elimination of foreign substances from the body, including drugs, pesticides, and other chemicals ingested in the food. When kidney function is compromised, metabolic waste products and foreign substances accumulate in the body because their excretion in the urine decreases.

Production and secretion of hormones (Chapters 6 and 9): The kidneys are important endocrine organs, producing and secreting renin, calcitriol (1,25-dihydroxyvitamin D_3), and erythropoietin. Renin activates the renin-angiotensin-aldosterone system, which is important in regulating blood pressure, as well as sodium and potassium balance. Calcitriol is necessary for normal reabsorption of Ca^{++} by the gastrointestinal tract and for its deposition in bone. With renal disease the ability of the kidneys to produce calcitriol is impaired, and levels of this hormone are reduced. As a result, Ca^{++} reabsorption by the intestine is decreased. This reduced intestinal Ca^{++} reabsorption contributes to the abnormalities in bone formation seen in patients with chronic renal disease. Erythropoietin stimulates red blood cell formation by the bone marrow. With many kidney diseases, erythropoietin production and secretion is reduced, which by decreasing erythrocyte production is a causal factor in the anemia seen in chronic renal failure.

In the following chapters various aspects of these important renal functions are considered. Where information is available, these functions are considered at several levels of organization: whole kidney, single nephron, individual tubular cell, cell membrane, and transport protein.

Adaptation to nephron loss (Chapter 11): An overriding theme of this book is the ability of the kidneys to respond to the homeostatic needs of the individual. The degree to which renal function can be regulated to meet these needs is truly impressive. For example, urine volume can vary from 0.5 to 18 L/day. However, the limits of renal function are infrequently reached in healthy individuals. It is useful to study diseased kidneys to appreciate the extremes to which kidneys can function. Consequently a brief discussion of the physiologic adaptation to nephron loss is presented. This section emphasizes the ability of the kidneys to maintain fluid, electrolyte, and acid-base balance as the number of functioning nephrons is reduced by disease processes.

Physiology of Body Fluids

OBJECTIVES

Upon completion of this chapter the student should be able to answer the following questions:

1. How do the body fluid compartments differ with respect to their volumes and ionic compositions?
2. What are the driving forces responsible for movement of water across cell membranes and the capillary wall?
3. How do the volumes of the intracellular and extracellular fluid compartments change under various pathophysiologic conditions?

In addition, the student should be able to define and understand the following properties of physiologically important solutions and fluids:

1. Molarity and equivalence
2. Osmotic pressure
3. Osmolarity and osmolality
4. Oncotic pressure
5. Tonicity

One of the major functions of the kidneys is to maintain the volume and composition of the body fluids despite wide variation in the daily intake of water and solutes. In this chapter the volume and composition of the body fluids is discussed to provide a background for the study of the kidneys as regulatory organs. Some of the basic principles, terminology, and concepts related to the properties of solutes in solution are also reviewed.

■ PHYSICOCHEMICAL PROPERTIES OF ELECTROLYTE SOLUTIONS

Molarity and Equivalence

The amount of a substance dissolved in a solution (i.e., its concentration) is expressed either in terms of **molarity** or **equivalence.** Molarity is the amount of a substance relative to its molecular weight. For example, glucose has a molecular weight of 180 g/mol. If 1 L of water contains 1 g of glucose, the molarity of this glucose solution would be determined as follows:

$$\frac{1 \text{ g/L}}{180 \text{ g/mol}} = 0.0056 \text{ mol/L or } 5.6 \text{ mmole/L} \qquad (1\text{-}1)$$

For uncharged molecules, such as glucose and urea, concentrations in the body fluids are usually expressed in terms of molarity.[1] Because many of the substances of biological interest are present at very low concentrations, units are more frequently expressed in the millimolar range (mmole/L or mM).

The concentration of solutes, which normally dissociate into more than one particle when dissolved in solution (e.g., NaCl), is usually expressed in terms of equivalence. Equivalence refers to the stoichiometry of the interaction between cation and anion and is determined by the valence of these ions. For example, consider a 1 L solution containing 9 g of NaCl (molecular weight = 58.4 g/mol). The molarity of this solution is 154 mmole/L. Because NaCl dissociates into Na^+ and Cl^- ions, and assuming complete dissociation, this solution contains 154 mmole/L of Na^+ and 154 mmole/L of Cl^-. Since the valence of these ions is 1, these concentrations can also be expressed as milliequivalents (mEq) of the ion per liter (i.e., 154 mEq/L for Na^+ and Cl^-, respectively).

For univalent ions, such as Na^+ and Cl^-, concentrations expressed in terms of molarity and equivalence are identical. However, this is not true for ions having valences greater than 1. Ac-

cordingly, the concentration of Ca^{++} (molecular weight = 40.1 g/mol and valence = 2) in a 1 L solution containing 0.1 g of this ion could be expressed as follows:

$$\frac{0.1 \text{ g/L}}{40.1 \text{ g/mol}} = 2.5 \text{ mmole/L} \qquad (1\text{-}2)$$

$$= 2.5 \text{ mmole/L} \times 2 \text{ mEq/mmole} = 5 \text{ mEq/L}$$

Although some exceptions exist, it is customary to express concentrations of ions in milliequivalents per liter.

Osmosis and Osmotic Pressure

The movement of water across cell membranes occurs by the process of **osmosis.** The driving force for this movement is the osmotic pressure difference across the cell membrane. Figure 1-1 illustrates the concept of osmosis and the measurement of the osmotic pressure of a solution.

Compartments A and B are separated by a semipermeable membrane (i.e., the membrane is highly permeable to water but impermeable to solute). Compartment A contains a solute, whereas compartment B contains only distilled water. Over time, water will move by osmosis from compartment B to compartment A.[2] This will raise the level of fluid in compartment A and decrease the level in compartment B. At equilibrium the hydrostatic pressure exerted by the column of water (h) will stop the movement of water from compartment B to A. This pressure will be equal and opposite to the osmotic pressure exerted by the solute particles in compartment A.

Osmotic pressure is determined solely by the number of solute particles in that solution. It is not dependent on such factors as the size of

---

1 The units used to express the concentrations of substances in various body fluids differ among laboratories. The system of international units (SI) is used in most countries and in most scientific and medical journals in the United States. Despite this convention, traditional units are still widely used. For urea and glucose the traditional units of concentration are mg/dl (i.e., mg per deciliter or 100 ml), whereas the SI units are mmol/L. Similarly, electrolyte concentrations are traditionally expressed as mEq/L, while the SI units are mmol/L (see Appendix B).

---

2 This water movement is driven by the concentration gradient for water. Because of the presence of solute particles in compartment A, its concentration of water is less than that in compartment B. Consequently, water moves across the semipermeable membrane from compartment B to compartment A down its gradient.

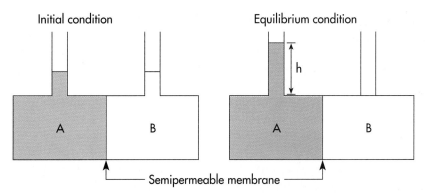

Initial condition

Equilibrium condition

A

B

A

B

h

Semipermeable membrane

Figure 1-1 ■ **Schematic representation of osmotic water movement and the generation of an osmotic pressure. The solute particles in compartment _A_ cause water to move by osmosis from compartment _B_ across the semipermeable membrane into compartment _A_. The water column in compartment A will rise until the hydrostatic pressure generated by the water column _(h)_ stops the flow of water from compartment _B_ into compartment _A_. This hydrostatic pressure is equal to the osmotic pressure generated by the solution in compartment _A_.**

the solute particles, their mass, or their chemical nature (e.g., valence). Osmotic pressure (π), measured in atmospheres (atm), is calculated by **van't Hoff's law** as follows:

$$\pi = nCRT \qquad (1\text{-}3)$$

where:

n = Number of dissociable particles per molecule
C = Total solute concentration
R = Gas constant
T = Temperature in degrees Kelvin (°K)

For a molecule that does not dissociate in water, such as glucose or urea, a solution containing 1 mmole/L of this solute at 37° C can exert an osmotic pressure of 2.54×10^{-2} atm as calculated by equation 1-3 using the following values:

n = 1
C = 0.001 mol/L
R = 0.082 atm L/mol °K
T = 310 °K

Because 1 atmosphere equals 760 mm Hg at sea level, π for this solution can also be expressed as 19.3 mm Hg.

Alternatively, osmotic pressure is expressed in terms of osmolarity (see below). Thus, a solution containing 1 mmole/L of solute particles exerts an osmotic pressure of 1 milliosmole/L (1 mOsm/L).

For substances that dissociate in a solution, n of equation 1-3 will have a value other than 1. For example, a 150 mmole/L solution of NaCl has an osmolarity of 300 mOsm/L, because each molecule of NaCl dissociates into a Na^+ and a Cl^- ion (i.e., n=2). If dissociation of a substance into its component ions is not complete, n will not be an integer. Accordingly, osmolarity for any solution can be calculated as follows:

$$(1\text{-}4)$$

Osmolarity = Concentration $\times$ # dissociable particles
mOsm/L = mmol/L $\times$ # particles/mole

Osmolarity and Osmolality

Osmolarity and **osmolality** are frequently confused and incorrectly interchanged. *Osmolarity* refers to the number of solute particles per 1 L of water, whereas *osmolality* is the number of solute particles in 1 kg of water. For dilute solutions the difference between osmolarity and osmolality is insignificant. Measurements of osmolarity are temperature dependent, because the volume of water varies with temperature (i.e., the volume is larger at higher temperatures). In contrast, osmolality, which is based on the mass of water, is temperature-independent. For this reason, *osmolality* is the preferred term for biologic systems and is used throughout this and subsequent chapters. Osmolality has the units of Osm/kg H_2O. Because of the dilute nature of physiologic solutions, osmolalities are expressed as milliosmoles per kilogram water (mOsm/kg H_2O).

Table 1-1 shows the relationship between molecular weight, equivalence, and osmoles for a number of physiologically significant solutes.

Tonicity

The **tonicity** of a solution is related to its effect on the volume of a cell. Solutions that do not change the volume of a cell are said to be **isotonic.** A **hypotonic** solution causes a cell to swell, whereas a **hypertonic** solution causes a cell to shrink. Although related to osmolality, tonicity also takes into consideration the ability of the solute to cross a cell membrane.

Consider two solutions: a 300 mmole/L solution of sucrose and a 300 mmole/L solution of urea. Both solutions have an osmolality of 300 mOsm/kg H_2O and are therefore isosmotic. When red blood cells, which for the purpose of this illustration also have an intracellular fluid osmolality of 300 mOsm/kg H_2O, are placed in the

TABLE 1-1

Units of measurement for physiologically significant substances

Substance	Atomic/molecular weight	Equivalents/mol	Osmoles/mol
Na^+	23.0	1	1
K^+	39.1	1	1
Cl^-	35.4	1	1
HCO_3^-	61.0	1	1
Ca^{++}	40.1	2	1
P_i	95.0	3	1
NH_4^+	18.0	1	1
NaCl	58.4	2[a]	2[b]
$CaCl_2$	111	4[c]	3
Glucose	180	—	1
Urea	60	—	1

a. One equivalent each for Na^+ and Cl^-.

b. NaCl does not dissociate completely in solution. The actual osmoles/mole is 1.88. However, for simplicity a value of 2 is often used.

c. Ca^{++} contributes two equivalents, as do the Cl^- ions.

two solutions, those in the sucrose solution maintain their normal volume, whereas those placed in urea swell and eventually burst. Thus the sucrose solution is isotonic, and the urea solution is hypotonic. The differential effect of these solutions on red cell volume is related to the permeability of the plasma membrane to sucrose and urea. The red cell membrane is highly permeable to urea but impermeable to sucrose.

To exert an osmotic pressure across a membrane, a solute must not permeate that membrane. Because the red cell membrane is impermeable to sucrose, sucrose exerts an osmotic pressure equal and opposite to the osmotic pressure generated by the contents of the red cell (in this case 300 mOsm/kg H_2O). In contrast, urea is readily able to cross the red blood cell membrane, and it cannot exert an osmotic pressure to balance that generated by the intracellular solutes of the red blood cell.[3] Consequently, sucrose is termed an *effective osmole,* whereas urea is referred to as an *ineffective osmole.*

To take into account the effect on osmotic pressure of a solute's ability to permeate the membrane, it is necessary to rewrite equation 1-3 as:

$$\pi = \sigma(nCRT) \qquad (1\text{-}5)$$

where sigma (σ) is termed the *reflection coefficient* or *osmotic coefficient* and is a measure of the relative ability of the solute to cross a cell membrane.

For a solute that can freely cross the cell membrane, such as urea, $\sigma=0$, and no effective osmotic pressure is exerted. A substance of this type is said to be an ineffective osmole. In con-

trast, $\sigma=1$ for a solute that cannot cross the cell membrane. Such a substance is said to be an effective osmole. Many solutes are neither completely able nor completely unable to cross cell membranes (i.e., $0<\sigma<1$) and generate an osmotic pressure that is only a fraction of what is expected from the total solute concentration.

Oncotic Pressure

Oncotic pressure is the osmotic pressure generated by large molecules (especially proteins) in solution. As illustrated in Figure 1-2, the magnitude of the osmotic pressure generated by a solution of protein does not conform to van't Hoff's law. The cause of this anomalous relationship between protein concentration and osmotic pressure is not completely understood but appears to be related to the size and shape of the molecule. For example, the correlation to van't Hoff's law is more precise with small, globular proteins than with larger protein molecules.

The oncotic pressure exerted by proteins in human plasma has a normal value of approximately 26-28 mm Hg. Although this pressure appears to be small when considered in terms of osmotic pressure (28 mm Hg $\approx$ 1.4 mOsm/kg H_2O), it is an important force involved in fluid movement across capillaries (details on this topic are presented below in the section of fluid exchange between body fluid compartments).

Specific Gravity

The total solute concentration in a solution can also be measured as **specific gravity.** *Specific gravity* is defined as the weight of a volume of solution divided by the weight of an equal volume of distilled water. Thus the specific gravity of distilled water is 1 g/ml. Because biological fluids contain a number of different substances, their specific gravities are greater than 1 g/ml. For example, normal human plasma has a specific gravity in the range of 1.008-1.010 g/ml.

---

3 Urea traverses the plasma membrane of red blood cells via a specific transport protein, with the driving force for movement being the urea concentration gradient. Thus, when the red cell is placed in the urea solution, urea enters the cell down its concentration gradient.

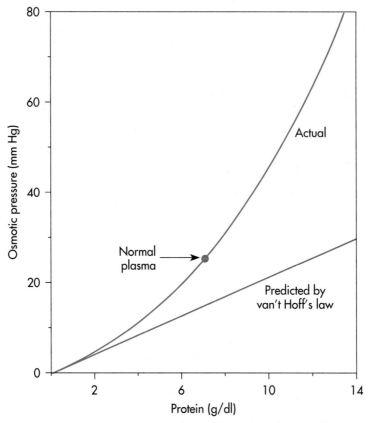

Figure 1-2 ■ **Relationship between the concentration of plasma proteins in solution and the osmotic pressure (oncotic pressure) they generate. Protein concentration is expressed as g/dl. Normal plasma protein concentration is indicated. Note how the actual pressure generated exceeds that predicted by van't Hoff's law.**

The specific gravity of urine is measured in clinical settings and used to assess the concentrating ability of the kidneys. The specific gravity of urine varies in proportion to its osmolality. However, because specific gravity depends on both the number and weight of solute particles, the relationship between specific gravity and osmolality is not always predictable. For example, patients who have been injected with radiocontrast dye (molecular weight > 500 g/mole) for x-ray studies can have high values of urine specific gravity (1.040-1.050) even though the urine osmolality is similar to that of plasma (e.g., 300 mOsm/kg H_2O).

■ **VOLUMES OF BODY FLUID COMPARTMENTS**

Water makes up approximately 60% of the body's weight, with variability among individuals being a function of the amount of adipose tissue. Because the water content of adipose tissue is lower than that of other tissue, increased amounts of adipose tissue reduce the fraction of total body weight due to water. The percentage of body weight attributed to water also varies with age. In newborns, it is approximately 75%. This decreases to the adult value of 60% by the age of 1 year.

As illustrated in Figure 1-3, **total body water** is distributed between two major compartments,

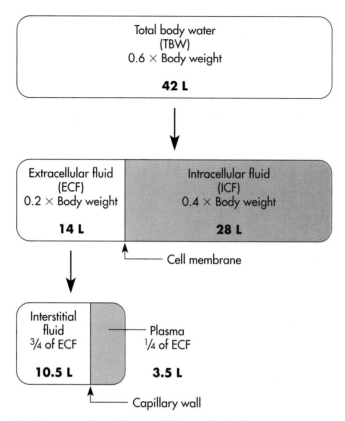

Figure 1-3 ■ **Relationship between the volumes of the major body fluid compartments. The actual values shown are calculated for a 70 kg individual.**

which are divided by the cell membrane.[4] The **intracellular fluid (ICF)** compartment is the larger compartment and contains approximately two thirds of the total body water. The remaining one third is contained in the **extracellular fluid (ECF)** compartment. Expressed as percentages of body weight, the volumes of total body water, ICF, and ECF are as follows:

Total body water $= 0.6 \times$ (Body weight)
ICF $= 0.4 \times$ (Body weight)
ECF $= 0.2 \times$ (Body weight)

The ECF compartment is further subdivided into **interstitial fluid** and **plasma,** which are separated by the capillary wall. The interstitial fluid surrounds the cells in the various tissues of the body and accounts for three fourths of the ECF volume. The ECF includes water contained within the bone and dense connective tissue. Plasma represents the remaining one fourth of the extracellular fluid.

---

4 In these and all subsequent calculations, it is assumed that 1 L of fluid (e.g., ICF and ECF) has a mass of 1 kg. This allows conversion from measurements of body weight to volume of body fluids.

■ COMPOSITION OF BODY FLUID COMPARTMENTS

Sodium is the major cation of the ECF, and Cl^- and HCO_3^- are the major anions. The ionic composition of the interstitial fluid and plasma in the ECF is similar, because these compartments are separated by only the capillary endothelium, a barrier that is freely permeable to small ions. The major difference between the interstitial fluid and plasma is that the latter contains significantly more protein. This differential concentration of protein can affect the distribution of cations and anions between these two compartments, because plasma proteins have a net negative charge and tend to increase the cation concentrations and reduce the anion concentrations in the plasma compartment. However, this effect is small, and the ionic compositions of the interstitial fluid and plasma can be considered identical. Because of its abundance, Na^+ (and its attendant anions, primarily Cl^- and HCO_3^-) is the major determinant of ECF osmolality. Accordingly, a rough estimate of the ECF osmolality can be obtained by simply doubling the sodium concentration $[Na^+]$. For example, if the plasma $[Na^+]$ is 145 mEq/L, the osmolality of plasma and ECF can be estimated as follows:

$$\text{Plasma Osmolality} = 2(\text{Plasma } [Na^+]) \qquad (1\text{-}6)$$
$$= 290 \text{ mOsm/kg } H_2O$$

Because water is in osmotic equilibrium across the capillary endothelium and the plasma membrane of cells, measurement of the plasma osmolality also provides a measure of the osmolality of ECF and ICF.

    In contrast to the ECF, the $[Na^+]$ of ICF is extremely low. K^+ is the predominant cation of this compartment. This asymmetric distribution of Na^+ and K^+ across the plasma membrane is maintained by the activity of the ubiquitous Na^+-K^+-ATPase. By its action, Na^+ is extruded from the cell in exchange for K^+. The anion composition of the ICF also differs markedly from that of the ECF, with the $[Cl^-]$ and $[HCO_3^-]$ of the ICF being lower in comparison. The major ICF anions are phosphates, organic anions, and protein. Figure 1-4 summarizes the ECF and ICF concentrations of some cations and anions.

■ FLUID EXCHANGE BETWEEN BODY FLUID COMPARTMENTS

Water moves freely between the various body fluid compartments. Two forces determine this movement: hydrostatic pressure and osmotic pressure. Hydrostatic pressure from the pumping of the heart and osmotic pressure by plasma proteins (oncotic pressure) are important determinants of fluid movement across the capillary wall. Because hydrostatic pressure gradients are not present across the cell membrane, only osmotic pressure differences between ICF and ECF cause fluid movement into and out of cells.

In clinical situations a more accurate estimate of the plasma osmolality is obtained by also considering the contribution of glucose and urea to the plasma osmolality. Accordingly, plasma osmolality can be estimated as follows:

$$\text{Plasma Osmolality} = 2(\text{Plasma } [Na^+]) \qquad (1\text{-}7)$$
$$+ \frac{[\text{glucose}]}{18} + \frac{[\text{BUN}]}{2.8}$$

The glucose and urea concentrations are expressed in units of mg/dl (dividing by 18 for glucose and 2.8 for urea[5] allows conversion from the units of mg/dl to mmole/L and thus to mOsm/kg H_2O). This estimation of plasma osmolality is especially useful when dealing with patients who have an elevated plasma [glucose] secondary to diabetes mellitus and patients with chronic renal failure, whose plasma [urea] is elevated.

---

5 The [urea] in plasma is measured as the nitrogen in the urea molecule, or blood urea nitrogen (BUN).

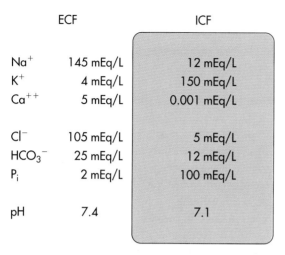

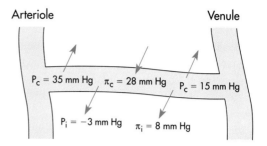

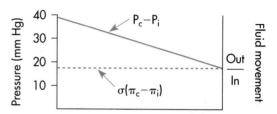

Figure 1-4 ■ Concentrations of some cations and anions between the extracellular fluid *(ECF)* and intracellular fluid *(ICF)*. The ICF concentrations are estimates from skeletal muscle and include amounts bound to intracellular proteins and free within the cytosol. Intracellular P_i is primarily in the form of organic molecules (e.g., ATP).

Capillary Fluid Exchange

The movement of fluid across a **capillary wall** is determined by the algebraic sum of the hydrostatic and oncotic pressures as expressed by the following equation **(Starling forces)**:

$$\text{Fluid Movement} = K_f[(P_c - P_i) - \sigma(\pi_c - \pi_i)] \quad (1\text{-}8)$$

where:

K_f = Filtration coefficient of the capillary wall
P_c = Hydrostatic pressure within the capillary lumen
π_c = Oncotic pressure of the plasma
P_i = Hydrostatic pressure of the interstitium
π_i = Oncotic pressure of the interstitial fluid
σ = Reflection coefficient for proteins across the capillary wall

The Starling forces for capillary fluid exchange vary between tissues and organs. Figure 1-5 illus-

Figure 1-5 ■ *Upper panel*, Schematic representation of the Starling forces responsible for the filtration and absorption of fluid across the wall of a typical skeletal muscle capillary. P_c = capillary hydrostatic pressure; P_i = interstitial hydrostatic pressure; π_c = capillary oncotic pressure; π_1 = interstitial oncotic pressure. Note that P_c decreases from the arteriole end to the venule end of the capillary, whereas all the other Starling forces are constant along the length of the capillary. Fluid filtered into the interstitium is taken up by the lymphatics and returned to the vascular system via the thoracic duct (not shown). *Lower panel*, Graph of hydrostatic and oncotic pressure differences along the capillary. (In this example $\sigma = 0.9$.) Net fluid movement across the wall of the capillary is also indicated. Note that fluid is filtered along the entire length of the capillary.

trates these forces as they have been estimated for a capillary bed located in skeletal muscle at rest.

The **filtration coefficient** (K_f) of a capillary reflects the intrinsic permeability of the capillary wall to the movement of fluid, as well as the surface area available for filtration. The K_f varies among different capillary beds. For example, the

K_f of glomerular capillaries in the kidneys is approximately 100 times greater in magnitude than that of skeletal muscle capillaries. This difference in K_f accounts for the large volume of fluid filtered across glomerular capillaries compared to the amount filtered across skeletal muscle capillaries (see Chapter 3).

The hydrostatic pressure within the lumen of a capillary (P_c) is a force for the movement of fluid from the lumen into the interstitium. Its magnitude depends upon arterial pressure, venous pressure, and precapillary (arteriolar) and postcapillary (venular and small vein) resistances. An increase in the arterial or venous pressures results in an increase in P_c, and a decrease in these pressures has the opposite effect. P_c increases with either a decrease in precapillary resistance or an increase in postcapillary resistance. Likewise, an increase in precapillary resistance or a decrease in postcapillary resistance decreases P_c. For virtually all capillary beds, precapillary resistance is greater than postcapillary resistance. Consequently, changes in venous pressure have a greater effect on P_c than do changes in arterial pressure. The magnitude of P_c varies among not only tissues but capillary beds within a given tissue, and it is also dependent upon the physiological state of the tissue.

The hydrostatic pressure within the interstitium (P_i) is difficult to measure, but in the absence of edema (abnormal accumulation of fluid in the interstitium), its value is near zero or slightly negative. Thus, under normal conditions, it will cause fluid to move out of the capillary. However, when there is edema, P_i is positive and it opposes the movement of fluid out of the capillary (see Chapter 6).

The oncotic pressure of plasma proteins (π_c) retards the movement of fluid out of the capillary lumen. At a normal plasma protein concentration, π_c has a value of approximately 26-28 mm Hg. The degree to which oncotic pressure influences capillary fluid movement depends on the permeability of the capillary wall to the protein molecules. If the capillary wall is highly permeable to protein, σ is near zero and the oncotic pressure generated by plasma proteins plays little or no role in capillary fluid exchange. This situation is seen in the capillaries of the liver (i.e., hepatic sinusoids), which are highly permeable to proteins. As a result the protein concentration of the interstitial fluid is essentially the same as that of plasma. In the capillaries of skeletal muscle $\sigma \approx 0.9$, whereas in the glomeruli of the kidneys the value is essentially 1. Therefore plasma protein oncotic pressure plays an important role in fluid movement across these capillary beds.

The protein that leaks across the capillary wall into the interstitium exerts oncotic pressure (π_i) and promotes the movement of fluid out of the capillary lumen. In skeletal muscle capillaries under normal conditions, π_i is small and has a value of only 8 mm Hg.

As depicted in Figure 1-5, the balance of Starling forces across muscle capillaries causes fluid to leave the lumen (filtration) along its entire length. This filtered fluid is then returned to the circulation via the lymphatics. The sinusoids of the liver also filter along their entire length. In contrast, the balance of forces across capillaries of the gastrointestinal tract and brain results in net fluid absorption.

Cellular Fluid Exchange

Osmotic pressure differences between ECF and ICF are responsible for fluid movement between these compartments. Because the plasma membranes of cells are highly permeable to water, a change in the osmolality of either the ICF or ECF results in rapid movement (i.e., minutes) of water between these compartments. Thus, **except for transient changes, the ICF and ECF compartments are in osmotic equilibrium.**

In contrast to water, the movement of ions across cell membranes is more variable and depends on the presence of specific membrane

Neurosurgical procedures and cerebral vascular accidents (strokes) frequently result in the accumulation of interstitial fluid in the brain (i.e., edema) and swelling of the neurons. Because the brain is enclosed within the skull, edema can raise intracranial pressure and thereby disrupt neuronal function, leading to coma and death. The blood-brain barrier, which separates the cerebral spinal fluid and brain interstitial fluid from blood, is freely permeable to water but not to most other substances. As a result, excess fluid in brain tissue can be removed by imposing an osmotic gradient across the blood-brain barrier. Mannitol can be used for this purpose. Mannitol is a sugar (molecular weight = 182 g/mole) that does not readily cross the blood-brain barrier and membranes of cells (neurons as well as other cells in the body). Therefore mannitol is an effective osmole, and intravenous infusion results in the movement of fluid from the brain tissue by osmosis.

transport proteins. Consequently, as a first approximation, fluid exchange between ICF and ECF under pathophysiological conditions can be analyzed by assuming that appreciable shifts of ions between the compartments do not occur.

A useful approach for understanding the movement of fluids between ICF and ECF is outlined on p. 12. To illustrate this approach, consider what happens when solutions containing various amounts of NaCl are added to the ECF.[6]

6 Fluids are usually administered intravenously. When electrolyte solutions are infused by this route there is rapid (i.e., minutes) equilibration between plasma and interstitial fluid, because of the high permeability of the capillary wall to water and electrolytes. Thus, these fluids are essentially added to the entire ECF.

Example #1 - Addition of Isotonic NaCl to the ECF Addition of an isotonic NaCl solution (e.g., intravenous infusion of 0.9% NaCl: osmolality ≈ 290 mOsm/kg H_2O)[7] to the ECF increases the volume of this compartment by the volume of fluid administered. Because this fluid has the same osmolality as the ECF and therefore also the ICF, there will be no driving force for fluid movement between these compartments, and the volume of the ICF will be unchanged. Although Na^+ can cross cell membranes, it is effectively restricted to the ECF by the activity of the Na^+-K^+-ATPase, which is present in all cells. There is therefore no net movement of the infused NaCl into the cells.

Example #2 - Addition of Hypotonic NaCl to the ECF Addition of a hypotonic NaCl solution to the ECF (e.g., intravenous infusion of 0.45% NaCl: osmolality ≈ 145 mOsm/kg H_2O) decreases the osmolality of this compartment, resulting in the movement of water into the ICF. After osmotic equilibration the osmolalities of the ICF and ECF are equal but lower than before the infusion, and the volume of each compartment is increased. The increase in ECF volume is greater than the increase in ICF volume.

Example #3 - Addition of Hypertonic NaCl to the ECF Addition of a hypertonic NaCl solution to the ECF (e.g., intravenous infusion of 3% NaCl: osmolality ≈ 1000 mOsm/kg H_2O) increases the osmolality of this compartment, resulting in the movement of water out of cells. After osmotic equilibration the osmolality of the ECF and ICF will be equal. The volume of the ECF is increased, whereas that of the ICF is decreased.

Table 1-2 summarizes the effects of various solutions on the volume and osmolality of the ECF and ICF.

7 A 0.9% NaCl solution has a concentration of 154 mEq/L. Because NaCl does not dissociate completely (i.e., 1.88 osmoles/mole), the osmolality of this solution is 290 mOsm/kg H_2O.

Principles for Analysis of Fluid Shifts between the ICF and ECF

- The volumes of the various body fluid compartments can be estimated in the normal adult by the following:

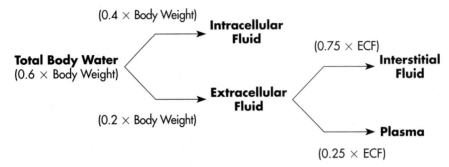

- All exchanges of water and solutes with the external environment occur through the ECF (e.g., intravenous infusion and intake or loss via the gastrointestinal tract). Changes in the ICF are secondary to fluid shifts between the ECF and ICF. Fluid shifts occur only if the perturbation of the ECF alters its osmolality.
- Except for brief periods of seconds to minutes, the ICF and ECF are in osmotic equilibrium. A measurement of plasma osmolality will provide a measure of both ECF and ICF osmolality.
- For the sake of simplification, it can be assumed that equilibration between the ICF and ECF occurs only by movement of water and not by movement of osmotically active solutes.
- Conservation of mass must be maintained, especially when considering either addition or removal of water and/or solutes from the body.

TABLE 1-2

Effects of NaCl solutions on body fluid volumes and osmolality

	ΔTBW (L)	ΔICF (L)	ΔECF (L)	ICF & ECF osmolality (mOsm/kg H$_2$O)
+ Isotonic NaCl (0.9%)	+1	0	+1	290
− Isotonic NaCl (0.9%)	−1	0	−1	290
+ Hypotonic NaCl (0.45%)	+1	+0.32	+0.68	287
− Hypotonic NaCl (0.45%)	−1	−0.33	−0.67	293
+ Hypertonic NaCl (3%)	+1	−1.6	+2.6	307
− Hypertonic NaCl (3%)	−1	+1.85	−2.85	272

Changes shown indicate the effect of addition to (+) or removal of (−) 1L of the indicated solution from the ECF of a 70 kg individual. Initial values: TBW = 42 L, ICF = 28 L, ECF = 14 L, and osmolality = 290 mOsm/kg H$_2$O.

Intravenous solutions are available in many formulations. The type of fluid administered to a particular patient is dictated by the patient's need. For example, if an increase in the patient's vascular volume is necessary, a solution containing substances that do not readily cross the capillary wall is infused (e.g., 5% albumin solution). The oncotic pressure generated by the albumin molecules retains fluid in the vascular compartment, expanding its volume. Expansion of the ECF is accomplished most often using isotonic saline solutions (e.g., 0.9% NaCl). As already noted, administration of an isotonic NaCl solution does not result in the development of an osmotic pressure gradient across the plasma membrane of cells. Therefore the entire volume of infused solution will remain in the ECF.

Patients whose body fluids are hyperosmotic need hypotonic solutions. These solutions may be hypotonic NaCl (e.g., 0.45% NaCl or 5% dextrose in water, D5W). Administration of the D5W solution is equivalent to infusion of distilled water, because the dextrose is metabolized to CO_2 and water. Administration of these fluids increases the volumes of both the ICF and ECF. Finally, patients whose body fluids are hypotonic need hypertonic solutions. These are typically NaCl-containing solutions (e.g., 3% and 5% NaCl). These solutions expand the volume of the ECF but decrease the volume of the ICF. Other constituents, such as electrolytes (e.g., K^+) or drugs, can be added to intravenous solutions to tailor the therapy to the patient's fluid, electrolyte, and metabolic needs.

■ SUMMARY

1. Water is a major constituent of the human body, composing 60% of the body weight. Body water is divided between two major compartments: the intracellular fluid (ICF) and the extracellular fluid (ECF). Two thirds of the water is in the ICF, and one third is in the ECF. Osmotic pressure gradients between the ICF and ECF drive water movement between these compartments. Because the plasma membrane of most cells is highly permeable to water, the ICF and ECF are in osmotic equilibrium.

2. The ECF is divided into a vascular compartment (plasma) and an interstitial fluid compartment. Starling forces across capillaries determine the exchange of fluid between these compartments.

3. Sodium is the major cation of the ECF. Potassium is the major ICF cation. This asymmetric distribution of Na^+ and K^+ is maintained by the activity of the Na^+-K^+-ATPase.

■ KEY WORDS AND CONCEPTS

- Molarity
- Equivalence
- Osmosis
- Osmotic pressure
- van't Hoff's law
- Osmolarity and osmolality
- Oncotic pressure
- Tonicity (isotonic, hypotonic, and hypertonic)
- Specific gravity
- Effective and ineffective osmole
- Total body water
- Intracellular fluid
- Extracellular fluid
- Interstitial fluid
- Plasma
- Capillary fluid exchange
- Starling forces
- Capillary filtration coefficient (K_f)
- Cellular fluid exchange

■ SELF-STUDY PROBLEMS

1. Calculate the molarity and osmolality of a 1 L solution containing the following solutes. Assume complete dissociation of all electrolytes.

		Molarity (mmole/L)	Osmolality (mOsm/kg H$_2$O)
9 g	NaCl	_____	_____
72 g	Glucose	_____	_____
22.2 g	CaCl$_2$	_____	_____
3 g	Urea	_____	_____
8.4 g	NaHCO$_3$	_____	_____

2. The intracellular contents of a cell generate an osmotic pressure of 300 mOsm/kg H$_2$O. The cell is placed in a solution containing 300 mmole/L of a solute (x). If solute x remains a single particle in solution and has a reflection coefficient of 0.5, what will happen to the volume of the cell in this solution? What would be the composition of an isotonic solution (i.e., a solution that will not cause a change in the volume of the cell) containing substance x?

3. An individual's plasma [Na$^+$] is measured and found to be 130 mEq/L (normal = 145 mEq/L). What is the individual's estimated plasma osmolality? What effect will the lower-than-normal plasma [Na$^+$] have on water movement across cell plasma membranes? Across the capillary endothelium?

4. Figure 1-5 illustrates the normal values for the Starling forces involved in fluid movement across a typical skeletal muscle capillary. Draw the new hydrostatic ($P_c - P_i$) and oncotic $\sigma(\pi_c - \pi_i)$ pressure curves if P_c at the venous end of the capillary was increased to 20 mm Hg. What effect would this have on fluid exchange across the capillary wall?

5. A 60 kg individual has an episode of gastroenteritis with vomiting and diarrhea. Over a 2-day period, this individual loses 4 kg of body weight. Before becoming ill, this individual had a plasma [Na$^+$] of 140 mEq/L, which was unchanged by the illness. Assuming the entire loss of body weight represents the loss of fluid (a reasonable assumption), estimate the following:

Initial conditions (before gastroenteritis)

Total body water:	_____	L
ICF volume:	_____	L
ECF volume:	_____	L
Total body osmoles:	_____	mOsm
ICF osmoles:	_____	mOsm
ECF osmoles:	_____	mOsm

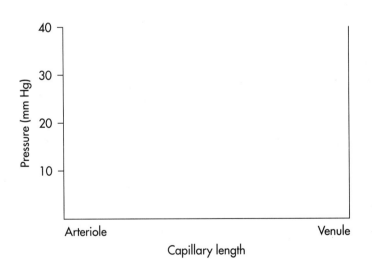

New equilibrium conditions (after gastroenteritis)

Total body water: _____ L
ICF volume: _____ L
ECF volume: _____ L
Total body osmoles: _____ mOsm
ICF osmoles: _____ mOsm
ECF osmoles: _____ mOsm

6. A 50 Kg individual with a plasma $[Na^+]$ of 145 mEq/L is infused with 5 g/kg of mannitol (molecular weight of mannitol = 182 g/mole) to reduce brain swelling following a stroke. After equilibration, estimate the following, assuming mannitol is restricted to the ECF compartment, no excretion occurs, and the infusion volume of the mannitol solution is negligible (total body water unchanged):

Initial conditions (before mannitol infusion)

Total body water: _____ L
ICF volume: _____ L
ECF volume: _____ L
Total body osmoles: _____ mOsm
ICF osmoles: _____ mOsm
ECF osmoles: _____ mOsm

**New equilibrium conditions
(after mannitol infusion)**

Total body water: _____ L
ICF volume: _____ L
ECF volume: _____ L
Total body osmoles: _____ mOsm
ICF osmoles: _____ mOsm
ECF osmoles: _____ mOsm
Plasma osmolality: _____ mOsm/kg H_2O
Plasma $[Na^+]$: _____ mEq/L

7. A 5% dextrose solution is isosmotic to plasma. What effect would infusion of 2 L of a 5% dextrose solution have on the volumes of the ECF and ICF and body fluid osmolality of a 65 kg individual, and why?

8. Two normal individuals, each weighing 70 kg with a P_{osm} = 290 mOsm/kg H_2O, excrete the following urine over the same time period:

Individual A: 1 L of urine having an osmolality of 1200 mOsm/kg H_2O.
Individual B: 3 L of urine having an osmolality of 300 mOsm/kg H_2O.

If neither individual has any fluid intake, who will have the higher plasma osmolality?

Structure and Function of the Kidneys and the Lower Urinary Tract

OBJECTIVES

Upon completion of this chapter the student should be able to answer the following questions:

1. Which structures in the renal corpuscle are filtration barriers to plasma proteins?
2. What is the physiologic significance of the juxtaglomerular apparatus?
3. What blood vessels supply the kidneys?
4. What nerves innervate the kidneys?
5. How does the urinary bladder store urine and eliminate it from the body?

In addition, the student should be able to describe the following:

1. The location of the kidneys and their gross anatomical features.
2. The different parts of the nephron and their location within the cortex and medulla.
3. The components of the renal corpuscle and the cell types located in each component.
4. The anatomy of the lower urinary tract.

■ STRUCTURE OF THE KIDNEYS

Structure and function are closely linked in the kidneys. Consequently, an appreciation of the gross anatomic and histologic features of the kidneys is a prerequisite for an understanding of their function.

Gross Anatomy

The kidneys are paired organs that lie on the posterior wall of the abdomen, behind the peritoneum on either side of the vertebral column. In the adult human, each kidney weighs between 115 and 170 g and is approximately 11 cm in length, 6 cm in width, and 3 cm thick.

The gross anatomical features of the human kidney are illustrated in Figure 2-1. The medial side of each kidney contains an indentation through which pass the renal artery and vein, nerves, and pelvis. On the cut surface of a bisected kidney, two regions are evident: an outer

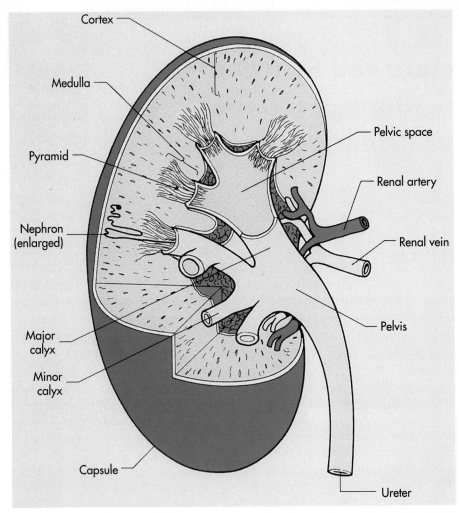

Cortex

Medulla

Pyramid

Nephron
(enlarged)

Major
calyx

Minor
calyx

Capsule

Pelvic space

Renal artery

Renal vein

Pelvis

Ureter

Figure 2-1 ■ Structure of the human kidney, cut open to show internal structures. (Modified from Marsh DJ: *Renal physiology,* New York, 1983, Raven.)

region called the **cortex,** and an inner region called the **medulla.** The cortex and medulla are composed of **nephrons** (the functional units of the kidney), blood vessels, lymphatics, and nerves. The medulla in the human kidney is divided into 8 to 18 conical masses, the **renal pyramids.** The base of each pyramid originates at the corticomedullary border, and the apex terminates in a papilla, which lies within a **calyx.** The **pelvis** represents the upper expanded region of the ureter, which carries urine from the pelvis to the urinary bladder. In the human kidney the pelvis divides into two or three open-ended pouches, the **major calyces,** which extend outward from the dilated end of the pelvis. Each major calyx divides into **minor calyces,** which collect the urine from each papilla. The walls of the calyces, pelvis, and ureters contain smooth muscle that contracts to propel the urine toward the **urinary bladder.**

The blood flow to the two kidneys is equal to about 25% (1.25 L/min) of the cardiac output in resting individuals. However, the kidneys constitute less than 0.5% of the total body weight. As illustrated in Figure 2-2 *(left panel),* the renal artery branches to form progressively the **interlobar artery, arcuate artery, interlobular artery** (cortical radial artery), and **afferent arteriole,** which leads into the glomerular capillaries (i.e., **glomerulus**). The glomerular capillaries coalesce to form the **efferent arteriole,** which leads into a second capillary network, the peritubular capillaries, which supply blood to the nephron. The vessels of the venous system run parallel to the arterial vessels and form progressively the interlobular vein (cortical radial vein), the arcuate vein, the interlobar vein, and the renal vein, which courses beside the ureter.

Ultrastructure of the Nephron
The functional unit of the kidneys is the nephron. Each human kidney contains approximately 1.2 million nephrons, which are hollow tubes composed of a single cell layer (Figure 2-2, *right panel).* The nephron consists of a renal corpuscle, proximal tubule, loop of Henle, distal tubule, and collecting duct system.[8] The **renal corpuscle** consists of glomerular capillaries and

Bowman's capsule. The **proximal tubule** initially forms several coils, followed by a straight piece that descends toward the medulla. The next segment is **Henle's loop,** which is composed of the straight part of the proximal tubule, the **descending thin limb** (which ends in a hairpin turn), the **ascending thin limb** (only in nephrons with long loops of Henle), and the **thick ascending limb.** Near the end of the thick ascending limb the nephron passes between the afferent and efferent arterioles of the same nephron. This short segment of the thick ascending limb is called the *macula densa.* The **distal tubule** begins a short distance beyond the macula densa and extends to the point in the cortex where two or more nephrons join to form a **cortical collecting duct.** The cortical collecting duct enters the medulla and becomes the **outer medullary collecting duct** and then the **inner medullary collecting duct.**

Each nephron segment is composed of cells that are uniquely suited to perform specific transport functions (Figure 2-3). Proximal tubule cells have an extensively amplified apical membrane (the urine side of the cell) called the *brush border,* which is only present in the proximal tubule. The basolateral membrane (the blood side of the cell) is highly invaginated. These invaginations contain many mitochondria. In contrast, the descending and ascending thin limbs of Henle's loop have poorly developed apical and basolateral surfaces and few mitochondria. The cells of the thick ascending limb and the distal tubule have abundant mitochondria and extensive infoldings of the basolateral membrane. The collecting duct is composed of two cell types: principal cells and intercalated cells. **Principal cells** have a moderately invaginated basolateral membrane and contain few mitochondria. **Intercalated cells** have a high density of mitochondria. The final segment of the nephron, the inner medullary collecting duct, is composed of inner medullary collecting duct cells. Cells of the

---

8 The organization of the nephron is actually more complicated than presented here. However, for simplicity and clarity of presentation in subsequent chapters the nephron is divided into five segments. For details on the subdivisions of the five nephron segments, consult the references by Kriz and Bankir, Kriz and Kaissling, and Tisher and Madsen. The collecting duct system is not actually part of the nephron. However, for simplicity, we consider the collecting duct system part of the nephron.

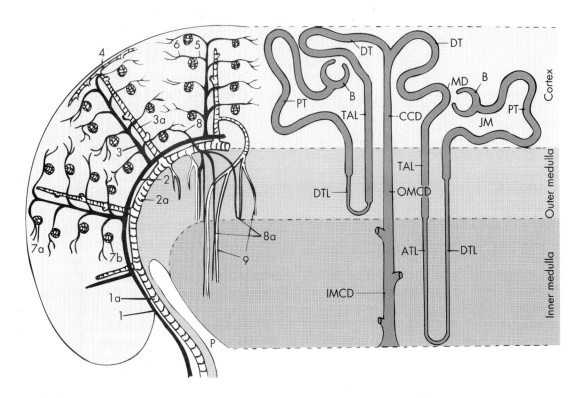

Figure 2-2 ■ *Left panel,* Organization of the vascular system of the human kidney (not drawn to scale). Scheme depicts the course and distribution of the intrarenal blood vessels; peritubular capillaries are not shown. The renal artery branches to form interlobar arteries *(1),* which give rise to arcuate arteries *(2).* Arcuate arteries lead to interlobular arteries *(3),* which radiate toward the renal capsule and branch to form afferent arterioles *(5).* Afferent arterioles branch to form glomerular capillary networks (i.e., glomeruli: *7A, 7B),* which then coalesce to form efferent arterioles *(6).* The efferent arterioles of the superficial nephrons form capillary networks (not shown) that suffuse the cells in the cortex. The efferent arterioles of the juxtamedullary nephrons divide into descending vasa recta *(8),* which form capillary networks that supply blood to the outer and inner medulla *(8a).* Blood from the peritubular capillaries enters consecutively the stellate vein *(4),* interlobular vein *(3a),* arcuate vein *(2a),* and interlobar vein *(1a).* Blood from the ascending vasa recta *(9)* enters the interlobular and arcuate veins. *P,* Pelvis. (Modified from Kriz W, Bankir LA: A standard nomenclature for structures of the kidney, *Am J Physiol* 254:F1, 1988.) *Right panel,* Organization of the human nephron. A superficial nephron is illustrated on the left, and a juxtamedullary nephron is illustrated on the right. Not drawn to scale. *B,* Bowman's capsule; *DT,* distal tubule; *PT,* proximal tubule; *CCD,* cortical collecting duct; *TAL,* thick ascending limb; *DTL,* descending thin limb; *OMCD,* outer medullary collecting duct; *ATL,* ascending thin limb; *IMCD,* inner medullary collecting duct; *MD,* macula densa. The loop of Henle includes the straight portion of the PT and the DTL, ATL, and TAL. (Modified from Koushanpour E, Kriz W: *Renal physiology: principles, structure, and function,* ed 2, New York, 1986, Springer-Verlag, and from Kriz W, Bankir L: A standard nomenclature for structures of the kidney, *Am Physiol* 254: F1, 1988.)

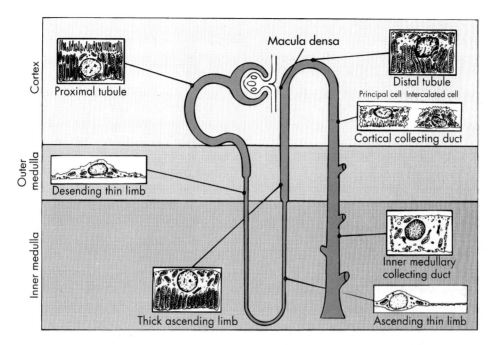

Figure 2-3 ■ Diagram of a nephron, including the cellular ultrastructure.

inner medullary collecting duct have poorly developed apical and basolateral surfaces and few mitochondria.

Nephrons may be subdivided into **superficial** and **juxtamedullary** types (Figure 2-2, *right panel)*. The renal corpuscle of each superficial nephron is located in the outer region of the cortex. Its loop of Henle is short, and its efferent arteriole branches into peritubular capillaries that surround the nephron segments of its own and adjacent nephrons. This capillary network conveys oxygen and important nutrients to the nephron segments, delivers substances to the nephron for secretion (i.e., the movement of a substance from the blood into the tubular fluid), and serves as a pathway for the return of reabsorbed water and solutes to the circulatory system. A few species, including humans, also possess very short **superficial nephrons** whose loops of Henle never enter the medulla.

The renal corpuscle of each juxtamedullary nephron is located in the region of the cortex adjacent to the medulla (Figure 2-2, *right panel)*. In comparison with the superficial nephrons the **juxtamedullary nephrons** differ anatomically in three important ways: (1) the renal corpuscle is larger, (2) the loop of Henle is longer and extends deeper into the medulla, and (3) the efferent arteriole forms not only a network of peritubular capillaries but also a series of vascular loops called the **vasa recta.** As illustrated in Figure 2-2 *(left panel)*, the vasa recta descend into the medulla where they form capillary networks that surround the **collecting ducts** and ascending limbs of Henle's loop. The blood returns to the cortex in the ascending vasa recta. **Although less than 0.7% of the renal blood flow enters the vasa recta, these vessels subserve important functions, including the following: conveying oxygen and impor-**

tant nutrients to nephron segments, delivering substances to the nephron for secretion, serving as a pathway for the return of
reabsorbed water and solutes to the circulatory system, and concentrating and diluting the urine. (You will learn more about urine
concentration and dilution in Chapter 5.)

Ultrastructure of the Renal Corpuscle

The first step in urine formation begins with the
ultrafiltration of plasma across the glomerular
capillaries (i.e., glomerulus). The term *ultrafiltration* refers to the passive movement of an essentially protein-free fluid from the glomerular
capillaries into Bowman's space. To appreciate
the process of ultrafiltration, it is important to describe the anatomy of the renal corpuscle. The
glomerulus consists of a network of capillaries
supplied by the afferent arteriole and drained by
the efferent arteriole (Figure 2-4). During development the glomerular capillaries press into the
closed end of the proximal tubule that forms
Bowman's capsule of a renal corpuscle. The capillaries are covered by epithelial cells, called
podocytes, which form the **visceral layer** of
Bowman's capsule (Figures 2-4 to 2-7). The visceral cells are reflected at the vascular pole to
form the **parietal layer** of Bowman's capsule.
The space between the visceral layer and the
parietal layer is called *Bowman's space,* which,
at the urinary pole of the glomerulus, becomes
the lumen of the proximal tubule.

The endothelial cells of glomerular capillaries
are covered by a basement membrane, which is
surrounded by podocytes (Figures 2-4 to 2-8).
The capillary endothelium, basement membrane,
and foot processes of podocytes form the so-
called **filtration barrier** (Figures 2-5 to 2-8).
The endothelium is fenestrated (i.e., contains 700
Å holes where $1 Å = 10^{-10}$ m) and is freely permeable to water; small solutes such as sodium,
urea, and glucose; and even small proteins, but
not to cells. Because endothelial cells express
negatively charged glycoproteins on their sur-

face, they can retard the filtration of large anionic
proteins. (See Chapter 3 for more details.) The
basement membrane, which is a porous matrix
of extracellular proteins, including type IV colla-
gen, laminin, fibronectin, and other negatively
charged proteins, is an important filtration barrier to plasma proteins. The podocytes, which
are endocytic (i.e., the process of endocytosis allows materials to enter the cell without passing
through the membrane), have long fingerlike processes that completely encircle the outer surface
of the capillaries (Figure 2-6). The processes of
the podocytes interdigitate to cover the basement membrane and are separated by gaps,
called **filtration slits.** Each filtration slit is
bridged by a thin diaphragm, which contains
pores with dimensions of 40 Å × 140 Å. Therefore the filtration slits retard the filtration of some
proteins and macromolecules that pass through
the endothelium and basement membrane. Because the endothelium, basement membrane,
and filtration slits contain negatively charged glycoproteins, some molecules are held back on the
basis of size and charge. For molecules with an
effective molecular radius between 20 Å and 42
Å, cationic molecules are filtered more readily
than anionic molecules. (See Chapter 3 for more
details.)

Nephrotic syndrome. The nephrotic syndrome is produced by a variety of disorders and
is characterized by an increase in the permeability of the glomerular capillaries to proteins.
The augmented permeability results in an increase in urinary protein excretion (proteinuria). Thus, the appearance of proteins in the
urine can indicate kidney disease. Individuals
with the nephrotic syndrome may also develop
edema and hypoalbuminemia as a result of the
proteinuria. (See Chapter 6.)

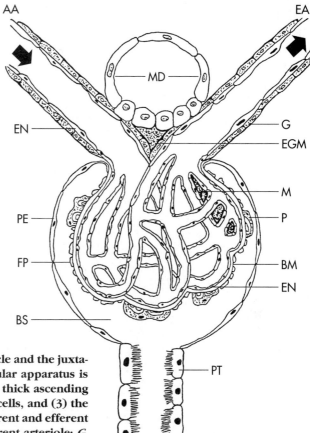

AA

EA

MD

EN

G

EGM

M

PE

P

FP

BM

EN

BS

PT

Figure 2-4 ■ **Anatomy of the renal corpuscle and the juxtaglomerular apparatus.** The juxtaglomerular apparatus is composed of (1) the macula densa of the thick ascending limb, (2) the extraglomerular mesangial cells, and (3) the renin-producing granular cells of the afferent and efferent arterioles. *AA,* Afferent arteriole; *EA,* efferent arteriole; *G,* granular cells of afferent and efferent arterioles; *MD,* macula densa; *BM,* basement membrane; *FP,* foot processes of podocyte; *P,* podocyte cell body (visceral cell layer); *M,* mesangial cells between capillaries; *EGM,* extraglomerular mesangial cells between the afferent and efferent arterioles; *EN,* endothelial cell; *PT,* proximal tubule cell; *BS,* Bowman's space; *PE,* parietal epithelium. (Modified from Koushanpour E, Kriz W: *Renal physiology: principles, structure, and function,* ed 2, Berlin, 1986, Springer-Verlag.)

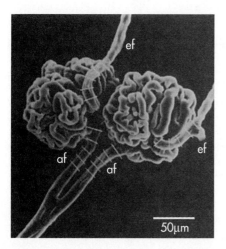

ef

af

ef

af

50μm

Figure 2-5 ■ **Scanning electron micrograph of interlobular artery *(IA),* afferent arteriole *(af);* efferent arteriole *(ef);* and glomerulus.** The white bars on the afferent and efferent arterioles indicate that they are about 15-20 μm in diameter. (From Kimura K and others: Effects of atrial natriuretic peptide on renal arterioles: morphometric analysis using microvascular casts, *Am J Physiol* 259:F936, 1990.)

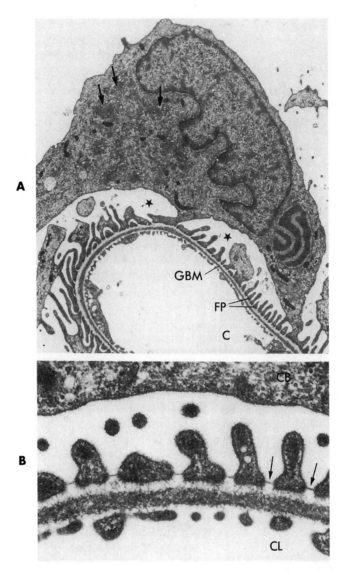

Figure 2-6 ■ A, Electron micrograph of a podocyte surrounding a glomerular capillary *(C)*. The cell body of the podocyte contains a large nucleus with three indentations. Cell processes of the podocyte form the interdigitating foot processes *(FP)*. The arrows in the cytoplasm of the podocyte indicate the well developed Golgi apparatus. *C*, Capillary lumen; *GBM*, glomerular basement membrane. *Stars* indicate Bowman's space. (Magnification ~ ×5700.) B, Electron micrograph of the filtration barrier of a glomerular capillary. *CL*, Capillary lumen; *CB*, cell body of a podocyte. The filtration barrier is composed of three layers: the endothelium, basement membrane, and foot processes of the podocytes. Note the diaphragm bridging the floor of the filtration slits *(arrows)*. (Magnification ~ ×42,700.) (Electron micrographs courtesy of Kriz W, Kaissling B: *Structural organization of the mammalian kidney.* In Seldin DW, Giebisch G, editors: *The kidney: physiology and pathophysiology,* ed 2, New York, 1992, Raven.)

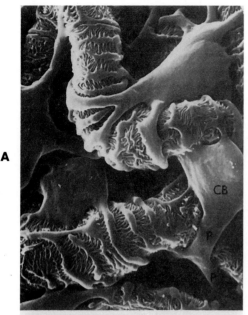

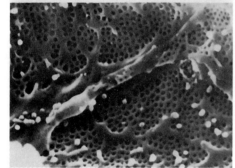

Figure 2-7 ■ A, Scanning electron micrograph showing the outer surface of glomerular capillaries. This is the view that would be seen from Bowman's space. Processes *(P)* of podocytes run from the cell body *(CB)* toward the capillaries, where they ultimately split into foot processes. Interdigitation of the foot processes creates the filtration slits. (Magnification ~ ×2500.) B, Scanning electron micrograph of the inner surface (blood side) of a glomerular capillary. This is the view that would be seen from the lumen of the capillary. The fenestrations of the endothelial cells are seen as small 700 Å holes. (Magnification ~ ×12000.) (Electron micrographs courtesy of Kriz W, Kaissling B: *Structural organization of the mammalian kidney.* In Seldin DW and Giebisch G, editors: *The kidney: physiology and pathophysiology,* ed 2, New York, 1992, Raven.)

> **Mesangial cells** are involved in the development of immune-complex–mediated glomerular disease. Because the glomerular basement membrane does not completely surround the glomerular capillaries (Figure 2-8), immune complexes can enter the mesangial area without crossing the glomerular basement membrane. Accumulation of immune complexes induces the infiltration of inflammatory cells into the mesangium and elicits the production of cytokines and autocoids by cells in the mesangium that enhance the inflammatory response. This inflammatory response can lead to scarring and eventually obliterates the glomerulus.

Another important component of the renal corpuscle is the **mesangium,** which consists of **mesangial cells** and the **mesangial matrix** (Figure 2-8). Mesangial cells are similar to monocytes and surround glomerular capillaries, provide structural support for the glomerular capillaries, secrete the extracellular matrix, exhibit phagocytic activity, and secrete prostaglandins and cytokines. Mesangial cells also contract, and because they are adjacent to glomerular capillaries, they may influence glomerular filtration rate by regulating blood flow through glomerular capillaries or altering the capillary surface area. (You will learn more about the factors that regulate glomerular filtration rate in Chapter 3.) Mesangial cells located outside the glomerulus (between the afferent and efferent arterioles) are called **extraglomerular mesangial cells** (or **lacis cells** or *Goormaghtigh cells*). Lacis cells, like mesangial cells, exhibit phagocytic activity.

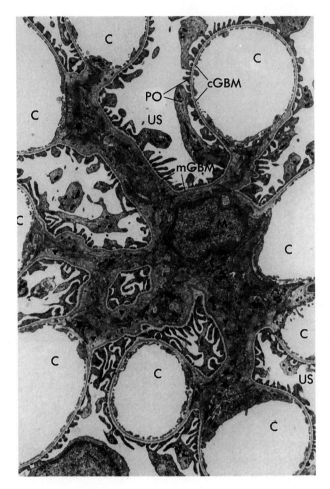

Figure 2-8 ■ Electron micrograph of the mesangium, the area between glomerular capillaries containing mesangial cells. *C,* **Glomerular capillaries;** *cGMB,* **capillary glomerular basement membrane surrounded by foot processes of podocytes** *(PO)* **and endothelial cells;** *mGMB,* **mesangial glomerular basement membrane surrounded by foot processes of podocytes and mesangial cells;** *M,* **mesangial cell that gives rise to several processes, some marked by stars;** *US,* **urinary space. Note the extensive extracellular matrix surrounded by mesangial cells (marked by** *triangles***). (Magnification ~ ×4100.)** (From Kriz W, Kaissling B: *Structural organization of the mammalian kidney.* In Seldin DW, Giebisch G, editors: *The kidney: physiology and pathophysiology,* ed 2, New York, 1992, Raven.)

Ultrastructure of the Juxtaglomerular Apparatus

The structures that compose the **juxtaglomerular apparatus** include:

1. The macula densa of the thick ascending limb
2. The extraglomerular mesangial cells
3. The renin-producing granular cells of the afferent and efferent arterioles (Figure 2-4).

Macula densa cells represent a morphologically distinct region of the thick ascending limb that passes through the angle formed by the afferent and efferent arterioles of the same nephron. The cells of the macula densa contact the extraglomerular mesangial cells and the granular cells of the afferent and efferent arterioles. Granular cells of the afferent and efferent arterioles are modified smooth muscle cells that manufacture, store, and release renin. Renin is involved in the formation of angiotensin II and ultimately in the secretion of aldosterone. (See Chapter 6.) The juxtaglomerular apparatus is one component of an important feedback mechanism (i.e., tubuloglomerular feedback mechanism) that is involved in the autoregulation of renal blood flow and the glomerular filtration rate. (You will learn more about this feedback mechanism in Chapter 3.)

Innervation of the Kidneys

Renal nerves help regulate renal blood flow, glomerular filtration rate, and salt and water reabsorption by the nephron. (Chapters 3 and 4 include a more complete discussion of the functional significance of renal nerves.) The nerve supply to the kidneys consists of sympathetic nerve fibers that originate mainly in the celiac plexus. There is no parasympathetic innervation. Adrenergic fibers that innervate the kidneys release norepinephrine and dopamine. The adrenergic fibers lie adjacent to the smooth muscle cells of the major branches of the renal artery (interlobar, arcuate, and interlobular arteries), and

the afferent and efferent arterioles. Moreover, the renin producing granular cells of the afferent and efferent arterioles are innervated by sympathetic nerves. Renin secretion is elicited by increased sympathetic activity. Nerve fibers also innervate the proximal tubule, loop of Henle, distal tubule, and collecting duct; activation of these nerves enhances sodium reabsorption by these nephron segments.

■ ANATOMY AND PHYSIOLOGY OF THE LOWER URINARY TRACT

Gross Anatomy and Histology

Once urine leaves the renal calyces and pelvis, it flows through the **ureters** and enters the urinary bladder, where urine is stored (Figure 2-9). The ureters are muscular tubes 30 cm long, and they enter the bladder on its posterior aspect near the base, above the bladder neck. The bladder is composed of two parts: the fundus, or body, which stores urine, and the neck, which is funnel-shaped and connects with the urethra. The bladder neck, which is 2 to 3 cm long, is also called the ***posterior urethra.*** In females the posterior urethra is the end of the urinary tract and the point of exit of urine from the body. In males, urine flows through the posterior urethra into the anterior urethra, which extends through the penis. Urine leaves the urethra through the external meatus.

The renal calyces, pelvis, ureter, and urinary bladder are lined with a transitional epithelium composed of several layers of cells: basal columnar cells, intermediate cuboidal cells, and superficial squamous cells. This epithelium is surrounded by a mixture of spiral and longitudinal smooth muscle fibers. The bladder is also lined with a transitional epithelium that is surrounded by a mixture of smooth muscle fibers, called the **detrusor muscle.** Detrusor muscle fibers are arranged at random. They form layers, except close to the bladder neck, where the fibers form three layers: inner longitudinal, middle circular, and

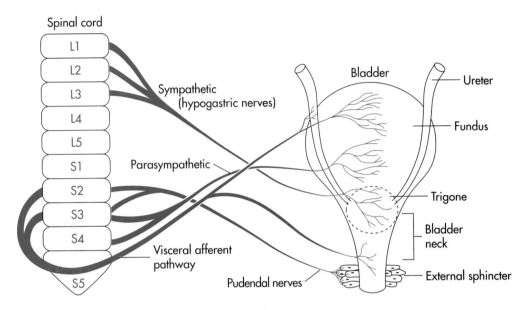

Figure 2-9 ■ Anatomy of the lower urinary tract and its innervation.

outer longitudinal. Muscle fibers in the bladder neck form the internal sphincter, which is not a true sphincter but a thickening of the bladder wall formed by converging muscle fibers. The internal sphincter is not under conscious control. Its inherent tone prevents emptying of the bladder until appropriate stimuli initiate urination. The urethra passes through the **urogenital diaphragm,** which contains a layer of skeletal muscle called the *external sphincter.* This muscle is under voluntary control and can be used to prevent or interrupt urination, especially in males. In females the external sphincter is poorly developed; thus, it is less important in voluntary bladder control. The smooth muscle cells in the lower urinary tract are electrically coupled, exhibit spontaneous action potentials, contract when stretched, and are under autonomic control.

The walls of the ureters, bladder, and urethra are highly folded and therefore very distensible. In the bladder and urethra these folds are called *rugae.* As the bladder fills with urine, the rugae flatten out and the volume of the bladder increases with very little change in intravesical pressure. The volume of this structure can increase from a minimum volume of 10 ml following urination to 400 ml, with a pressure change of only 5 cm H_2O, illustrating the highly compliant nature of the bladder.

Innervation of the Bladder

Innervation of the bladder and urethra is important in controlling urination. The smooth muscle of the bladder neck receives sympathetic innervation from the hypogastric nerves. α-adrenergic receptors, located mainly in the bladder neck and the urethra, cause contraction. Stimulation of these receptors facilitates storage of urine by inducing closure of the urethra. Sacral parasympathetic fibers (muscarinic) innervate the body of the bladder and cause a sustained bladder contraction. Sensory fibers of the pelvic nerves (visceral afferent pathway) also innervate the fun-

Nephrolithiasis (i.e., **kidney stones**) is a common medical problem. Five to ten percent of Americans have kidney stones sometime during their lives. Most stones (80%-90%) are composed of calcium salts. The remaining stones are composed of uric acid, magnesium-ammonium acetate, or cysteine. Stones are formed by crystallization in a supersaturated urinary milieu. When the ureter is blocked with a kidney stone, reflex constriction of the ureter around the stone elicits severe flank pain. The pain is perceived by sensory nerve fibers (pelvic nerves), which innervate the ureter.

dus. These sensory fibers carry input from receptors that detect bladder fullness, pain, and temperature sensation. The sacral pudendal nerves innervate the skeletal muscle fibers of the external sphincter, and excitatory impulses cause contraction.

Passage of Urine from the Kidneys to the Bladder

As urine collects in the renal calyces, stretch promotes their inherent pacemaker activity. The pacemaker activity initiates a peristaltic contraction that begins in the calyces and spreads to the pelvis and along the length of the ureter, thereby forcing urine from the renal pelvis toward the bladder. Transmission of the peristaltic wave is caused by action potentials that are generated by the pacemaker and pass along the smooth muscle syncytium.

Micturition

Micturition is the process of emptying the urinary bladder. Two processes are involved: (1) progressive filling of the bladder until the pressure rises to a critical value and (2) a neuronal reflex called the **micturition reflex** that empties the bladder. The micturition reflex is an automatic spinal cord reflex. However, it can be in-

hibited or facilitated by centers in the brain stem and the cerebral cortex.

Filling of the bladder stretches the bladder wall and causes it to contract. Contractions are the result of a reflex initiated by stretch receptors in the bladder. Sensory signals from the bladder fundus enter the spinal cord via pelvic nerves and return directly to the bladder through parasympathetic fibers in the same nerves. Stimulation of parasympathetic fibers causes intense stimulation of the detrusor muscle. The smooth muscle in the bladder is a syncytium; accordingly, stimulation of the detrusor also causes the muscle cells in the neck of the bladder to contract. Because the muscle fibers of the bladder outlet are oriented both longitudinally and radially, contraction opens the bladder neck and allows urine to flow through the posterior urethra. A voluntary relaxation of the external sphincter, by cortical inhibition of the pudendal nerve, permits the flow of urine through the external meatus. Voluntary relaxation of the external sphincter is required and may be the event that initiates micturition. Interruption of the hypogastric sympathetic nerves and the pudendal nerves to the lower urinary tract does not alter the micturition reflex. In contrast, destruction of the parasympathetic nerves results in complete bladder dysfunction.

■ SUMMARY

1. The functional unit of the kidney is the nephron, which consists of a renal corpuscle, proximal tubule, loop of Henle, distal tubule, and collecting duct.
2. The renal corpuscle is composed of glomerular capillaries and Bowman's capsule.
3. The juxtaglomerular apparatus is one component of an important feedback mechanism that regulates renal blood flow and the glomerular filtration rate. The structures that compose the juxtaglomerular apparatus include the macula densa, extraglomerular

mesangial cells, and renin-producing granular cells.

4. The lower urinary tract is composed of the ureters, bladder, and urethra. Micturition is the process of emptying the urinary bladder. The micturition reflex is an automatic spinal cord reflex. However, it can be inhibited or facilitated by centers in the brain stem and cortex.

KEY WORDS AND CONCEPTS

- Cortex
- Nephrons
- Pelvis
- Major calyces
- Urinary bladder
- Interlobar artery
- Interlobular artery
- Glomerular capillaries
- Peritubular capillaries
- Glomerulus
- Henle's loop
- Collecting duct system
- Bowman's space
- Superficial nephrons
- Vasa recta
- Visceral layer
- Filtration slits
- Filtration barrier
- Mesangial cells
- Extraglomerular mesangial cells
- Juxtaglomerular apparatus
- Detrusor muscle
- Ureters
- Urogenital diaphragm
- Medulla
- Renal pyramids
- Pelvic space
- Minor calyces

- Renal artery
- Arcuate artery
- Afferent arteriole
- Efferent arteriole
- Renal corpuscle
- Proximal tubule
- Distal tubule
- Bowman's capsule
- Macula densa
- Juxtamedullary nephrons
- Podocytes
- Parietal layer
- Ultrafiltration
- Mesangium
- Mesangial matrix
- Lacis cells
- Micturition reflex
- Trigone
- Urethra
- Pudendal nerves

■ SELF-STUDY PROBLEMS

1. Identify the structures that are filtration barriers to plasma proteins.

2. What is the functional significance of the juxtaglomerular apparatus?

3. What are the voluntary and involuntary components of micturition?

4. A man receives a knife wound to the spinal cord at the level of the 12th thoracic vertebra. Following recovery, his legs are paralyzed and he has no sensation below the waist. With regard to urinary bladder function, he has no sensation of bladder fullness and is incontinent (i.e., unable to control micturition). Studies of his bladder function show spontaneous contractions of the detrusor muscle, especially as the bladder fills with urine. How do you explain his urinary bladder function?

3

Glomerular Filtration and Renal Blood Flow

OBJECTIVES

Upon completion of this chapter the student should be able to answer the following questions:

1. How can the concepts of mass balance be used to measure the glomerular filtration rate and renal blood flow?
2. Why can inulin clearance and creatinine clearance be used to measure the glomerular filtration rate?
3. Why can P-aminohippuric acid (PAH) clearance be used to measure renal plasma flow?
4. What are the factors that determine which molecules cross the glomerulus and enter Bowman's space?

5. Why does a loss of negative charges on the glomerulus result in proteinuria (loss of protein in the urine)?
6. What Starling forces are involved in the formation of the glomerular ultrafiltrate and how do changes in each force affect the glomerular filtration rate?
7. What is autoregulation of renal blood flow and glomerular filtration rate and which factors are responsible for autoregulation?
8. Which hormones regulate renal blood flow?
9. Why do hormones influence renal blood flow despite autoregulation?

The first step in the formation of urine by the kidneys is the production of an ultrafiltrate of plasma across the glomerulus. The process of glomerular filtration and the regulation of glomerular filtration rate and renal blood flow are discussed in this chapter. The concept of renal clearance, which is the theoretical basis for the measurements of glomerular filtration rate and renal blood flow, is also presented in this chapter.

Knowledge of the glomerular filtration rate (GFR) is essential in evaluating the severity and course of kidney disease. The GFR is equal to the sum of the filtration rates of all the functioning nephrons. Thus, GFR is an index of kidney function. A fall in GFR means that disease is progressing, whereas an increase in GFR generally suggests recovery.

■ RENAL CLEARANCE

The concept of renal **clearance** is based on the Fick principle (i.e., mass balance or conservation of mass). Figure 3-1 illustrates the various factors required to describe the **mass balance** relationships of a kidney. The renal artery is the single input source to the kidney, whereas the renal vein and ureter constitute the two output routes. The following equation defines the mass balance relationship:

$$P^a_x \times RPF^a = (P^v_x \times RPF^v) + (U_x \times \dot{V}) \qquad (3\text{-}1)$$

where: P^a_x and P^v_x are the concentrations of substance x in the renal artery and renal vein plasma, respectively; RPF^a and RPF^v are the **renal plasma flow** (RPF) rates in the artery and vein, respectively; U_x is the concentration of x in the urine; and $\dot{V}$ is the urine flow rate. This relationship permits the quantification of the amount of x excreted in the urine versus the amount returned to the systemic circulation in the renal venous blood. Thus, for any substance that is neither synthesized nor metabolized, the amount that enters the kidneys is equal to the amount that leaves the kidneys in the urine plus the amount that leaves the kidneys in the renal venous blood.

The principle of renal clearance emphasizes the excretory function of the kidney; it considers only the rate at which a substance is excreted into the urine, and not its rate of return to the systemic circulation in the renal vein. Therefore, in terms of mass balance (Equation 3-1), the urinary excretion rate of x ($U_x \times \dot{V}$) is proportional to the plasma concentration of x (P^a_x).

$$P^a_x \propto U_x \times \dot{V} \qquad (3\text{-}2)$$

In order to equate the urinary excretion rate of x to its renal arterial plasma concentration, it is necessary to determine the rate at which x is re-

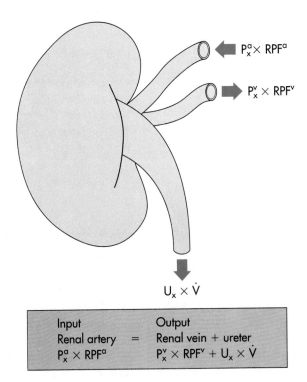

$$P^a_x \times RPF^a$$

$$P^v_x \times RPF^v$$

$$U_x \times \dot{V}$$

Input		Output	
Renal artery	=	Renal vein + ureter	
$P^a_x \times RPF^a$		$P^v_x \times RPF^v + U_x \times \dot{V}$	

Figure 3-1 ■ Mass balance relationships for the kidney. See text for definition of symbols.

moved from the plasma by the kidneys. This removal rate is the clearance (C_x).

$$Pa_x \times C_x = U_x \times \dot{V} \qquad (3\text{-}3)$$

If Equation 3-3 is rearranged and the concentration of x in the renal artery plasma (P_x) is assumed to be identical to its concentration in a plasma sample from any peripheral blood vessel, the following relationship is obtained:

$$C_x = \frac{U_x \times \dot{V}}{P_x} \qquad (3\text{-}4)$$

Clearance has the dimensions of volume/time, and it represents a volume of plasma from which all the substance has been removed and excreted into the urine per unit time. This last point is best illustrated by considering the following example:

If a substance is present in the urine at a concentration of 100 mg/ml, and the urine flow rate is 1 ml/min, then the excretion rate for this substance is calculated as follows:

$$\textbf{Excretion Rate} = U_x \times \dot{V} = 100 \text{ mg/ml} \qquad (3\text{-}5)$$
$$\times \text{ (1 ml/min)} = 100 \text{ mg/min}$$

If this substance is present in the plasma at a concentration of 1 mg/ml, then its clearance according to Equation 3-4 is as follows:

$$C_x = \frac{(U_x \times \dot{V})}{P_x} = \frac{100 \text{ mg/min}}{1 \text{ mg/ml}} = 100 \text{ ml/min} \qquad (3\text{-}6)$$

In other words, 100 ml of plasma will be completely cleared of substance x each minute. The definition of clearance as a volume of plasma from which all the substance has been removed and excreted into the urine per unit time is somewhat misleading because it is not a real volume of plasma; rather, it is an idealized volume.[9] The concept of clearance is important because it can be used to measure the glomerular filtra-

tion rate and renal plasma flow and determine whether a substance is reabsorbed or secreted along the nephron.

Glomerular Filtration Rate: Clearance of Inulin

Inulin is a polymer of fructose (molecular weight approximately 5000) that can be used to measure the **glomerular filtration rate** (GFR). It is not produced by the body and therefore must be administered intravenously. Inulin is freely filtered across the glomerulus into Bowman's space and is not reabsorbed, secreted, or metabolized by the cells of the nephron. Accordingly, **the amount of inulin excreted in the urine per minute equals the amount of inulin filtered at the glomerulus each minute** (Figure 3-2):

$$\textbf{Amount Filtered = Amount Excreted} \qquad (3\text{-}7)$$
$$\text{GFR} \times P_{in} = U_{in} \times \dot{V}$$

where: GFR is the glomerular filtration rate, P_{in} and U_{in} are the plasma and urine concentrations of inulin, and $\dot{V}$ is the urine flow. If Equation 3-7 is solved for the GFR

$$\text{GFR} = \frac{U_{in} \times \dot{V}}{P_{in}} \qquad (3\text{-}8)$$

This equation is the same form as that for clearance (Equation 3-4). **Thus, the clearance of inulin provides a means for determining the GFR.**

Inulin is not the only substance that can be used to measure the GFR. Any substance that meets the following criteria will serve as an appropriate marker for the measurement of GFR:

1. The substance must be freely filtered across the glomerulus into Bowman's space.
2. The substance must not be reabsorbed or secreted by the nephron.
3. The substance must not be metabolized or produced by the kidney.
4. The substance must not alter GFR.

---

[9] For most substances cleared from the plasma by the kidneys, only a portion is actually removed and excreted in a single pass through the kidneys.

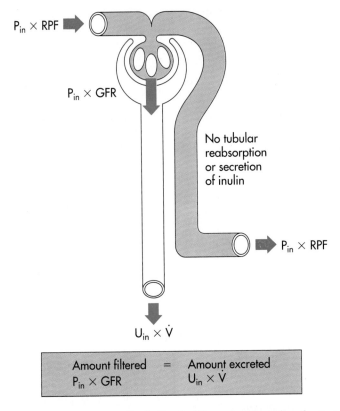

$$P_{in} \times RPF$$

$$P_{in} \times GFR$$

No tubular
reabsorption
or secretion
of inulin

$$P_{in} \times RPF$$

$$U_{in} \times \dot{V}$$

Amount filtered	=	Amount excreted
$P_{in} \times GFR$		$U_{in} \times V$

Figure 3-2 ■ Renal handling of inulin. Inulin is freely filtered across the glomerulus and is not reabsorbed, secreted, or metabolized by the nephron. P_{in}, Plasma inulin concentration; RPF, renal plasma flow; GFR, glomerular filtration rate; U_{in}, urinary concentration of inulin; $\dot{V}$, urine flow rate. Note that all the inulin coming to the kidney in the renal artery does not get filtered at the glomerulus (normally 15%-20% of plasma and inulin are filtered). The portion that is not filtered is returned to the systemic circulation in the renal vein.

Whereas inulin is used extensively in experimental studies, the fact that it must be infused intravenously limits its clinical use. Consequently, **creatinine** is used to estimate the GFR in clinical practice. Creatinine is a by-product of skeletal-muscle creatine metabolism. It is produced at a relatively constant rate, and the amount produced is proportional to the muscle mass. With regard to the measurement of GFR, creatinine has an advantage over inulin because it is produced endogenously and thus obviates the need for an intravenous infusion, as is required for inulin. However, creatinine is not a perfect substance to measure GFR because it is secreted to a small extent by the organic cation secretory system in the proximal tubule (see Chapter 4). The error introduced by this secretory component is approximately 10%. Thus, the amount of creatinine excreted in the urine exceeds the amount expected from filtration alone by 10%. However, the method used to quantitate the plasma creatinine concentration overestimates the true value by 10%. Consequently, the two errors cancel, and in most clinical situations **creatinine clearance** provides a reasonably accurate measure of the GFR.

As illustrated in Figure 3-2, not all the inulin (or any substance used to measure GFR) that enters the kidney in the renal arterial plasma is filtered at the glomerulus. Likewise, not all of the plasma coming into the kidney is filtered.[10] The portion of plasma that is filtered is termed the **filtration fraction** and is determined as follows:

$$\text{Filtration Fraction} = \frac{\text{GFR}}{\text{RPF}} \qquad (3\text{-}9)$$

where, again, RPF is renal plasma flow. Under normal conditions the filtration fraction averages 0.15 to 0.20. **This means that only 15%-20% of the plasma that enters the glomerulus is actually filtered.** The remaining 80%-85% continues on through the glomerulus into the efferent arterioles and peritubular capillaries and is finally returned to the systemic circulation in the renal vein.

---

10 Nearly all the plasma that enters the kidney in the renal artery passes through the glomerulus. Approximately 10% does not.

A fall in GFR may be the first and only clinical sign of kidney disease. Thus, a measurement of GFR is important when kidney disease is suspected. For example, a 50% loss of functioning nephrons will reduce the GFR by approximately 20%-30%. This smaller-than-anticipated decline in GFR is caused by compensation of the remaining nephrons. Because measurements of GFR are cumbersome, kidney function is usually assessed in the clinical setting by measuring plasma [creatinine] (P_{cr}), which is inversely related to GFR (Figure 3-3). It is evident from inspection of Figure 3-3, however, that GFR must decline substantially before an increase in P_{cr} can be detected in a clinical setting. For example, a fall in GFR from 120 ml/min to 100 ml/min is accompanied by an increase in P_{cr} from 1.0 mg/dl to 1.2 mg/dl. This does not appear to be a significant change in P_{cr}, yet GFR has fallen by almost 20%.

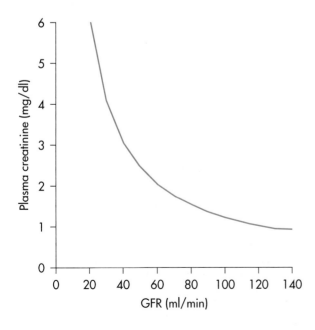

Figure 3-3 ▪ **Relationship between GFR and plasma creatinine concentration. As with inulin the amount of creatinine filtered by the kidneys is essentially equal to the amount that is excreted (i.e., amount filtered = amount excreted; thus, GFR $\times$ P_{cr} = U_{cr} $\times$ $\dot{V}$). Because production of creatinine by skeletal muscle is constant, excretion must also be constant to maintain steady-state creatinine balance. Thus, if GFR falls from 120 to 60 ml/min, P_{cr} must increase from 1 to 2 mg/dl to keep the filtration of creatinine and thus its excretion equal to the production rate.**

Renal Plasma Flow: Clearance of PAH

P-aminohippuric acid (PAH) is an organic anion filtered across the glomerulus that can be used to measure RPF (Figure 3-4). As with inulin, PAH is not produced in the body and therefore must be infused intravenously. PAH is an organic anion that is excreted into the urine by the processes of glomerular filtration and tubular secretion. For this discussion it is sufficient to recognize that the PAH secretory mechanism in the proximal tubule has a maximum rate of approx-

imately 80 mg/min. Delivery of PAH to the peritubular capillaries at a rate less than this will cause virtually all of the PAH to be secreted into the tubular fluid, and thus little PAH will remain in the renal vein plasma. When the plasma PAH concentration is low and the secretory mechanism is not overwhelmed (generally at plasma [PAH] below 0.12 mg/ml), the clearance of PAH can be used to measure the RPF. However, when the PAH secretory mechanism is overwhelmed, the clearance of PAH cannot be used to measure

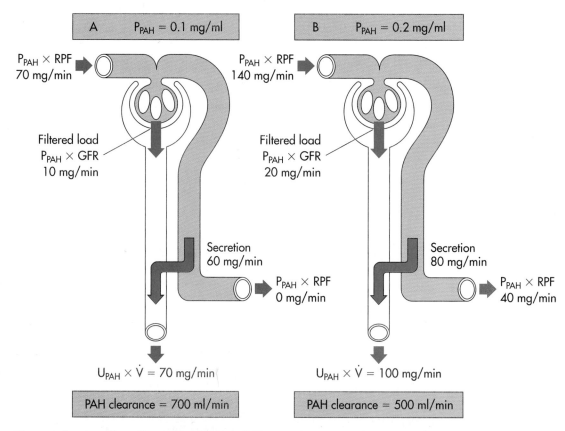

Figure 3-4 ■ **Renal handling of PAH at two different plasma concentrations (P_{PAH}). A,** The P_{PAH} is less than the value that would lead to saturation of the PAH secretory mechanism (i.e., <80 mg/min.). **B,** The elevated P_{PAH} results in the delivery of more PAH to the secretory mechanism than can be secreted (i.e., >80 mg/min). For both cases the RPF is 700 ml/min and the GFR is 100 ml/min. U_{PAH}, urine PAH concentration; $\dot{V}$, urine flow rate. The clearance of PAH is calculated from Equation 3-4.

RPF. Figure 3-5 depicts the renal handling of PAH in terms of whole kidney mass balance, and illustrates why, when PAH delivery to the peritubular capillaries is less than approximately 80 mg/min, PAH clearance is a reliable estimate of the RPF. The amount of PAH that arrives at the kidneys per minute is simply the product of the plasma PAH concentration (P^a_{PAH}) and the RPF. Because all the PAH is excreted into the urine (when PAH delivery to the peritubular capillaries is less than ~80 mg/min) and none is returned to the systemic circulation via the renal vein, the following mass balance relationship holds true:

$$RPF \times P^a_{PAH} = U_{PAH} \times \dot{V} \qquad (3\text{-}10)$$

where: U_{PAH} is urine PAH concentration and $\dot{V}$ is urine flow. Rearranging and solving for the RPF, the following equation is obtained:

$$RPF = \frac{U_{PAH} \times \dot{V}}{P^a_{PAH}} \qquad (3\text{-}11)$$

This equation conforms to the general clearance equation (Equation 3-4). **Thus, at low plasma PAH concentrations, the PAH clearance is equal to the RPF.** At high plasma PAH concentrations, however, the PAH secretory mechanism will be saturated, and a significant amount of PAH will appear in the renal venous blood. Under this condition, Equations 3-10 and 3-11 do not hold; the clearance of PAH does not equal the RPF.

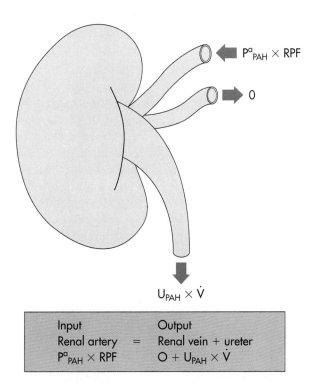

Input		Output
Renal artery	=	Renal vein + ureter
$P^a_{PAH} \times RPF$		$0 + U_{PAH} \times \dot{V}$

Figure 3-5 ■ **Mass balance relationships for the use of PAH clearance to measure the renal plasma flow (RPF).** P^a_{PAH}, Plasma PAH concentration; U_{PAH}, urine PAH concentration; $\dot{V}$, urine flow rate.

The relationship between PAH clearance and RPF described here is idealized. Even at plasma PAH concentrations that do not exceed the capability of the secretory mechanism, some PAH still appears in the renal venous blood. The reason for this is related to the anatomy of the nephron and renal blood vessels. The PAH secretory mechanism is located in the proximal tubule. The PAH entering the peritubular capillaries surrounding proximal tubules is secreted. However, some capillaries perfuse the medulla (i.e., vasa recta), the renal capsule, and parts of the renal hilum rather than form peritubular capillaries. Thus, the PAH in this plasma cannot be secreted, and this PAH will be returned to the systemic circulation in the renal vein plasma. In recognition of the fact that the clearance of PAH does not provide an accurate measure of the RPF (i.e., it underestimates the true value by approximately 10%), it is more appropriate to refer to the clearance of PAH as providing a measure of the **effective RPF (ERPF).** It is effective in the sense that this represents plasma flow past portions of the nephron able to secrete PAH effectively.

The clearance of PAH can also be used to estimate RBF. Normally the plasma fraction of blood accounts for 50%-60% of the blood volume, and the cells account for the remainder. To determine what fraction of the blood is composed of cells, the **hematocrit (HCT)** is measured. Normally the HCT is in the range of 0.40-0.50. Once the HCT is known, the renal blood flow can be calculated as follows:

$$RBF = \frac{RPF}{1 - HCT} \qquad (3\text{-}12)$$

Thus, if the HCT of an individual is 0.40 and the RPF is 700 ml/min, RBF is 1167 ml/min. (i.e., RBF = 700 ml/min/1 − 0.4 = 1167 ml/min.). However, measurement of RPF provides little useful information and is rarely performed in clinical situations. Kidney function is usually assessed by measuring plasma (creatinine) (P_{cr}), which, as discussed above, is inversely related to GFR.

■ GLOMERULAR FILTRATION

The first step in the formation of urine is the production of an ultrafiltrate of the plasma by the glomerulus. The ultrafiltrate is devoid of cellular elements and essentially protein-free. The concentrations of salts and organic molecules such as glucose and amino acids are similar in the plasma and ultrafiltrate. Ultrafiltration is driven by Starling forces across the glomerular capillaries, and changes in these forces alter the glomerular filtration rate. Glomerular filtration rate and RPF are normally held within very narrow ranges by a phenomenon called **autoregulation.** This section will review the composition of the glomerular filtrate, the dynamics of its formation, and the relationship between RPF and glomerular filtration rate. In addition, the factors that contribute to the autoregulation of glomerular filtration rate and renal blood flow will be discussed.

Determinants of Ultrafiltrate Composition

The unique structure of the glomerular filtration barrier (capillary endothelium, basement membrane, and filtration slits of the podocytes) determines the composition of the ultrafiltrate of plasma. The glomerular filtration barrier restricts the filtration of molecules on the basis of size and electrical charge (Figure 3-6). In general, neutral molecules with a radius less than 20 angstroms (Å, where Å = 10^{-10} meters) are filtered freely, molecules larger than 36 Å are not filtered, and molecules between 20 and 42 Å are filtered to various degrees. For example, serum albumin, an anionic protein that has an effective molecular radius of 35.5 Å, is filtered poorly (approximately 7 grams of albumin are filtered each day[11]). Because albumin is reabsorbed avidly by the proximal tubule, however, almost none appears in the urine.

---

11 Approximately 70,000 g/day of albumin passes through the glomeruli. Therefore the filtration of 7 g/day represents only 0.01% of the albumin that passes through the glomeruli. This is well below the filtration fraction for substances that are freely filtered (15%-20%).

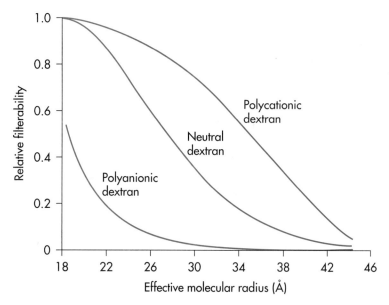

Figure 3-6 ■ Influence of size and electrical charge of dextran on its filterability. A value of one indicates that it is filtered freely, whereas a value of zero indicates that it is not filtered. The filterability of neutral dextrans between approximately 20 Å and 42 Å depends on charge. Dextrans larger than 42 Å are not filtered, regardless of charge and polycationic dextrans, and neutral dextrans smaller than 20 Å are freely filtered.

Figure 3-6 illustrates how electrical charge affects the filtration of macromolecules (e.g., dextrans) by the glomerulus. Dextrans are a family of exogenous polysaccharides that are manufactured in various molecular weights. They take an electrically neutral form or have negative charges (polyanionic) or positive charges (polycationic). At constant charge, filtration decreases as the size (i.e., effective molecular radius) increases. For any given molecular radius, cationic molecules are more readily filtered than anionic molecules. The restriction of anionic molecules is explained by the presence of negatively charged glycoproteins on the surface of all components of the glomerular filtration barrier. These charged glycoproteins repel similarly charged molecules. Because most plasma proteins are negatively charged, the negative charge on the filtration barrier restricts the filtration of proteins that have a molecular radius of 20 to 42 Å.

The importance of the negative charges on the filtration barrier in restricting the filtration of plasma proteins is illustrated in Figure 3-7. Removal of negative charges from the filtration barrier causes proteins to be filtered solely on the basis of their effective molecular radius. Hence, at any molecular radius between approximately 20 and 42 Å, the filtration of polyanionic proteins will increase compared with the normal state, in which the filtration barrier has anionic charges. In a number of glomerular diseases the negative charge on the filtration barrier is lost secondarily to immunologic damage and inflammation. As a result, filtration of proteins is increased, and proteins appear in the urine (proteinuria).

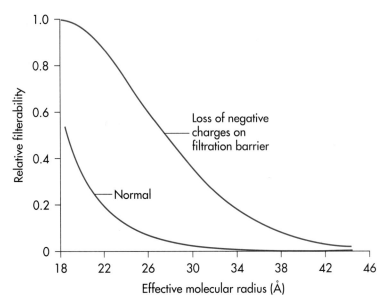

**Figure 3-7 ■ Reduction of the negative charges on the filtration barrier of the glomerulus, as can oc-
cur in many immunologically mediated renal diseases, results in the filtration of proteins on the basis of size only. In this situation the relative filterability of proteins is dependent only on the molecular radius. Accordingly, the excretion of polyanionic proteins (20 to 42 Å) in the urine increases
because more proteins of this size are filtered.**

Dynamics of Ultrafiltration

The forces responsible for the glomerular filtration of plasma are the same as those involved in fluid exchange across all capillary
beds (see Chapter 1). Ultrafiltration occurs because the **Starling forces** (i.e., hydrostatic and
oncotic pressures) drive fluid from the lumen
of glomerular capillaries, across the filtration
barrier, into Bowman's space (Figure 3-8). The
hydrostatic pressure in the glomerular capillary
(P_{GC}) is oriented to promote the movement of
fluid from the glomerular capillary into Bowman's space. Because the glomerular ultrafiltrate is essentially protein-free, the oncotic
pressure in Bowman's space (π_{BS}) is near zero.
Therefore P_{GC} is the only force that favors filtration, and it is opposed by the hydrostatic

pressure in Bowman's space (P_{BS}) and the
oncotic pressure in the glomerular capillary
(π_{GC}).

As illustrated in Figure 3-8, a net ultrafiltration
pressure (P_{UF}) of 17 mm Hg exists at the afferent
end of the glomerulus, whereas at the efferent
end the P_{UF} is 8 mm Hg (where $P_{UF} = P_{GC} - P_{BS}
- \pi_{GC}$). Two additional points concerning Star-
ling forces are important. First, P_{GC} decreases
slightly along the length of the capillary because
of the resistance to flow in the capillary. Second,
π_{GC} increases along the length of the glomerular
capillary because water is filtered and protein is
retained in the glomerular capillary; accordingly,
the protein concentration in the capillary rises
and π_{GC} increases.

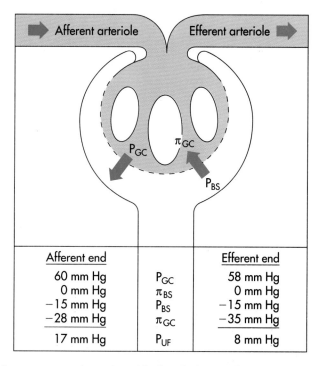

Afferent end		Efferent end
60 mm Hg	P_{GC}	58 mm Hg
0 mm Hg	π_{BS}	0 mm Hg
−15 mm Hg	P_{BS}	−15 mm Hg
−28 mm Hg	π_{GC}	−35 mm Hg
17 mm Hg	P_{UF}	8 mm Hg

Figure 3-8 ■ Schematic representation of an idealized glomerular capillary and the Starling forces across the glomerular capillary. P_{UF}, Net ultrafiltration pressure; P_{GC}, glomerular capillary hydrostatic pressure; P_{BS}, Bowman's space hydrostatic pressure; π_{GC}, glomerular capillary oncotic pressure; π_{BS}, Bowman's space oncotic pressure.

The glomerular filtration rate (GFR) is proportional to the sum of the Starling forces that exists across the capillaries [$(P_{GC} - P_{BS}) - (\pi_{GC} - \pi_{BS})$] times the ultrafiltration coefficient, K_f:

$$\text{GFR} = K_f \left[(P_{GC} - P_{BS}) - (\pi_{GC} - \pi_{BS}) \right] \quad (3\text{-}13)$$

The K_f is the product of the intrinsic permeability of the glomerular capillary and the glomerular surface area available for filtration. The rate of glomerular filtration is considerably greater in glomerular capillaries, versus systemic capillaries, mainly because the K_f is approximately 100 times higher. However, the hydrostatic pressure within the glomerular capillaries is approximately twice as high as that in systemic capillaries.

The GFR can be altered by changing K_f or any of the Starling forces. In normal individuals, under physiologic conditions, GFR is regulated by alterations in P_{GC} that are mediated primarily by changes in glomerular arteriolar resistance. P_{GC} is affected in three ways:

1. **Changes in afferent arteriolar resistance:** a fall in resistance increases P_{GC} and GFR, whereas an increase in resistance decreases P_{GC} and GFR.
2. **Changes in efferent arteriolar resistance:** a fall in resistance reduces P_{GC} and GFR, whereas an increase in resistance elevates P_{GC} and GFR.
3. **Changes in renal arteriolar pressure:** an increase in blood pressure transiently increases P_{GC}, which enhances GFR, whereas a decrease in blood pressure decreases P_{GC} and GFR.

Pathologic conditions and drugs may also affect GFR. A reduction in GFR in disease states is most often due to decreases in K_f, which result from the loss of filtration surface area (see Chapter 11). GFR also changes in pathophysiologic conditions because of changes in P_{GC}, π_{GC}, and P_{BS}.

1. **Changes in K_f:** Increased K_f enhances GFR, whereas decreased K_f reduces GFR. Some kidney diseases reduce K_f by reducing the number of filtering glomeruli (i.e., surface area). Some drugs and hormones that dilate the glomerular arterioles also increase K_f. Similarly, drugs and hormones that constrict the glomerular arterioles also decrease K_f.
2. **Changes in P_{GC}:** In acute renal failure, GFR declines because P_{GC} falls. As discussed above, a reduction in P_{GC} is caused by a decline in renal arterial pressure and an increase in afferent arteriolar or a decrease in efferent arteriolar resistance.
3. **Changes in π_{GC}:** An inverse relationship exists between π_{GC} and GFR. Alterations in π_{GC} result from changes in protein synthesis outside of the kidneys. In addition, protein loss in the urine caused by some renal diseases can lead to a decrease in plasma [protein] and thus π_{GC}.
4. **Changes in P_{BS}:** Increased P_{BS} reduces GFR, whereas decreased P_{BS} facilitates GFR. Acute obstruction of the urinary tract (e.g., a kidney stone occluding the ureter) increases P_{BS}.

■ RENAL BLOOD FLOW

In resting subjects the blood flow to the kidneys (about 1.25 L/min) is equal to about 25% of the cardiac output. However, the kidneys constitute less than 0.5% of the total body weight. Blood flow through the kidneys serves several important functions, including the following:

1. Indirectly determining the GFR
2. Modifying the rate of solute and water reabsorption by the proximal tubule
3. Participating in the concentration and dilution of the urine
4. Delivering oxygen, nutrients, and hormones to the cells of the nephron and returning carbon dioxide and reabsorbed fluid and solutes to the general circulation
5. Delivering substrates for excretion in the urine

The blood flow through any organ may be represented by the following equation:

$$Q = \Delta P/R \qquad (3\text{-}14)$$

where: Q equals blood flow, ΔP equals mean arterial pressure minus venous pressure for that organ, and R equals the resistance to flow through that organ. Accordingly, RBF is equal to the pressure difference between the renal artery and the renal vein divided by the renal vascular resistance:

$$RBF = \frac{\text{aortic pressure} - \text{renal venous pressure}}{\text{renal vascular resistance}} \qquad (3\text{-}15)$$

The afferent arteriole, efferent arteriole, and interlobular artery are the major resistance vessels in the kidney and thereby determine renal vascular resistance. The kidneys, like most other organs, regulate their blood flow by adjusting the vascular resistance in response to changes in arterial pressure. As illustrated in Figure 3-9, this adjustment in resistance is so precise that blood flow remains relatively constant as arterial blood pressure changes between 90 and 180 mm Hg. GFR is also regulated over the same range of arterial pressures. The phenomenon whereby RBF and GFR are maintained relatively constant is called **autoregulation.** As the term indicates, autoregulation is achieved by changes in vascular

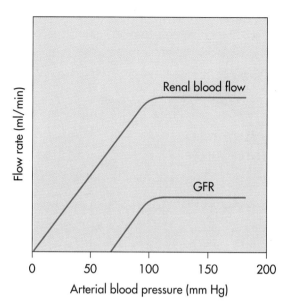

Figure 3-9 ■ **Relationships between arterial blood pressure and renal blood flow (RBF) and glomerular filtration rate (GFR). Autoregulation maintains RBF and GFR relatively constant as blood pressure changes from 90 to 180 mm Hg.**

resistance—primarily through the afferent arterioles of the kidneys. Because both GFR and RBF are regulated over the same range of pressures, it is not surprising that the same mechanisms regulate both flows.

Two mechanisms are responsible for autoregulation of RBF and GFR: one that responds to changes in arterial pressure and another that responds to changes in the flow rate of tubular fluid. Both regulate the tone of the afferent arteriole. The pressure-sensitive mechanism, the so-called **myogenic mechanism,** is related to an intrinsic property of vascular smooth muscle—the tendency to contract when it is stretched. Accordingly, when arterial pressure rises and the renal afferent arteriole is stretched, the smooth muscle contracts. Because the increase in the resistance of the arteriole offsets the increase in pressure, RBF and therefore GFR remain constant (i.e., RBF is constant if the ratio of $\Delta P/R$ is kept constant; see Equation 3-14).

The second mechanism responsible for autoregulation of GFR and RBF, the flow-dependent mechanism, is known as **tubuloglomerular feedback** (Figure 3-10). This mechanism involves a feedback loop in which the flow of tubular fluid (or some other factor, such as the rate of NaCl reabsorption, which increases in direct proportion to flow) is sensed by the macula densa of the **juxtaglomerular apparatus (JGA)** and converted into a signal that affects afferent arteriolar resistance and thus GFR. When GFR increases and causes the flow of tubular fluid at the macula densa to rise, the JGA sends a signal that causes vasoconstriction to return RBF and GFR to normal levels. In contrast, when GFR and tubular flow past the macula densa decrease, the JGA sends a signal causing RBF and GFR to increase to normal levels. The signal affects RBF and GFR mainly by changing the resistance of the afferent arteriole, but the mediator for this effect is controversial. Questions remain about tubuloglomerular feedback concerning the variable sensed at the macula densa and the effector substance that alters the resistance of the afferent arteriole. It has been suggested that flow-dependent changes in NaCl reabsorption are sensed by the macula densa. The effector mechanism may be adenosine, which constricts the afferent arteriole (in contrast to its vasodilator effect on most other vasculature beds), ATP, which selectively vasoconstricts the afferent arteriole, or even a metabolite or arachidonic acid. Nitric oxide, a vasodilator, produced by the macula densa, may also play a role in tubuloglomerular feedback but is not essential for autoregulation. The macula densa may release both a vasoconstrictor and a vasodilator (e.g., nitric oxide),

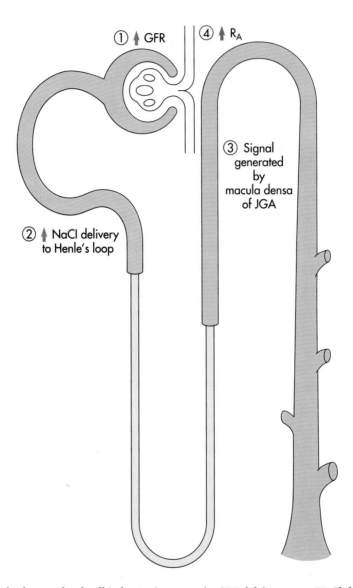

Figure 3-10 ■ **Tubuloglomerular feedback. An increase in GFR (1) increases NaCl delivery to the loop of Henle (2), which is sensed by the macula densa and converted into a signal (3) that increases R_A (4: the resistance of the afferent arteriole), which decreases GFR.** (Modified from Cogan MG: *Fluid and electrolytes: physiology and pathophysiology,* Norwalk, Conn., 1991, Appleton & Lange.)

which oppose each other's actions at the level of the afferent arteriole.

Because animals engage in many activities that can change arterial blood pressure, mechanisms that maintain RBF and GFR at relatively constant levels despite changes in arterial pressure are highly desirable. If RBF and GFR were to rise or fall suddenly in proportion to changes in blood pressure, urinary excretion of fluid and solute would also change suddenly because alterations in GFR influence water and solute excretion (the reason for which will be discussed in the next chapter). Such changes in water and solute excretion without comparable alterations in intake would alter fluid and electrolyte balance. Accordingly, autoregulation of GFR and RBF provides an effective means for uncoupling renal function from arterial pressure and ensures that fluid and solute excretion remain constant.

Three points concerning autoregulation should be made:

1. Autoregulation is absent below arterial pressures of 90 mm Hg
2. Autoregulation is not perfect; RBF and GFR do change slightly as arterial blood pressure rises
3. Despite autoregulation, GFR and RBF can be changed under appropriate conditions by several hormones (see Table 3-1).

Individuals with renal artery stenosis (a narrowing of the artery lumen) caused by atherosclerosis, for example, can have an elevated systemic blood pressure mediated by stimulation of the renin-angiotensin system (see Chapter 6 for details). The pressure in the artery proximal to the stenosis is increased, but it is normal or reduced distal to the stenosis. Autoregulation plays an important role in maintaining RBF, P_{GC}, and GFR in the presence of this stenosis. The administration of drugs to lower systemic blood pressure also lowers pressure distal to the stenosis; accordingly RBF, P_{GC}, and GFR fall.

■ REGULATION OF RENAL BLOOD FLOW AND GFR

Several factors and hormones have a major effect on RBF and GFR (Table 3-1). As discussed in the previous section, the myogenic mechanism and tubuloglomerular feedback play a key role in maintaining constant RBF and GFR. **Sympathetic nerves, angiotensin II, prostaglandins, nitric oxide** (i.e., **NO**), **endothelin, bradykinin,** and perhaps **adenosine** exert the major control over RBF and GFR. The physiologic and pathophysiologic roles of the other hormones discussed later in this chapter are under investigation. Figure 3-11 illustrates the ways in which changes in the resistance of the afferent and efferent arterioles, mediated by changes in hormone concentration, modulate RBF and GFR.

Sympathetic Nerves

The afferent and efferent arterioles are innervated by sympathetic neurons; however, sympathetic tone is minimal when effective circulating volume (ECV) is normal. Norepinephrine, released by sympathetic nerves, and circulating epinephrine, secreted by the adrenal medulla, cause vasoconstriction by binding to α_1-adrenoceptors, which are located mainly on the afferent arterioles and thereby decrease RBF and GFR. A reduction in the ECV or strong emotional stimuli such as fear and pain activate sympathetic nerves and reduce RBF and GFR.

Angiotensin II

Produced systematically and within the kidneys, angiotensin II constricts the afferent and efferent arterioles[12] and decreases RBF and GFR (see

---

12 The efferent arteriole is more sensitive to angiotensin II than the afferent arteriole. Therefore, with low concentrations of angiotensin II, constriction of the efferent arteriole predominates. However, with high concentrations of angiotensin II, constriction of both afferent and efferent arterioles occurs.

TABLE 3-1

Major hormones that influence GFR and RBF

	Stimulus	Effect on GFR	Effect on RBF
Vasoconstrictors			
Sympathetic nerves	↓ ECV, shear stress	↓	↓
Angiotensin II	↓ ECV, renin	↓	↓
Endothelin	Shear stress, AII, BK, epinephrine	↓	↓
Vasodilators			
Prostaglandins (PGI_2, PGE_2)	↓ ECV, shear stress, AII	NC	↑
Nitric oxide	Shear stress, Ach, His, BK, ATP	↑	↑
Bradykinin	PG, ↓ ACE	↑	↑

ECV, Extracellular fluid volume; *Ach,* acetylcholine; *His,* histamine; *BK,* bradykinin; *AII,* angiotensin II; *ACE,* angiotensin-converting enzyme; *PG,* prostaglandins.

Hemorrhage decreases arterial blood pressure, which activates the sympathetic nerves to the kidneys via the baroreceptor reflex. Norepinephrine elicits an intense vasoconstriction of the afferent and efferent arterioles and thereby decreases RBF and GFR. The rise in sympathetic activity also increases the release of epinephrine and angiotensin II, which cause further vasoconstriction and a fall in RBF. The rise in the vascular resistance of the kidney and other vascular beds increases total peripheral resistance, which, by increasing blood pressure (BP = cardiac output × total peripheral resistance), offsets the fall in mean arterial blood pressure elicited by hemorrhage. Hence, this system works to preserve arterial pressure at the expense of maintaining a normal RBF and GFR. This example illustrates the important point that, although autoregulatory mechanisms can prevent the effects of changes in arterial pressure on RBF and GFR, when needed, sympathetic nerves and angiotensin II have important salutary effects on RBF and GFR.

Chapter 6 for details on the renin-angiotensin system). Figure 3-12 illustrates how norepinephrine, epinephrine, and angiotensin II act together to decrease RBF and GFR, as would occur, for example, with hemorrhage.

Prostaglandins

Prostaglandins may not regulate RBF or GFR in healthy, resting people. However, during pathophysiologic conditions such as hemorrhage, prostaglandins (i.e., PGI_2, PGE_2) are produced locally within the kidneys and increase RBF without changing GFR. Prostaglandins dampen the vasoconstrictor effects of sympathetic nerves and angiotensin II. This effect of prostaglandins is important because it prevents severe and potentially harmful vasoconstriction and renal ischemia. Prostaglandin synthesis is stimulated by decreased ECV and stress (i.e., surgery, anesthesia), angiotensin II, and sympathetic nerves.

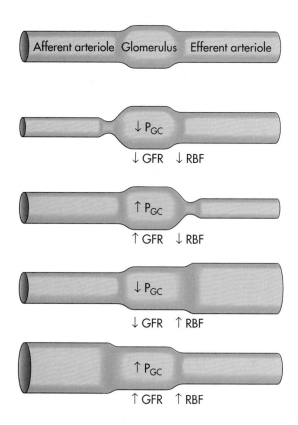

Figure 3-11 ■ Relationship between selective changes in the resistance of either the afferent arteriole or efferent arteriole on RBF and GFR. Constriction of either the afferent or efferent arteriole increases resistance, and according to Equation 3-14 (Q = ΔP/R) an increase in resistance (R) will decrease flow (Q) (i.e., RBF). Dilatation of either the afferent or efferent arteriole will increase flow (i.e., RBF). Constriction of the afferent arteriole decreases P_{GC} (because less of the arterial pressure is transmitted to the glomerulus) and thereby reduces GFR. In contrast, constriction of the efferent arteriole elevates P_{GC} and thus increases GFR. Dilatation of the afferent arteriole increases P_{GC} (because more of the arteriole pressure is transmitted to the glomerulus) and thereby increases GFR. In contrast, dilatation of the efferent arteriole decreases P_{GC} and thus decreases GFR. (Modified from Rose BD, Rennke HG: Renal pathophysiology: the essentials, Baltimore, 1994, Williams & Wilkins.)

Nitric Oxide

Nitric oxide, an endothelium-derived relaxing factor, plays an important vasodilatory role in basal conditions and counteracts vasoconstriction produced by angiotensin II and catecholamines. An increase in shear stress acting on endothelial cells in the arterioles and a number of hormones including acetylcholine, histamine, bradykinin, and ATP increase the production of NO, which causes vasodilatation of the afferent and efferent arterioles in the kidneys. In addition, NO also decreases total peripheral resistance, and inhibition of NO production increases blood pressure.

Abnormal production of NO is observed in individuals with diabetes and hypertension. Excess NO production in diabetes may be responsible for glomerular hyperfiltration and damage of the glomerulus, which are characteristics of the disease. Elevated NO levels increase glomerular capillary pressure secondary to a fall in the resistance of the afferent arteriole. The ensuing hyperfiltration is thought to cause glomerular damage. The normal response to an increase in dietary salt intake includes stimulation of NO production, which maintains blood pressure. In some individuals, NO production may not increase appropriately in response to an increase in salt intake, and blood pressure therefore rises.

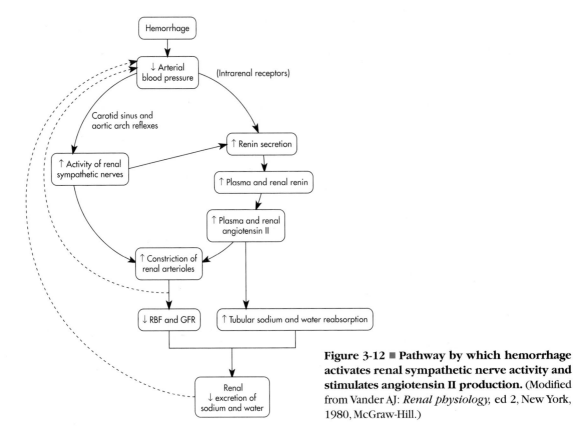

Figure 3-12 ■ **Pathway by which hemorrhage activates renal sympathetic nerve activity and stimulates angiotensin II production.** (Modified from Vander AJ: *Renal physiology,* ed 2, New York, 1980, McGraw-Hill.)

Endothelin

Endothelin is a potent vasoconstrictor secreted by endothelial cells of renal vessels, mesangial cells, and distal tubular cells in response to angiotensin II, bradykinin, epinephrine, and shear stress. Endothelin causes profound vasoconstriction of the afferent and efferent arterioles and decreases GFR and RBF. Although this potent vasoconstrictor may not influence GFR and RBF in the basal state, endothelin production is elevated in a number of glomerular disease states (e.g., renal disease associated with diabetes mellitus).

Bradykinin

Kallikrein is a proteolytic enzyme produced in the kidneys that cleaves circulating kininogen to bradykinin, which is a vasodilator that acts by stimulating the release of NO and prostaglandins. Bradykinin increases GFR and RBF.

Adenosine

Adenosine is produced within the kidneys and causes vasoconstriction of the afferent arteriole, thereby reducing RBF and GFR. As previously mentioned, adenosine may play a role in tubuloglomerular feedback.

Atrial Natriuretic Peptide (ANP)

The secretion of ANP by the heart rises with hypertension and expansion of ECV, causing vasodilatation of the afferent arteriole and vasoconstriction of the efferent arteriole. The net effect of ANP, therefore, is to produce a modest increase in GFR with little change in RBF.

ATP

Various cells release ATP into the renal interstitial fluid. ATP has dual effects on GFR and RBF. Under some conditions, ATP constricts the afferent arteriole, reduces RBF and GFR, and may play a role in tubuloglomerular feedback. In contrast, ATP may stimulate NO production and increase GFR and RBF in other situations.

Glucocorticoids

Administration of therapeutic doses of glucocorticoids increases GFR and RBF.

Histamine

Local release of histamine may play a role in modulating RBF during the basal state and during inflammation and injury. Histamine increases RBF without elevating GFR by decreasing the resistance of the afferent and efferent arterioles.

Angiotensin–converting enzyme (ACE) degrades and thereby inactivates bradykinin and converts angiotensin I, an inactive hormone, to angiotensin II. Thus, ACE increases AII levels and decreases bradykinin levels. Administration of ACE inhibitors, to reduce systemic blood pressure in patients with hypertension, reduces AII levels and elevates bradykinin levels. These effects lower systemic vascular resistance, reduce blood pressure, and decrease renal vascular resistance, thereby increasing RBF and GFR. (Chapter 6 presents a more complete discussion of the renin–angiotensin system and ACE.)

Dopamine

The proximal tubule produces the vasodilator hormone dopamine, which has several actions within the kidney, such as increasing RBF and inhibiting renin secretion.

As illustrated in Figure 3-13, endothelial cells play an important role in regulating the resistance of the afferent and efferent arterioles by producing a number of paracrine hormones including NO, PGI_2, endothelin, and angiotensin II that regulate contraction or relaxation of smooth muscle cells in afferent and efferent arterioles or mesangial cells. Shear stress, acetylcholine, histamine, bradykinin, and ATP stimulate the production of NO, which causes vasorelaxation of the afferent and efferent arterioles and thereby increases GFR and RBF. Angiotensin–converting enzyme, which occurs primarily on the surface of endothelial cells lining the afferent arteriole and glomerular capillaries, converts angiotensin I to angiotensin II, a hormone that causes vasoconstriction of the afferent and efferent arterioles and thereby decreases GFR and RBF. Angiotensin II may also be produced in juxtaglomerular cells and proximal tubular cells. PGI_2 and PGE_2 secretion by endothelial cells, stimulated by sympathetic nerve activity or angiotensin II, causes relaxation of the afferent arterioles and increases GFR and RBF. Finally, endothelin release from endothelial cells causes profound vasoconstriction of the afferent and efferent arterioles and decreases GFR and RBF.

■ SUMMARY

1. The rate of glomerular filtration is calculated by measuring the clearance of inulin or creatinine. Changes in GFR can be monitored by measuring the plasma [creatinine].
2. Effective RPF is determined by the clearance of P-aminohippuric acid (PAH).
3. Starling forces across the glomerular capillaries provide the driving force for the ultrafiltration of plasma from the glomerular capillaries into Bowman's space.

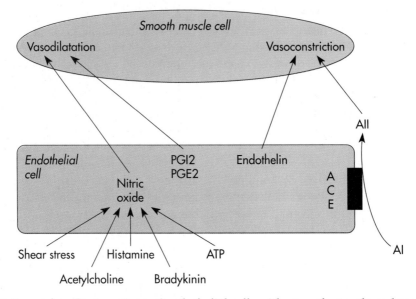

Figure 3-13 ■ **Examples of interactions of endothelial cells with smooth muscle and mesangial cells.** *ACE,* Angiotensin-converting enzyme; *AI,* angiotensin I; *AII,* angiotensin II. (Modified from Arendshorst WJ, Navar LG: *Renal circulation and glomerular hemodynamics.* In Schrier RW and Gottschalk CW, editors: *Diseases of the kidney,* ed 6, Boston, Little, Brown & Co [in press].)

4. The glomerular ultrafiltrate is devoid of cellular elements, contains very little protein, but is otherwise identical to plasma. Neutral proteins with a molecular radius smaller than 20 Å are readily filtered; proteins between 20 and 42 Å are filtered at rates that depend on size and charge (anionic proteins are less readily filtered); and proteins with molecular radii greater than 42 Å are not filtered.

5. Renal blood flow (1.25 L/min) is about 25% of the cardiac output, yet the kidneys constitute less than 0.5% of the body weight. Renal blood flow serves several important functions, including determining the glomerular filtration rate; modifying solute and water reabsorption by the proximal tubule; participating in concentration and dilution of the urine; delivering oxygen, nutrients, and hormones to the cells of the nephron; returning carbon dioxide and reabsorbed fluid and solutes to the general circulation; and delivering substrates for excretion in the urine.

6. Autoregulation maintains constant renal blood flow and glomerular filtration rate, despite changes in arterial blood pressure between 90 and 180 mm Hg. Autoregulation is achieved by changes in renal vascular resistance mediated by the myogenic reflex and tubuloglomerular feedback.

7. Sympathetic nerves, angiotensin II, prostaglandins, NO, endothelin, bradykinin, and perhaps adenosine exert the most control over RBF and GFR.

KEY WORDS AND CONCEPTS

- Clearance
- Mass balance
- Inulin
- Inulin clearance
- Glomerular filtration rate (GFR)
- Creatinine
- Creatinine clearance
- Filtration fraction
- P-aminohippuric acid (PAH)
- PAH clearance
- Renal plasma flow (RPF)
- Effective renal plasma flow (ERPF)
- Hematocrit
- Renal blood flow (RBF)
- Autoregulation
- Starling forces
- Myogenic mechanism
- Tubuloglomerular feedback
- Sympathetic nerves, angiotensin II, prostaglandins, NO, endothelin, bradykinin, and adenosine
- Juxtaglomerular apparatus (JGA)

■ SELF-STUDY PROBLEMS

1. Pflorizin is a drug that completely inhibits the reabsorption of glucose by the kidneys. The following data are obtained in order to assess the effect of pflorizin on the clearance of glucose. Fill in the missing data.

Before pflorizin

Plasma (inulin):	1 mg/ml
Plasma (glucose):	1 mg/ml
Inulin excretion rate:	100 mg/min
Glucose excretion rate:	0 mg/min
Inulin clearance:	_____ ml/min
Glucose clearance:	_____ ml/min

After pflorizin

Plasma (inulin):	1 mg/ml
Plasma (glucose):	1 mg/ml
Inulin excretion rate:	100 mg/min
Glucose excretion rate:	_____ mg/min
Inulin clearance:	_____ ml/min
Glucose clearance:	_____ ml/min

How do you explain the change in glucose excretion and clearance seen with pflorizin?

2. Finding which of the following substances in the urine would indicate damage to the glomerular ultrafiltration barrier?
   a. Red blood cells
   b. Glucose
   c. Sodium
   d. Proteins

3. Explain how hormones (e.g., sympathetic agonists, angiotensin II, and prostaglandins) change renal blood flow.

4. Explain why the use of nonsteroidal antiinflammatory drugs (e.g., indomethacin for arthritis) does not affect GFR or RBF in patients with normal renal function and why administration of nonsteroidal antiinflammatory agents is not recommended for patients with severe reductions in GFR and RBF.

Renal Transport Mechanisms: NaCl and Water Reabsorption Along the Nephron

OBJECTIVES

Upon completion of this chapter the student should be able to answer the following questions:

1. What three processes are involved in the production of urine?
2. What is the composition of "normal" urine?
3. What transport mechanisms are responsible for NaCl reabsorption by the nephron? Where are they located along the nephron?
4. How is water reabsorption "coupled" to NaCl reabsorption in the proximal tubule?
5. Why are solutes, but not water, reabsorbed by the thick ascending limb of Henle's loop?
6. What is glomerulotubular balance, and what is its physiologic importance?
7. What are the major hormones that regulate NaCl and water reabsorption in the kidneys? What is the nephron site of action of each hormone?

Formation of urine involves three basic processes: ultrafiltration of plasma by the glomerulus, reabsorption of water and solutes from the ultrafiltrate, and secretion of selected solutes into the tubular fluid. Although 180 L of essentially protein-free fluid is filtered by the human glomeruli each day,[13] less than 1% of the filtered water and NaCl and variable amounts of the other solutes are excreted in the urine (Table 4-1). By the processes of reabsorption and secretion the renal tubules modulate the volume and composition of the urine (Table 4-2). Consequently the tubules control precisely the volume, osmolality, composition, and pH of the intracellular and extracellular fluid compartments.

Because of the importance of tubular reabsorption and secretion, the first part of this chapter defines some basic transport mechanisms used by kidney cells to reabsorb and secrete solutes. Then, NaCl and water reabsorption and some of the factors and hormones that regulate

---

13 The normal glomerular filtration rate (GFR) averages 127-184 L/day in women and 140-197 L/day in men. Thus, the volume of the ultrafiltrate represents a volume that is 10 times that of the extracellular fluid volume. For simplicity, we will assume throughout the remainder of this book that the GFR is 180 L/day.

53

TABLE 4·1

Filtration, excretion, and reabsorption of water, electrolytes, and solutes

Substance	Measure	Filtered	Excreted	Reabsorbed	% Filtered load reabsorbed
Water	L/day	180	1.5	178.5	99.2
Na^+	mEq/day	25,200	150	25,050	99.4
K^+	mEq/day	720	100	620	86.1
Ca^{++}	mEq/day	540	10	530	98.2
HCO_3^-	mEq/day	4320	2	4318	99.9+
Cl^-	mEq/day	18,000	150	17,850	99.2
Glucose	mmol/day	800	0	800	100.0
Urea	g/day	56	28	28	50.0

The filtered amount of any substance is calculated by multiplying the concentration of that substance in the ultrafiltrate by the glomerular filtration rate. For example, the filtered load of Na^+ is calculated as follows: $[Na^+]$ultrafiltrate (140 mEq/L) $\times$ glomerular filtration rate (180 L/day) = 25,200 mEq/day.

reabsorption are discussed. Details on acid-base transport, K^+, Ca^{++}, and Pi transport and their regulation are provided in Chapters 7-9.

■ GENERAL PRINCIPLES OF MEMBRANE TRANSPORT

Solutes may be transported across cell membranes by **passive mechanisms, active transport mechanisms, or endocytosis. In mammals, solute movement occurs by both passive and active mechanisms, whereas all water movement is passive.**

The movement of a solute across a membrane is passive if it develops spontaneously and does not require direct expenditure of metabolic energy. **Passive transport (diffusion)** of uncharged solutes occurs from an area of higher concentration to one of lower concentration (i.e., down its chemical concentration gradient). In addition to concentration gradients, the passive diffusion of ions (but not uncharged solutes, such as glucose and urea) is affected by the electrical potential difference (i.e., electrical gradient) across cell membranes and the renal

> ### *Mechanisms of Solute Transport*
>
> **Passive:**
>
> Spontaneous, down an electrochemical gradient (no energy requirement)
> > Diffusion
> > Facilitated diffusion
> > > Channels
> > > Uniport
> > > Coupled transport: antiport or symport
> > Solvent drag
>
> **Active:**
>
> Against an electrochemical gradient (requires direct input of energy). Includes endocytosis.

tubules. Cations (Na^+, K^+, etc.) move to the negative side of the membrane, whereas anions (Cl^-, HCO_3^-, etc.) move to the positive side of the membrane. Diffusion of lipid-soluble substances, such as the gases O_2, CO_2, and NH_3, occurs across the lipid bilayer of plasma membranes. Diffusion of water (osmosis) occurs

TABLE 4-2

Composition of urine

Substance	Concentration
Na$^+$	50-130 mEq/L
K$^+$	20-70 mEq/L
NH$_4$$^+$	30-50 mEq/L
Ca^{++}	5-12 mEq/L
Mg^{++}	2-18 mEq/L
Cl$^-$	50-130 mEq/L
Pi	20-40 mEq/L
Urea	200-400 mM
Creatinine	6-20 mM
pH	5.0-7.0
Osmolality	500-800 mOsm/kg H$_2$O
Glucose*	0
Amino acids*	0
Protein*	0
Blood*	0
Ketones*	0
Leukocytes*	0
Bilirubin*	0

These values represent average ranges. Asterisks indicate that the presence of these substances in freshly voided urine is measured with dipstick reagent strips. These small strips of plastic contain reagents that change color in a semi-quantitative manner in the presence of specific compounds. Water excretion ranges between 0.5 and 1.5 L/day. (Table modified from Valtin HV: Renal physiology, ed 2, Boston, 1983, Little, Brown & Co.)

through channels in the cell membrane and is driven by osmotic pressure gradients. When water is reabsorbed across tubule segments, the solutes dissolved in the water are also carried along with the water. This process is called **solvent drag** and can account for a substantial amount of solute reabsorption across the proximal tubule.

In **facilitated diffusion,** transport depends on the interaction of the solute with a specific protein in the membrane that facilitates its move-

ment across the membrane. If defined broadly, the term *facilitated diffusion* can be used to describe several different types of membrane transporters. For example, one form of facilitated diffusion is the diffusion of ions, such as Na$^+$ and K$^+$, through aqueous-filled channels created by proteins that span the plasma membrane. Also, the movement of a single molecule across the membrane by means of a transport protein (**uniport**), as occurs with urea and glucose, is a form of facilitated diffusion.[14] Another form of facilitated diffusion is **coupled transport,** in which the movement of two or more solutes across a membrane depends on their interaction with a specific transport protein. Coupled transport of two or more solutes in the same direction is mediated by a **symport** mechanism. Examples of symport mechanisms in the kidneys include Na$^+$-glucose, Na$^+$-amino acid, and Na$^+$-phosphate symporters in the proximal tubule, and 1Na$^+$-1K$^+$-2Cl$^-$ symport in the thick ascending limb of Henle's loop. Coupled transport of two or more solutes in opposite directions is mediated by an **antiport** mechanism. A Na$^+$-H$^+$ antiporter in the proximal tubule mediates Na$^+$ reabsorption and H$^+$ secretion. With coupled transporters, at least one of the solutes is usually transported against its electrochemical gradient. The energy for this uphill movement is derived from the passive downhill movement of at least one of the other solutes into the cell. For example, in the proximal tubule, operation of the Na$^+$-H$^+$ antiporter in the apical membrane of the cell results in the movement of H$^+$ against its electrochemical gradient, out of the cell into the tubular lumen. This uphill movement of H$^+$ is driven by the movement of Na$^+$ from the tubular lumen into the cell, down its electrochemical gradient. The uphill

---

14 Some authors restrict the term *facilitated diffusion* to this type of transport and use as the classic example the glucose uniporter that brings glucose into a wide variety of cells (e.g., skeletal muscle cells).

movement of H$^+$ is termed **secondary active transport** to reflect the fact that the movement of H$^+$ is not directly coupled to the hydrolysis of ATP (see below). Instead, the energy is derived from the gradient of the other coupled ion (in this example, Na$^+$).

Transport is active if it is coupled directly to energy derived from metabolic processes (i.e., it consumes ATP). **Active transport** of solutes usually takes place from an area of lower concentration to an area of higher concentration. In the kidney **the most prevalent active transport mechanism is the Na$^+$-K$^+$-ATPase** (or sodium pump), which is located in the basolateral membrane. The Na$^+$-K$^+$-ATPase is composed of several proteins that together actively move Na$^+$ out of the cell and K$^+$ into the cell. Other active transport mechanisms in the kidneys include the H$^+$-ATPase and H$^+$-K$^+$-ATPase, which are responsible for H$^+$ secretion in the collecting duct system (see Chapter 8), and the Ca^{++}-ATPase, which is responsible for Ca^{++} movement from the cytoplasm into the blood (see Chapter 9).

Endocytosis is the movement of a substance across the plasma membrane by a process involving the invagination of a piece of membrane until it completely pinches off and forms a vesicle in the cytoplasm. This is an important mechanism for the reabsorption of small proteins and macromolecules by the proximal tubule and the retrieval of water channels from the apical membrane of collecting duct cells. Because endocytosis requires ATP, it is a form of active transport.

■ GENERAL PRINCIPLES OF TRANSEPITHELIAL SOLUTE AND WATER TRANSPORT

As illustrated in Figure 4-1, renal cells are held together by **tight junctions.** Below the tight junctions the cells are separated by lateral intercellular spaces. The tight junctions separate the apical membranes from the basolateral membranes. An epithelium can be compared to a six-pack of soda, wherein the cans are the cells and the plastic holder represents the tight junctions.

In the nephron a substance can be reabsorbed or secreted through cells, the so-called **transcellular pathway,** or between cells, the so-called **paracellular pathway** (Figure 4-1). Na$^+$ reabsorption by the proximal tubule is a good example of transport by the transcellular pathway. Na$^+$ reabsorption in this nephron segment depends on the operation of the Na$^+$-K$^+$-ATPase pump (Figure 4-1). The Na$^+$-K$^+$-ATPase pump, which is located exclusively in the basolateral membrane, moves Na$^+$ out of the cell into the blood and K$^+$ into the cell. Thus, the operation of the Na$^+$-K$^+$-ATPase pump lowers intracellular Na$^+$ concentration and increases intracellular K$^+$ concentration. Because intracellular [Na$^+$] is low (12 mEq/L) and the [Na$^+$] in tubular fluid is high (145 mEq/L), Na$^+$ moves across the apical cell membrane, down a chemical concentration gradient from the tubular lumen into the cell. The Na$^+$-K$^+$-ATPase pump senses the addition of Na$^+$ to the cell and is stimulated to increase its rate of Na$^+$ extrusion into the blood, thereby returning intracellular Na$^+$ to normal levels. Thus, transcellular Na$^+$ reabsorption by the proximal tubule is a two-step process:

1. Movement across the apical membrane into the cell, down an electrochemical gradient established by the Na$^+$-K$^+$-ATPase pump
2. Movement across the basolateral membrane against an electrochemical gradient via the Na$^+$-K$^+$-ATPase pump

The reabsorption of Ca^{++} and K$^+$ across the proximal tubule is a good example of paracellular transport. Some of the water reabsorbed across the proximal tubule traverses the paracellular pathway. Some solutes dissolved in this water, particularly Ca^{++} and K$^+$, are entrained in the reabsorbed fluid and thereby reabsorbed by the process of solvent drag.

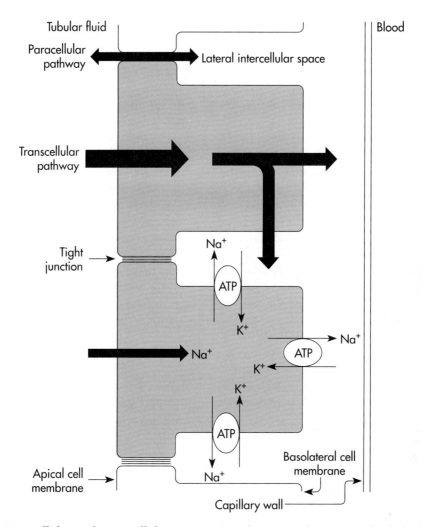

Figure 4-1 ■ Paracellular and transcellular transport pathways in the proximal tubule. See text for details.

■ NaCl, SOLUTE, AND WATER REABSORPTION ALONG THE NEPHRON

Quantitatively the reabsorption of NaCl and water represents the major function of the nephrons (approximately 25,000 mEq/day of Na^+ and 179 L/day of water are reabsorbed). In addition, the transport of many other physiologically important solutes is linked either directly or indirectly to Na^+ reabsorption. In the follow-

ing sections the NaCl and water transport properties of each nephron segment and its regulation by hormones, among other factors, are presented.

Proximal Tubule

The proximal tubule reabsorbs approximately 67% of the filtered water, Na^+, Cl^-, K^+, and other solutes. In addition, virtually all the glucose and amino acids filtered by the glomerulus are reabsorbed. **The key element in proximal tubule reabsorption is the Na$^+$-K$^+$-ATPase pump in the basolateral membrane.** The reabsorption of every substance, including water, is linked in some manner to the operation of the Na$^+$-K$^+$-ATPase pump.

Na$^+$ Reabsorption Na$^+$ is reabsorbed by different mechanisms in the early (first half of the proximal tubule) and late (second half of the proximal tubule) segments of the proximal tubule. In the early segment, Na$^+$ is reabsorbed primarily with HCO$_3$$^-$ and a number of organic molecules (e.g., glucose, amino acids, Pi, lactate). By contrast, Na$^+$ is reabsorbed mainly with Cl$^-$ in the second half of the proximal tubule. This occurs because of differences in the Na$^+$ transport systems present in the early and late segments of the proximal tubule, as well as differences in the composition of tubular fluid at these sites.

In the early segment of the proximal tubule, Na$^+$ uptake into the cell is coupled with either H$^+$ or organic solutes (Figure 4-2). Na$^+$ entry into the cell across the apical membrane is mediated by specific symporter and antiporter proteins and not by diffusion through channels. For example, Na$^+$ entry is coupled with H$^+$ extrusion from the cell by the Na$^+$-H$^+$ antiporter (Figure 4-2, A). H$^+$ secretion, by the Na$^+$-H$^+$ antiporter, results in NaHCO$_3$ reabsorption. (Chapter 8 has more details on this mechanism.) Na$^+$ also enters proximal cells by several symporter mechanisms, including Na$^+$-glucose, Na$^+$-amino acid, Na$^+$-Pi, and Na$^+$-lactate symporters (Figure 4-2, *B*). The glucose (and other organic solutes) that enters the cell with Na$^+$ leaves the cell across the basolateral membrane by passive transporter mechanisms. The Na$^+$ that enters the cell across the apical membrane, by either a symport or antiport mechanism, leaves the cell and enters the blood via the Na$^+$-K$^+$-ATPase. In summary, in the early segment of the proximal tubule the reabsorption of Na$^+$ is coupled to that of HCO$_3$$^-$ and a num-

ber of organic molecules. Reabsorption of many of these organic molecules is so avid that these solutes are almost completely removed from the tubular fluid in the first half of the proximal tubule (Figure 4-3). The reabsorption of NaHCO$_3$ and Na$^+$-organic solutes across the proximal tubule establishes a transtubular osmotic gradient that provides the driving force for the passive reabsorption of water by osmosis. Because water is reabsorbed in excess of Cl$^-$ in the early segment of the proximal tubule, the Cl$^-$ concentration in tubular fluid rises along the length of the early proximal tubule (Figure 4-3).

In the second half of the proximal tubule, Na$^+$ is primarily reabsorbed with Cl$^-$ across both the transcellular and paracellular pathways (Figure 4-4). Na$^+$ is reabsorbed with Cl$^-$, rather than with organic solutes or HCO$_3$$^-$ as the accompanying anion. This occurs because the cells lining the second half of the proximal tubule have different Na$^+$ transport mechanisms than the early segment of the proximal tubule and because the tubular fluid that enters the second half of the proximal tubule contains very little glucose and amino acids and has a high concentration of Cl$^-$ (140 mEq/L versus 105 mEq/L in the first half of the proximal tubule). The Cl$^-$ concentration is high because, in the first half of the proximal tubule, Na$^+$ is preferentially reabsorbed with HCO$_3$$^-$ and organic solutes (Figure 4-2).

The mechanism of transcellular Na$^+$ reabsorption in the second half of the proximal tubule is illustrated in Figure 4-4. Na$^+$ enters the cell across the luminal membrane by the parallel operation of Na$^+$-H$^+$ and one or more Cl$^-$-Anion antiporters. Because the secreted H$^+$ and Anion combine in the tubular fluid and reenter the cell, the operation of the Na$^+$-H$^+$ and Cl$^-$-Anion antiporters is equivalent to NaCl uptake from tubular fluid into the cell. Na$^+$ leaves the cell by the Na$^+$-K$^+$-ATPase pump, and Cl$^-$ leaves the cell and enters the blood by a KCl symport protein in the basolateral membrane.

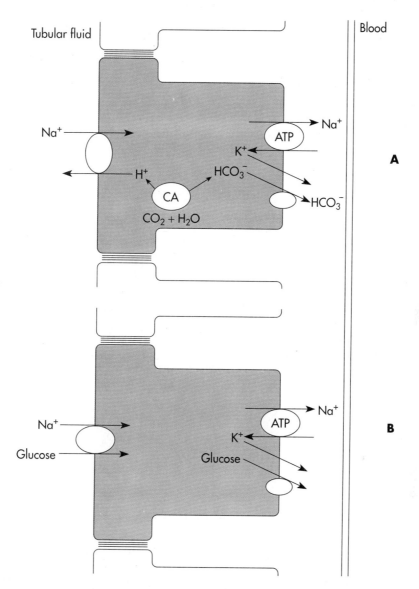

Figure 4-2 ■ Na$^+$ transport processes in the first half of the proximal tubule. The transport mechanisms depicted are present in all cells in the first half of the proximal tubule. They are separated into different cells to simplify the discussion. **A,** The operation of the Na$^+$-H$^+$-transporter in the apical membrane and the Na$^+$-K$^+$-ATPase and the HCO$_3^-$ transporter in the basolateral membrane mediate NaHCO$_3$ reabsorption. CO$_2$ and H$_2$O combine inside the cells to form H$^+$ and HCO$_3^-$ in a reaction facilitated by the enzyme carbonic anhydrase (CA). **B,** The operation of the Na$^+$-glucose transporter, in the apical membrane, in conjunction with the Na$^+$-K$^+$-ATPase and the glucose transporter, in the basolateral membrane, mediate Na$^+$-glucose reabsorption. Na$^+$ reabsorption is also coupled with other solutes, including amino acids, Pi, and lactate. Reabsorption of these solutes is mediated by Na$^+$-amino acid, Na$^+$-phosphate, and Na$^+$-lactate symporters located in the apical membrane and the Na$^+$-K$^+$-ATPase and the amino acid, Pi, and lactate transporters in the basolateral membrane.

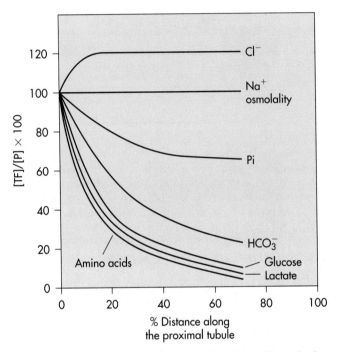

Figure 4-3 ■ Concentration of solutes in tubule fluid as a function of length along the proximal tubule. *[TF]* is the concentration of the substance in tubular fluid; *[P]* is the concentration of the substance in plasma. Values above 100 indicate that relatively less of the solute than water was reabsorbed, and values below 100 indicate that relatively more of the substance than water was reabsorbed. (Modified from Vander AJ: Renal physiology, ed 4, New York, 1991, McGraw-Hill.)

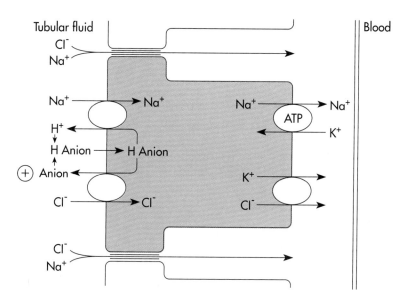

Figure 4-4 ■ Na$^+$ transport processes in the second half of the proximal tubule. Na$^+$ and Cl$^-$ enter the cell across the apical membrane by the operation of parallel Na$^+$-H$^+$ and Cl$^-$-Anion antiporters. More than one Cl$^-$-Anion antiporter may be involved in this process, but only one is depicted here. The secreted H$^+$ and Anion combine in the tubular fluid to form an HAnion complex that can recycle across the plasma membrane. Accumulation of HAnion in tubular fluid establishes an HAnion concentration gradient that favors HAnion recycling across the apical plasma membrane into the cell. Inside the cell H$^+$ and the Anion dissociate and recycle back across the apical plasma membrane. The net result is NaCl uptake across the apical membrane. The Anion may be OH$^-$, formate (HCO$_2$$^-$), oxalate$^-$, HCO$_3$$^-$, or sulfate. The lumen-positive transepithelial voltage, indicated by the plus sign inside the circle in the tubular lumen, is generated by the diffusion of Cl$^-$ (lumen-to-blood) across the tight junction. The high [Cl$^-$] of tubular fluid provides the driving force for Cl$^-$ diffusion.

NaCl is also reabsorbed across the second half of the proximal tubule by a paracellular route. **Paracellular NaCl reabsorption occurs because the rise in [Cl$^-$] in the tubule fluid in the early segment of the proximal tubule creates a concentration gradient of Cl$^-$ (140 mEq/L in the tubule lumen and 105 mEq/L in the interstitium) that favors the diffusion of Cl$^-$ from the tubular lumen across the tight junctions into the lateral intercellular space.** Movement of the negatively charged Cl$^-$ generates a positive transepithelial voltage (tubular fluid positive relative to the blood), which causes the diffusion of positively charged Na$^+$ out of the tubular fluid, across the tight junction into the blood. Thus,

in the second half of the proximal tubule some Na$^+$ and Cl$^-$ is reabsorbed across the tight junctions by passive diffusion. The reabsorption of NaCl establishes a transtubular osmotic gradient that provides the driving force for the passive reabsorption of water by osmosis (see below).

In summary, reabsorption of Na$^+$ and Cl$^-$ in the proximal tubule occurs across the paracellular and transcellular pathways. Approximately 17,000 mEq of the 25,200 mEq of NaCl filtered each day is reabsorbed in the proximal tubule (~67% of the filtered load). Of this, two thirds moves across the transcellular pathway, and the remaining one third moves across the paracellular pathway (Tables 4-3 and 4-4).

T A B L E   4 - 3

NaCl transport along the nephron

Segment	Percent of filtered load reabsorbed	Mechanism of Na⁺ entry across the apical membrane	Major regulatory hormones
Proximal tubule	67	Na^+-H^+ exchange, Na^+-cotransport with amino acids and organic solutes, Na^+/H^+-Cl^-/anion exchange Paracellular	Angiotensin II Norepinephrine Epinephrine Dopamine
Loop of Henle	25	$1Na^+$-$1K^+$-$2Cl^-$ symport	Aldosterone
Distal tubule	~4	Na^+-Cl^- symport	Aldosterone
Late distal tubule and collecting duct	~3	Na^+ channels	Aldosterone ANP Urodilatin

T A B L E   4 - 4

Water transport along the nephron

Segment	Percent of filtered load reabsorbed	Mechanism of water reabsorption	Hormones that regulate water permeability
Proximal tubule	67	Passive	None
Loop of Henle	15	DTL only. Passive	None
Distal tubule	0	No water reabsorption	None
Late distal tubule and collecting duct	~8-17	Passive	ADH, ANP*

*ANP inhibits the ADH-stimulated water permeability.

Water Reabsorption The proximal tubule reabsorbs 67% of the filtered water. Figure 4-5 illustrates the mechanism of water reabsorption in the proximal tubule. **The driving force for water reabsorption is a transtubular osmotic gradient established by solute reabsorption (i.e., NaCl, Na⁺ glucose).** The reabsorption of Na⁺ with organic solutes, HCO_3^-, and Cl^- from the tubular fluid into the lateral intercellular spaces reduces the osmolality of the tubular fluid and increases the osmolality of the lateral intercellular space. Because the proximal tubule is highly permeable to water, water will flow by osmosis across both the tight junctions and the proximal tubular cells. Accumulation of fluid and solutes within the lateral intercellular

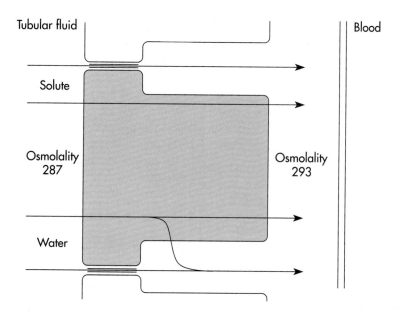

Figure 4-5 ■ Routes of water and solute reabsorption across the proximal tubule. Transport of solutes including Na⁺, Cl⁻, and organic solutes into the lateral intercellular space increases the osmolality of this compartment, which establishes the driving force for osmotic water reabsorption across the proximal tubule. This occurs because some Na⁺-K⁺-ATPase pumps and organic solute and HCO₃⁻ and Cl⁻ transporters are located on the lateral cell membranes and deposit these solutes between cells. Furthermore, some NaCl also enters the lateral intercellular space by diffusion across the tight junction (i.e., paracellular pathway). An important consequence of osmotic water flow across the transcellular and paracellular pathways in the proximal tubule is that some solutes, especially K⁺ and Ca⁺⁺, are entrained in the reabsorbed fluid and thereby reabsorbed by the process of solvent drag.

space increases the hydrostatic pressure in this compartment which, in turn, forces fluid and solutes to move into the capillaries. Thus, water reabsorption follows solute reabsorption in the proximal tubule. The reabsorbed fluid is slightly hyperosmotic to plasma. An important consequence of osmotic water flow across the proximal tubule is that some solutes, especially K⁺ and Ca⁺⁺, is entrained in the reabsorbed fluid and thereby reabsorbed by the process of solvent drag (Figure 4-5). Because the reabsorption of virtually all organic solutes, Cl⁻, other ions, and water is coupled to Na⁺ reabsorption, changes in

Na⁺ reabsorption influence the reabsorption of water and other solutes by the proximal tubule.

The **Fanconi syndrome** is a renal disease that is either hereditary or acquired and results from an impaired ability of the proximal tubule to reabsorb amino acids, glucose, and low molecular weight proteins. Because other segments of the nephron cannot reabsorb these solutes, Fanconi syndrome results in an increase in the excretion of amino acids, glucose, Pi, and low molecular weight proteins in the urine.

Protein Reabsorption Proteins that are filtered are also reabsorbed in the proximal tubule. As mentioned previously, peptide hormones, small proteins, and even small amounts of larger proteins, such as albumin, are filtered by the glomerulus. Although filtration of proteins is small (the concentration of proteins in the ultrafiltrate is only 40 mg/L), the amount of protein filtered per day is significant because the GFR is so high.

filtered protein = GFR × [protein] in the ultrafiltrate
filtered protein = 180 L/day × 40 mg/L = 7.2 g/day

These proteins are partially degraded by enzymes on the surface of the proximal tubule cells and are then taken up into the cell by endocytosis. Once inside the cell, enzymes digest the proteins and peptides into their constituent amino acids, which leave the cell across the basolateral membrane and are returned to the blood. Normally this mechanism reabsorbs virtually all of the protein filtered, leaving the urine essentially protein free. However, because the mechanism is easily saturated, protein will appear in the urine if the amount of protein filtered increases. Disruption of the glomerular filtration barrier to proteins increases the filtration of proteins and results in proteinuria (appearance of protein in the urine). Proteinuria is frequently seen with kidney disease.

During routine urinalysis it is not abnormal to find traces of protein in the urine. It is important to realize that protein in the urine can be derived from two potential sources: (1) filtration and incomplete reabsorption by the proximal tubule and (2) synthesis by the thick ascending limb of Henle's loop. Cells in the thick ascending limb produce Tamm-Horsfall glycoprotein and secrete the protein into the tubular fluid. Because the mechanism for protein reabsorption is upstream of the thick ascending limb, the secreted Tamm-Horsfall glycoprotein appears in the urine.

Organic Anion and Organic Cation Secretion In addition to reabsorbing solutes and water, cells of the proximal tubule also secrete organic cations and organic anions (see Tables 4-5 and 4-6 for a partial listing). Many of the substances are end-products of metabolism that circulate in the plasma. The proximal tubule also secretes numerous exogenous organic compounds, including P-aminohippuric acid (PAH), and drugs such as penicillin and pollutants. Because many of these organic compounds can be

T A B L E   4 - 5

Some organic anions secreted by the proximal tubule

Endogenous anions	Drugs
cAMP	Acetazolamide
Bile salts	Chlorothiazide
Hippurates	Furosemide
Oxalate	Penicillin
Prostaglandins	Probenecid
Urate	Salicylate (Aspirin)
	Hydrochlorothiazide
	Bumetanide

T A B L E   4 - 6

Some organic cations secreted by the proximal tubule

Endogenous cations	Drugs
Creatinine	Atropine
Dopamine	Isoproterenol
Epinephrine	Cimetidine
Norepinephrine	Morphine
	Quinine
	Amiloride
	Procainamide

bound to plasma proteins, they are not readily filtered. Therefore excretion by filtration alone eliminates only a small portion of these potentially toxic substances from the body. Excretion rates of these substances are high because they are both filtered and secreted from the peritubular capillaries into the tubular fluid. Because the kidneys remove virtually all organic anions and cations from the plasma entering the kidneys, it is evident that these secretory mechanisms are very powerful and serve a vital function by clearing these substances from the plasma.

Figure 4-6 illustrates the mechanism of PAH transport across the proximal tubule as an example of organic anion secretion. This secretory pathway has a maximum transport rate, a low specificity (i.e., it transports a variety of organic

anions), and is responsible for the secretion of all organic anions listed in Table 4-5. The organic anion PAH, which can be used to measure RPF, has been used to unravel the details of this pathway. PAH is taken up into the cell, across the basolateral membrane, against its chemical gradient in exchange for α-ketoglutarate (αKG) via a PAH-αKG antiport mechanism. αKG accumulates inside the cells via metabolism of glutamate and by a Na$^+$-αKG symporter, also present in the basolateral membrane. Thus, PAH uptake into the cell against its electrochemical gradient is coupled to the exit of αKG out of the cell, down its chemical gradients generated by the Na$^+$-αKG antiport mechanism and metabolism of glutamate. The resulting high intracellular concentration of PAH provides the driving force for PAH exit across the

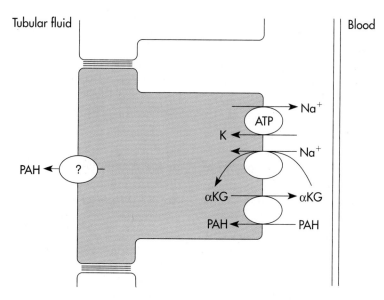

Figure 4-6 ■ Organic anion secretion (e.g., PAH) across the proximal tubule. PAH enters the cell across the basolateral membrane by a PAH-α-ketoglutarate (αKG) antiport mechanism. The uptake of αKG into the cell, against its chemical gradients, is driven by the movement of Na$^+$ into the cell. The αKG recycles across the basolateral membrane. PAH leaves the cell across the apical membrane, down its chemical concentration gradient by an unknown mechanism.

luminal membrane into the tubular fluid via a PAH-anion antiporter (Figure 4-6).

Figure 4-7 illustrates the mechanism of organic cation (OC^+) transport across the proximal tubule. Organic cations are taken up into the cell, across the basolateral membrane, by a mechanism that involves facilitated diffusion (i.e., uniport mechanism) and is driven by the magnitude of the cell-negative potential difference across the basolateral membrane. Organic cation transport across the luminal membrane into the tubular fluid is mediated by an OC^+-H^+ antiporter. The transport mechanisms for organic cation secretion are nonspecific (see Table 4-6), and several cations compete for the transport pathway.

Henle's Loop

Henle's loop reabsorbs approximately 25% of the filtered NaCl and K^+. Ca^{++} and HCO_3^- are also reabsorbed in the loop of Henle (see Chapters 8 and 9 for more details). This reabsorption occurs almost exclusively in the thick ascending limb. By comparison, the ascending thin limb has a much lower reabsorptive capacity, and the descending thin limb does not reabsorb significant amounts of solutes. The loop of Henle reabsorbs approximately 15% of the filtered water. This reabsorption, however, occurs exclusively in the descending thin limb. **The ascending limb is impermeable to water.**

The key element in solute reabsorption by the thick ascending limb is the Na^+-K^+-ATPase pump in the basolateral membrane (Figure 4-8). As with reabsorption in the proximal tubule the reabsorption of every solute by the thick ascending limb is in some manner linked to the Na^+-K^+-ATPase pump. The operation of the Na^+-K^+-ATPase pump maintains a low cell [Na^+]. This low [Na^+] provides a favorable chemical gradient for the movement of Na^+ from the tubular fluid into the cell. The movement of Na^+ across the apical membrane into the cell is mediated by the $1Na^+$- $1K^+$-$2Cl^-$-symporter, which couples the movement of $1Na^+$ with $1K^+$ and $2Cl^-$. This sym-

Because all organic anions compete for the same transporter, elevated plasma levels of one anion inhibit the secretion of the others. For example, a reduction of penicillin secretion by the proximal tubule can be produced by infusing PAH. Because the kidneys are responsible for eliminating penicillin from the body, the infusion of PAH into individuals receiving penicillin reduces urinary penicillin excretion and thereby extends the biologic half life of the drug. When penicillin was in short supply during World War II, hippurates were given with the penicillin to extend the drug's therapeutic effect.

The histamine H_2-antagonist cimetidine, used to treat gastric ulcers, is secreted by the organic cation pathway in the proximal tubule. Cimetidine reduces the urinary excretion of the antiarrhythmic drug procainamide, also an organic cation, by competing with procainamide for the secretory pathway. It is important to recognize that coadministration of organic cations can often increase the plasma concentration of both drugs to levels that are much higher than the plasma concentration of the drugs when given alone, and it can often lead to drug toxicity.

port protein uses the potential energy released by the downhill movement of Na^+ and Cl^- to drive the uphill movement of K^+ into the cell. A Na^+-H^+ antiporter in the apical cell membrane also mediates Na^+ reabsorption as well as H^+ secretion (HCO_3^- reabsorption) in the thick ascending limb. (Chapter 8 contains details on HCO_3^- reabsorption by the thick ascending limb.) Na^+ leaves the cell across the basolateral membrane via the Na^+-K^+-ATPase pump, and K^+, Cl^-, and HCO_3^- leave the cell across the basolateral membrane by separate pathways.

The voltage across the thick ascending limb is oriented with the tubular fluid positive relative to the blood because of the unique location of

Tubular fluid

Blood

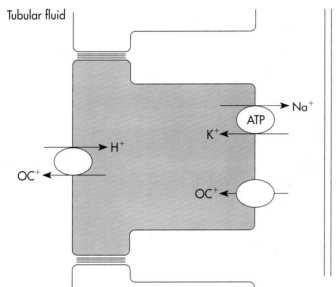

Figure 4-7 ■ Organic cation (OC$^+$) secretion across the proximal tubule. OC$^+$ enter the cell across the basolateral membrane by facilitated diffusion. The uptake of OC$^+$ into the cell, against their chemical gradient, is driven by the cell-negative potential difference. OC$^+$ leave the cell across the apical membrane in exchange with H$^+$ by an OC$^+$-H$^+$ antiport mechanism.

transport proteins in the apical and basolateral membranes. **The important points to recognize are that increased salt transport by the thick ascending limb increases the magnitude of the positive voltage in the lumen and that this voltage is an important driving force for the reabsorption of several cations, including Na$^+$, K$^+$ and Ca^{++} across the paracellular pathway** (Figure 4-8). Thus, salt reabsorption across the thick ascending limb occurs by transcellular and paracellular pathways. Fifty percent of solute transport is transcellular, and the other half is paracellular.

Because the thick ascending limb is impermeable to water, reabsorption of NaCl and other solutes reduces the osmolality of tubular fluid to less than 150 mOsm/kg H$_2$O.

Inhibition of the 1Na$^+$-1K$^+$-2Cl$^-$ symporter in the thick ascending limb by loop diuretics such as furosemide (i.e., Lasix) inhibits NaCl reabsorption by the thick ascending limb and thereby increases urinary NaCl excretion. Furosemide also inhibits K$^+$ and Ca^{++} reabsorption by reducing the lumen-positive voltage that drives the paracellular reabsorption of these ions. Thus, furosemide increases urinary K$^+$ and Ca^{++} excretion. Furosemide also increases water excretion by reducing the osmolality of the interstitial fluid in the medulla. Because water reabsorption by the descending thin limb (DTL) of Henle's loop is passive and driven by the osmotic gradient between the tubular fluid in the DTL (which is ~290 mOsm/kg H$_2$O at the beginning of the DTL) and the interstitial fluid (which is ~1200 mOsm/kg H$_2$O in the medulla), a reduction of the osmolality of the interstitial fluid reduces water reabsorption.

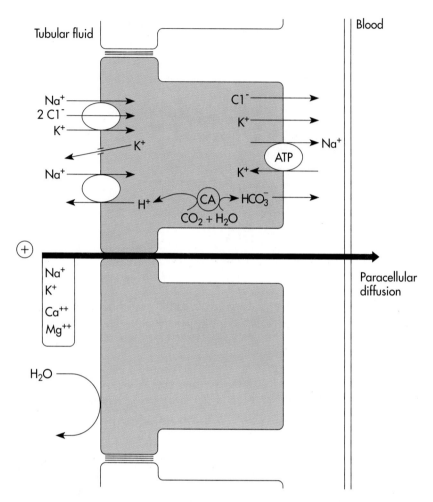

Figure 4-8 ■ **Transport mechanisms for NaCl reabsorption in the thick ascending limb of Henle's loop. The lumen-positive transepithelial voltage plays a major role in driving passive paracellular reabsorption of cations.** *CA*, Carbonic anhydrase.

Distal Tubule and Collecting Duct

The distal tubule and the collecting duct reabsorb approximately 7% of the filtered NaCl, secrete variable amounts of K^+ and H^+, and reabsorb a variable amount of water (~8%-17%). Water reabsorption depends on the plasma concentration of ADH. The initial segment of the distal tubule (early distal tubule) reabsorbs Na^+, Cl^-, and Ca^{++} and, like the thick ascending limb,

is impermeable to water (Figure 4-9). NaCl entry into the cell across the apical membrane is mediated by a Na^+-Cl^- symporter (Figure 4-9). Na^+ leaves the cell via the Na^+-K^+-ATPase pump, and Cl^- leaves the cell by diffusion via channels. NaCl reabsorption is reduced by thiazide diuretics, which inhibit the Na^+-Cl^- symporter (see Chapter 10). Thus, the active dilution of the tubular fluid begins in the thick ascending limb

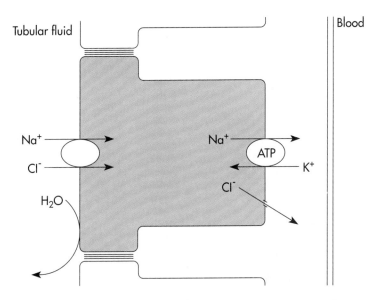

Figure 4-9 ■ **Transport mechanism for Na⁺ and Cl⁻ reabsorption in the early segment of the distal tubule. This segment is impermeable to water. See the text for details.**

and continues in the early segment of the distal tubule.

The last segment of the distal tubule (late distal tubule) and the collecting duct are composed of two cell types, principal cells and intercalated cells. As illustrated in Figure 4-10, **principal cells reabsorb Na⁺ and water and secrete K⁺. Intercalated cells secrete either H⁺ (reabsorb HCO₃⁻) or HCO₃⁻ and are therefore important in regulating acid-base balance.** (Chapter 8 contains details on H⁺ secretion and HCO₃⁻ reabsorption by intercalated cells.) **Intercalated cells also reabsorb K⁺.** Both Na⁺ reabsorption and K⁺ secretion by principal cells depend on the activity of the Na⁺-K⁺-ATPase pump in the basolateral membrane (Figure 4-10). This enzyme maintains a low cell [Na⁺], which provides a favorable chemical gradient for the movement of Na⁺ from the tubular fluid into the cell. Because Na⁺ enters the cell across the apical membrane by diffusion through channels in the membrane, the negative

potential inside the cell facilitates Na⁺ entry. Na⁺ leaves the cell across the basolateral membrane and enters the blood via the Na⁺-K⁺-ATPase pump. Sodium reabsorption generates a lumen-negative voltage across the late distal tubule and collecting duct. Cells in the collecting duct reabsorb significant amounts of Cl⁻, most likely across the paracellular pathway. Reabsorption of Cl⁻ is driven by the lumen-negative transepithelial voltage.

K⁺ is secreted from the blood into the tubular fluid by principal cells in two steps (Figure 4-10). K⁺ uptake across the basolateral membrane is mediated by the Na⁺-K⁺-ATPase pump. Because the [K⁺] inside the cells is high (150 mEq/L) and the [K⁺] in tubular fluid is low (~10 mEq/L), K⁺ diffuses down its concentration gradient, across the apical cell membrane and into the tubular fluid. Although the negative potential inside the cells tends to retain K⁺ within the cell, the electrochemical gradient across the apical membrane favors K⁺ secretion from the cell into the tubular

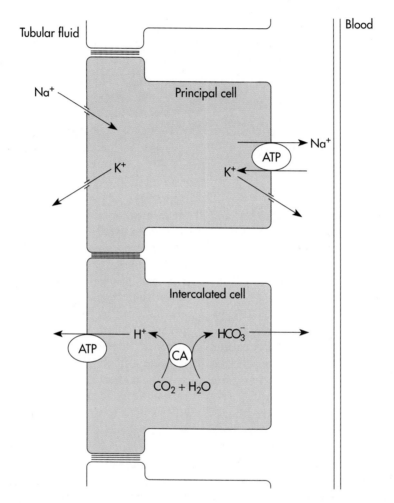

Figure 4-10 ■ **Transport pathways in principal cells and intercalated cells of the distal tubule and collecting duct. See the text for details.** *CA,* **Carbonic anhydrase. Consult Chapter 7 for details on K+ reabsorption by intercalated cells.**

fluid. Additional details of K^+ secretion and its regulation are considered in Chapter 7.

> Amiloride is a diuretic that inhibits Na^+ reabsorption by the distal tubule and collecting duct by directly inhibiting Na^+ channels in the luminal cell membrane. Amiloride also inhibits Cl^- reabsorption indirectly by its effect on inhibiting Na^+ reabsorption. Inhibition of Na^+ reabsorption reduces the lumen-negative voltage, the driving force for paracellular Cl^- reabsorption. Because of amiloride's effect on reducing the magnitude of the lumen-negative voltage, amiloride also acts to inhibit K^+ secretion. By inhibiting K^+ secretion across the distal tubule and collecting duct, amiloride reduces the amount of K^+ excreted in the urine (see Chapter 10). Consequently, amiloride is frequently referred to as a *K^+-sparing diuretic.* It is most often used in patients who excrete too much K^+ in their urine.

The mechanism of K^+ reabsorption by intercalated cells is not completely understood but is thought to be mediated by an H^+-K^+-ATPase located in the apical cell membrane (see Chapter 8).

■ REGULATION OF NACL AND WATER REABSORPTION

Several hormones and factors regulate NaCl reabsorption. Table 4-7 summarizes each hormone's major stimulus for secretion, the nephron site of action, and the effect on transport. Quantitatively, angiotensin II, aldosterone, ANP, urodilatin, epinephrine, and norepinephrine released by sympathetic nerves are the most important hormones that regulate NaCl reabsorption and therefore urinary NaCl excretion. However, other hormones (including dopamine and glucocorticoids), Starling forces, and the phenomenon of glomerulotubular balance also influence NaCl reabsorption. ADH is the only major hormone that directly regulates the amount of water excreted by the kidneys.

TABLE 4-7

Hormones that regulate NaCl and water reabsorption

Hormone	Major stimulus	Nephron site of action	Effect on transport
Angiotensin II	↑ Renin	PT	↑ NaCl & H_2O reabsorption
Aldosterone	↑ Angiotensin II, ↑ $[K^+]_p$	TAL, DT/CD	↑NaCl & H_2O reabsorption*
ANP	↑ BP, ↑ ECV	CD	↓ H_2O & NaCl reabsorption
Urodilatin	↑ BP, ↑ ECV	CD	↓H_2O & NaCl reabsorption
Sympathetic nerves	↓ ECV	PT, TAL, DT/CD	↑NaCl & H_2O reabsorption*
Dopamine	↑ ECV	PT	↓H_2O & NaCl reabsorption
ADH	↑ P_{osm}, ↓ ECV	DT/CD	↑H_2O reabsorption

PT, Proximal tubule; *TAL*, thick ascending limb; *DT/CD*, distal tubule and collecting duct; *ECV*, effective circulating volume; *BP*, blood pressure; *$[K^+]_p$* plasma $[K^+]$; *P_{osm}* plasma osmolality. All of the hormones listed act within minutes, except aldosterone, which exerts its action on NaCl reabsorption with a delay of one hour. Asterisk indicates that the effect on H_2O reabsorption does not include the TAL; ↓ indicates a decrease, and ↑ indicates an increase.

1. Angiotensin II: Angiotensin II is one of the most potent hormones that stimulate NaCl and water reabsorption in the proximal tubule. A decrease in the extracellular fluid volume activates the renin-angiotensin-aldosterone system (discussed in Chapter 6) and thereby increases plasma angiotensin II concentration.

2. Aldosterone: Aldosterone is synthesized by the glomerulosa cells of the adrenal cortex and stimulates NaCl reabsorption by the thick ascending limb of Henle's loop and the distal tubule and collecting duct. Aldosterone also stimulates K^+ secretion by the distal tubule and collecting duct (see Chapter 7). **The two most important stimuli to aldosterone secretion are an increase in angiotensin II concentration and an increase in plasma [K^+].** By acting to stimulate NaCl reabsorption in the collecting duct, aldosterone also increases water reabsorption by this nephron segment.

Some individuals with an expanded extracellular fluid volume and elevated blood pressure are treated with drugs that inhibit angiotensin-converting enzyme (ACE inhibitors, such as Captopril) to lower fluid volume and blood pressure. Inhibition of angiotensin-converting enzyme blocks the degradation of angiotensin I to angiotensin II and thereby lowers plasma angiotensin levels (see Chapter 6). The decline in plasma angiotensin II concentration has three effects: (1) NaCl and water reabsorption by the proximal tubule falls; (2) aldosterone secretion falls, which reduces NaCl reabsorption in the distal tubule and collecting duct; and (3) because angiotensin is a potent vasoconstrictor, the systemic arterioles dilate and arterial blood pressure falls. In addition, ACE degrades the vasodilating hormone bradykinin. ACE inhibitors therefore increase the concentrations of bradykinin. Thus, ACE inhibitors decrease the extracellular fluid volume and the arterial blood pressure by promoting renal NaCl and water excretion and depressing total peripheral resistance.

---

3. Atrial natriuretic peptide (ANP) and urodilatin: ANP and urodilatin are encoded by the same gene and have very similar amino acid sequences. ANP is a 28-amino-acid peptide hormone secreted by the cardiac atria, and its secretion is stimulated by a rise in blood pressure and an increase in the extracellular fluid volume. ANP decreases blood pressure by decreasing total peripheral resistance and enhancing urinary NaCl and water excretion. The hormone inhibits NaCl reabsorption by the medullary portion of the collecting duct, inhibits ADH-stimulated water reabsorption across the collecting duct, and inhibits the secretion of ADH from the posterior pituitary.

   Urodilatin is a 32-amino-acid peptide that differs from ANP by the addition of four amino acids to the amino terminus. Urodilatin is secreted by the distal tubule and collecting duct and is not present in the systemic circulation; thus, urodilatin influences only the function of the kidneys. Stimulated by a rise in blood pressure and an increase in the extracellular fluid volume, urodilatin secretion inhibits NaCl and water reabsorption across the medullary portion of the collecting duct. Urodilatin is a more potent natriuretic and diuretic hormone than ANP because ANP entering the kidneys in the blood is degraded by a neutral endopeptidase that has no effect on urodilatin.

4. Sympathetic nerves: Catecholamines released from sympathetic nerves (norepinephrine) and the adrenal medulla (epinephrine) stimulate NaCl and water reabsorption by the proximal tubule, thick ascending limb of Henle's loop, distal tubule, and collecting duct. Activation of sympathetic nerves (e.g., after hemorrhage or a decrease in the extracellular fluid volume) stimulates NaCl and water reabsorption by the proximal tubule, thick ascending limb of Henle's loop, distal tubule, and collecting duct.

5. Dopamine: Dopamine, a catecholamine, is released from dopaminergic nerves in the kidney and may also be synthesized by cells of the proximal tubule. The action of dopamine is opposite to that of norepinephrine and epinephrine. Dopamine secretion is stimulated by an increase in extracellular fluid volume, and its secretion directly inhibits NaCl and water reabsorption in the proximal tubule.

6. Antidiuretic hormone (ADH): **Antidiuretic hormone is the most important hormone that regulates water balance** (see Chapter 5). This hormone is secreted by the posterior pituitary in response to an increase in plasma osmolality or a decrease in the extracellular fluid volume. ADH increases the permeability of the collecting duct to water, and because an osmotic gradient exists across the wall of the collecting duct, the hormone increases water reabsorption by the collecting duct (see Chapter 5 for details). ADH has little effect on urinary NaCl excretion.

7. Starling forces: Starling forces[15] regulate NaCl and water reabsorption across the proximal tubule (Figure 4-11). As described above, Na^+, Cl^-, HCO_3^-, amino acids, glucose, and water are transported into the intercellular space of the proximal tubule. Starling forces between this space and the peritubular capillaries facilitate the movement of the reabsorbate into the capillaries. Starling forces that favor movement from the interstitium into the peritubu-

lar capillaries are the capillary oncotic pressure (π_c) and the hydrostatic pressure in the intercellular space (P_i). The opposing Starling forces are the interstitial oncotic pressure (π_i) and the capillary hydrostatic pressure (P_c). Normally the sum of the Starling forces favors movement of solute and water from the interstitium into the capillary. However, some of the solutes and fluid that enter the lateral intercellular space leak back into the proximal tubular fluid. Starling forces do not affect transport by the loop of Henle, distal tubule, and collecting duct because these segments are less permeable to H_2O than is the proximal tubule.

Starling forces across the peritubular capillaries surrounding the proximal tubule are readily altered. For example, dilation of the efferent arteriole increases the hydrostatic pressure in the peritubular capillaries (P_c), whereas constriction of the efferent arteriole decreases P_c. An increase in P_c inhibits solute and water reabsorption by increasing the backleak of NaCl and water across the tight junction, whereas a decrease in P_c stimulates reabsorption by decreasing backleak across the tight junction.

The oncotic pressure in the peritubular capillary is determined in part by the rate of formation of the glomerular ultrafiltrate. For example, if one assumes a constant plasma flow in the afferent arteriole, as less ultrafiltrate is formed (i.e., as GFR decreases) the plasma proteins become less concentrated in the plasma that enters the efferent arteriole and peritubular capillary. Hence the peritubular oncotic pressure decreases. Thus, the peritubular oncotic pressure is directly related to the filtration fraction (FF = GFR/RPF). A fall in the FF, owing to a decrease in GFR at constant RPF, decreases the peritubular capillary oncotic pressure. This in turn increases the backflux of NaCl and water from the lateral intercellular space into the tubular fluid and thereby decreases net solute and water reabsorption across

---

15 Starling forces across the wall of the peritubular capillaries are the hydrostatic pressure in the peritubular capillary (P_c) and lateral intercellular space (P_i) and the oncotic pressure in the peritubular capillary (π_c) and the lateral intercellular space (π_i). Thus, the reabsorption of water, resulting from sodium transport from tubular fluid into the lateral intercellular space, will be modified by the Starling forces. Thus:

$$Q = K_f \{(P_i - P_c) + (\pi_c - \pi_i)\}$$

Where Q equals flow (positive numbers indicate flow from the intercellular space into blood).

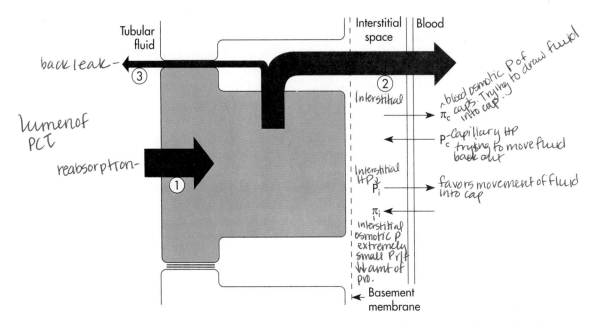

Handwritten annotations on figure:

back leak —

lumen of PCT

reabsorption —

blood osmotic P of cap. Trying to draw fluid into cap.

π_c

P-Capillary HP trying to move fluid back out

favors movement of fluid into cap

Interstitial osmotic P extremely small P r/t ↓ amt of pro.

Figure 4-11 ■ **Routes of solute and water transport across the proximal tubule and the Starling forces that modify reabsorption.** *1,* Solute and water are reabsorbed across the apical membrane. This solute and water then cross the lateral cell membrane. Some solute and water reenter the tubule fluid (indicated by arrow labeled *3*), and the remainder enters the interstitial space and then flows into the capillary (indicated by arrow labeled *2*). The width of the arrows is directly proportional to the amount of solute and water moving by the pathways labeled *1-3.* Starling forces across the capillary wall determine the amount of fluid flowing through pathways *2* versus *3.* Transport mechanisms in the apical cell membranes determine the amount of solute and water entering the cell (pathway *1*). π_c, Capillary oncotic pressure; P_c, capillary hydrostatic pressure; π_i, interstitial fluid oncotic pressure; P_i, interstitial hydrostatic pressure. Thin arrows across the capillary wall indicate direction of water movement in response to each force.

the proximal tubule. An increase in the FF has the opposite effect.

The importance of Starling forces in regulating solute and water reabsorption by the proximal tubule is underscored by the phenomenon of **glomerulotubular balance (G-T balance).** Spontaneous changes in GFR markedly alter the filtered load of sodium (filtered load = GFR × [Na⁺]). Unless such changes were rapidly accompanied by adjustments in Na⁺ reabsorption, urine Na⁺ excretion would fluctuate widely and disturb the Na⁺ balance of the whole body. However, spontaneous changes in GFR do not alter

Na⁺ balance because of the phenomenon of G-T balance. **G-T balance refers to the fact that when body Na⁺ balance is normal, Na⁺ and water reabsorption increase in parallel with an increase in GFR and filtered load of Na⁺. Thus, a constant fraction of the filtered Na⁺ and water is reabsorbed from the proximal tubule despite variations in GFR.** The net result of G-T balance is to reduce the impact of GFR changes on the amount of Na⁺ and water excreted in the urine.

Two mechanisms are responsible for G-T balance. One is related to the oncotic and hydrostatic pressures between the peritubular capillaries and lateral intercellular space (i.e., Starling forces), and the other is related to the filtered load of glucose and amino acids. As an example of the first mechanism, an increase in GFR (at constant RPF) raises the protein concentration above normal in the glomerular capillary plasma. This protein-rich plasma leaves the glomerular capillaries, flows through the efferent arteriole, and enters the peritubular capillaries. The increased oncotic pressure in the peritubular capillaries augments the movement of solute and fluid from the lateral intercellular space into the peritubular capillaries and thereby increases net solute and water reabsorption by the proximal tubule.

The second mechanism responsible for G-T balance is initiated by an increase in the filtered load of glucose and amino acids. As discussed earlier in this chapter, the reabsorption of Na^+ in the early segment of the proximal tubule is coupled to that of glucose and amino acids. The rate of Na^+ reabsorption therefore depends in part on the filtered load of glucose and amino acids. As GFR and the filtered load of glucose and amino acids increase, Na^+ and water reabsorption also rises.

In addition to G-T balance, another physiologic mechanism operates to minimize changes in the filtered load of Na^+. As described on page 43, an increase in GFR (and thus in the amount of Na^+ filtered by the glomerulus) activates the tubuloglomerular feedback mechanism, which returns GFR and the filtration of Na^+ to normal values. Thus, spontaneous changes in GFR (e.g., those caused by changes in posture) only increase the amount of Na^+ filtered for a few minutes. Until GFR returns to normal values, the mechanisms that underlie G-T balance maintain a constant rate of urinary sodium excretion and thereby maintain Na^+ homeostasis.

■ SUMMARY

1. The four major segments of the nephron (proximal tubule, Henle's loop, distal tubule, and collecting duct) determine the composition and volume of the urine by the processes of selective reabsorption of solutes and water and secretion of solutes.

2. Tubular reabsorption allows the kidneys to retain those substances that are essential and regulate their levels in the plasma by altering the degree to which they are reabsorbed. The reabsorption of Na^+, Cl^-, other anions, and organic solutes together with water constitutes the major function of the nephron. Approximately 25,200 mEq of Na^+ and 178 L of water are reabsorbed each day. The proximal tubule cells reabsorb 67% of the glomerular ultrafiltrate, and cells of the loop of Henle reabsorb about 25% of the NaCl that was filtered and about 15% of the water that was filtered. The distal segments of the nephron (distal tubule and collecting duct system) have a more limited reabsorptive capacity. However, the final adjustments in the composition and volume of the urine and most of the regulation by hormones and other factors occur in distal segments.

3. Secretion of substances into tubular fluid is a means for excreting various by-products of metabolism, and it also serves to eliminate exogenous organic anions and cations (e.g., drugs) and pollutants from the body. Many organic compounds are bound to plasma proteins and are therefore unavailable for ultrafiltration. Thus, secretion is their major route of excretion in the urine.

4. Various hormones (including angiotensin II, aldosterone, ADH, ANP, and urodilatin), sympathetic nerves, dopamine, and Starling forces regulate NaCl reabsorption by the kidneys. ADH is the major hormone that regulates water reabsorption.

■ KEY WORDS AND CONCEPTS

- Reabsorption
- Secretion
- Passive diffusion
- Facilitated transport
- Uniport, symport, and antiport
- Secondary active transport
- Active transport
- Endocytosis
- Solvent drag
- Coupled transport
- Tight junctions
- Lateral intercellular space
- Transcellular pathway
- Paracellular pathway
- Water reabsorption is secondary to solute transport
- Glomerulotubular balance
- Starling forces
- Atrial natriuretic peptide (ANP) and urodilatin
- Sympathetic nerves
- Renin-angiotensin-aldosterone system
- Dopamine
- Antidiuretic hormone (ADH)

■ SELF-STUDY PROBLEMS

1. Consider the amount of water and NaCl filtered and reabsorbed by the kidneys each day. What does this tell you about the amount of energy (ATP) expended by the kidneys? Could this explain why the blood flow is so high relative to the size of the kidneys?

2. What are the composition and volume of a normal 24-hour urine?

3. Compare and contrast passive and active transport.

4. If it were possible to completely inhibit the Na^+-K^+-ATPase in the kidney, what would happen to transcellular and paracellular NaCl reabsorption across the proximal tubule? If GFR was unchanged, how much water and NaCl would appear in the urine every day?

5. Describe the mechanisms and pathways of Na^+, glucose, amino acid, Cl^-, and water reabsorption by the proximal tubule. Which pathways occur in the first phase of reabsorption, and which occur in the second phase? How do Starling forces affect solute and water reabsorption?

6. Describe how Na^+ and Cl^- are reabsorbed by the thick ascending limb of Henle's loop. If a diuretic that inhibits NaCl reabsorption (e.g., furosemide) in the thick ascending limb was given to an individual, what would happen to water reabsorption by this segment?

7. What is glomerulotubular balance, and what is the physiologic importance of this phenomenon? What would happen to Na^+ balance if glomerulotubular balance did not exist?

8. List the hormones and factors that regulate NaCl and water reabsorption by each segment of the nephron.

5

Regulation of Body Fluid Osmolality: Regulation of Water Balance

OBJECTIVES

Upon completion of this chapter the student should be able to answer the following questions:

1. Why do changes in water balance result in alterations in the [Na$^+$] of the extracellular fluid (ECF)?
2. How is the secretion of antidiuretic hormone (ADH) controlled by changes in the osmolality of the body fluids and in effective circulating volume and blood pressure?
3. What are the cellular events associated with the action of ADH on the collecting duct, and how do they lead to an increase in the water permeability of this segment?
4. What is the role of Henle's loop in the production of both dilute and concentrated urine?
5. What is the composition of the medullary interstitial fluid, and how does it participate in the process of producing a concentrated urine?
6. What are the roles of the vasa recta in the process of diluting and concentrating the urine?
7. How is the diluting and concentrating ability of the kidneys quantitated?

As described in Chapter 1, water constitutes approximately 60% of the healthy adult human body. The body water is divided into two compartments (i.e., intracellular fluid [ICF] and ECF), which are in osmotic equilibrium. Water intake into the body generally occurs orally. However, in clinical situations, intravenous infusion is an important route of water entry. Regardless of the route of entry (oral versus intravenous), water first enters the ECF and then equilibrates with the ICF. **The kidneys are responsible for regulating water balance and under most conditions are the major route for elimination of water from the body** (Table 5-1). Other routes of water loss from the body include evaporation from the cells of the skin and respiratory passages. Collectively, water loss by these routes is termed *insensible water loss* because the individual is unaware of its occurrence. The production of sweat accounts for the loss of additional water. Water loss by this mechanism can increase dramatically in a hot environment, with exercise, or in the presence of fever (Table 5-2).

T A B L E   5 - 1

Normal routes of water gain and loss in adults at room temperature (23° C)

Route	ml/day
Water Intake:	
Fluid*	1200
In food	1000
Metabolically produced from food	300
Total	2500
Water Output:	
Insensible	700
Sweat	100
Feces	200
Urine	1500
Total	2500

*Fluid intake varies widely for both social and cultural reasons.

Finally, water can be lost from the gastrointestinal tract. Fecal water loss is normally small, but it increases with diarrhea. Vomiting can cause gastrointestinal water losses.

Water loss in sweat, feces, and evaporation from the lungs and skin is not regulated. In contrast, the renal excretion of water is tightly regulated to maintain whole body water balance. The maintenance of water balance requires that water intake and loss from the body are precisely matched. If intake exceeds losses, positive water balance exists. Conversely, when intake is less than losses, negative water balance exists.

When water intake is low or water losses increase, the kidneys conserve water by producing a small volume of urine that is hyperosmotic with respect to plasma. When water intake is high, a large volume of hypoosmotic urine is produced. In a normal individual the urine osmolality can vary from approximately 50 to 1200 mOsm/kg H_2O, and the corresponding urine volume can vary from approximately 18 L/day to 0.5 L/day.

T A B L E   5 - 2

Effect of environmental temperature and exercise on water loss and intake in adults (in ml/day)

	Normal temperature	Hot weather	Prolonged heavy exercise
Water loss			
Insensible loss:			
Skin	350	350	350
Lungs	350	250	650
Sweat	100	1400	5000
Feces	200	200	200
Urine	1500	1200	500
Total loss	2500	3400	6700
Water intake to maintain water balance	2500	3400	6700

In hot weather and during prolonged heavy exercise, water balance is maintained only if the individual increases water intake to match the increased loss of water in sweat. Decreased water excretion by the kidneys alone is insufficient to maintain water balance.

It is important to recognize that disorders of water balance are manifested by alterations in the body fluid osmolality, which are usually measured by changes in plasma osmolality (P_{osm}). Because the major determinant of plasma osmolality is Na^+ (with its anions Cl^- and HCO_3^-), these disorders result in alterations in the plasma $[Na^+]$. It is tempting to suspect a problem in Na^+ balance when evaluating an abnormal plasma $[Na^+]$ in an individual. However, the problem relates to water balance, not Na^+ balance. As described in Chapter 6, changes in Na^+ balance result in alterations in the volume of ECF, not its osmolality.

The kidneys control water excretion independently of their ability to control the excretion of various other physiologically important substances (e.g., Na^+, K^+, H^+, urea). Indeed, this ability is necessary for survival because it allows water balance to be achieved without upsetting the other homeostatic functions of the kidneys.

This chapter discusses the mechanisms by which the kidneys excrete either hypoosmotic (dilute) or hyperosmotic (concentrated) urine. The control of vasopressin secretion and its important role in regulating the excretion of water by the kidneys are also explained.

In the clinical setting, hypoosmolality (a reduction in plasma osmolality) shifts water into cells, and this process results in cell swelling. Symptoms associated with hypoosmolality are related primarily to swelling of brain cells. For example, a rapid fall in P_{osm} can alter neurologic function and thereby cause nausea, malaise, headache, confusion, lethargy, seizures, and coma. When P_{osm} is increased (i.e., hyperosmolality), water is lost from cells. The symptoms of an increase in P_{osm} are also primarily neurologic and include lethargy, weakness, seizures, coma, and even death.

■ ANTIDIURETIC HORMONE

Antidiuretic hormone (ADH), or **vasopressin,** acts on the kidneys to regulate the volume and osmolality of the urine. When plasma ADH levels are low, a large volume of urine is excreted **(diuresis),** and the urine is dilute.[16] When plasma levels are high, a small volume of urine is excreted **(antidiuresis),** and the urine is concentrated. Figure 5-1 illustrates the effect of ADH on the urine flow rate and osmolality. The excretion of total solute (e.g., Na^+, K^+, H^+, urea) by the kidneys is also shown. Note that ADH does not appreciably alter the excretion of solute. This underscores the fact that ADH controls water excretion and maintains water balance without altering the excretion and homeostatic control of other substances.

ADH is a small peptide that is 9 amino acids in length. It is synthesized in neuroendocrine cells located within the **supraoptic** and **paraventricular nuclei** of the hypothalamus. The synthesized hormone is packaged in granules that are transported down the axon of the cell and stored in the nerve terminals located in the **neurohypophysis (posterior pituitary).** The anatomies of the hypothalamus and pituitary gland are shown in Figure 5-2.

The secretion of ADH by the posterior pituitary can be influenced by several factors. **The two primary physiologic regulators of ADH secretion are the osmolality of the body fluids (osmotic) and volume and pressure of the vascular system (hemodynamic).** Other factors that can alter ADH secretion include nausea (stimulates), atrial natriuretic peptide (inhibits), and angiotensin II (stimulates). A number of drugs, prescription and nonprescription, also

---

16 Diuresis is simply a large urine output. When the urine contains primarily water, it is referred to as a *water diuresis.* This is in contrast to the diuresis seen with diuretic agents (see Chapter 10). In this latter case, there is a large urine output, but the urine contains solute plus water.

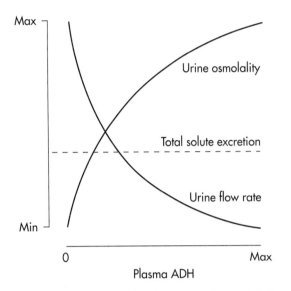

Figure 5-1 ■ **Relationship between plasma ADH levels and urine osmolality, urine flow rate, and total solute excretion.**

affect ADH secretion. For example, nicotine stimulates secretion, whereas ethanol inhibits secretion.

Osmotic Control of ADH Secretion

Changes in the osmolality of body fluids play the most important role in regulating ADH secretion; changes as minor as 1% are sufficient to alter it significantly. Cells located in the hypothalamus, distinct from those that synthesize ADH, sense changes in body fluid osmolality. These cells, termed *osmoreceptors,* appear to behave as osmometers and sense changes in body fluid osmolality by either shrinking or swelling. It is important to recognize that the osmoreceptors respond only to solutes in plasma that are **effective osmoles** (see Chapter 1). For

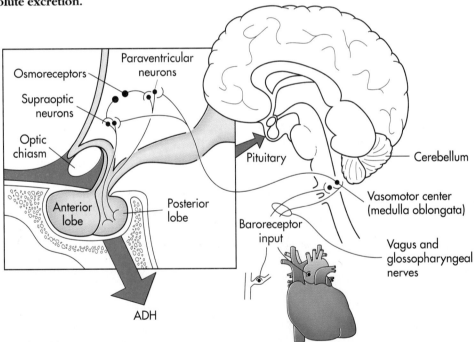

Figure 5-2 ■ **Anatomy of the hypothalamus and pituitary gland (midsagittal section) depicting the pathways for ADH section. Also shown are pathways involved in regulating ADH secretion. Afferent fibers from the baroreceptors are carried in the vagus and glossopharyngeal nerves. The closed box illustrates expanded view of the hypothalamus and pituitary gland.**

example, urea is an **ineffective osmole** when the function of the osmoreceptors is considered. Thus, elevation of the plasma urea concentration alone has little effect on ADH secretion.

When the effective osmolality of the plasma increases, the osmoreceptors send signals to the ADH synthesizing/secreting cells located in the supraoptic and paraventricular nuclei of the hypothalamus, and ADH synthesis and secretion are stimulated. Conversely, when the effective osmolality of the plasma is reduced, secretion is inhibited. Because ADH is rapidly degraded in the plasma, circulating levels can be reduced to zero within minutes after secretion is inhibited. As a result the ADH system can respond rapidly to fluctuations in body fluid osmolality.

Figure 5-3, *A* illustrates the effect of changes in plasma osmolality on circulating ADH levels. The slope of the relationship is quite steep and accounts for the sensitivity of this system. The **set point** of the system is the plasma osmolality value at which ADH secretion begins to increase. Below this set point, virtually no ADH is released. The set point varies among individuals and is genetically determined. In healthy adults, it varies from 275 to 295 mOsm/kg H_2O. Several physiologic factors can also change the set point in a given individual. As discussed later, alterations in blood volume and pressure can shift it. In addition, pregnancy is associated with a decrease in the set point.

Hemodynamic Control of ADH Secretion

A decrease in blood volume or pressure also stimulates ADH secretion. The receptors responsible for this response are located in both the low-pressure (left atrium and pulmonary vessels) and the high-pressure (aortic arch and carotid sinus) sides of the circulatory system. These receptors, called **baroreceptors,** respond to stretch (see Chapter 6). Signals from baroreceptors are relayed to the ADH secretory cells of the supraoptic and paraventricular hypothalamic nuclei via afferent fibers in the vagus and

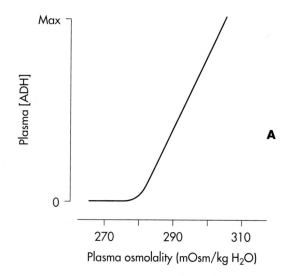

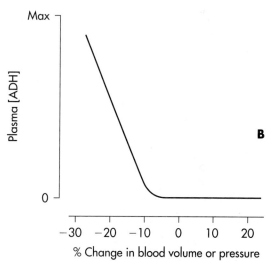

Figure 5-3 ■ Osmotic and hemodynamic control of ADH secretion. Depicted are the relationships between plasma ADH levels and plasma osmolality (A) and blood volume and pressure (B).

glossopharyngeal nerves. The sensitivity of the baroreceptor system is less than that of the osmoreceptors, and a 5% to 10% decrease in blood volume or pressure is required before ADH secretion is stimulated. This is illustrated in Figure 5-3, *B.*

Inadequate release of ADH from the posterior pituitary results in excretion of large volumes of dilute urine **(polyuria).** To compensate for this loss of water, the individual must ingest large volumes of water **(polydipsia)** to maintain constant body fluid osmolality. If the individual is deprived of water, the body fluids will become hyperosmotic. This condition is called ***central diabetes insipidus*** or ***pituitary diabetes insipidus.*** Central diabetes insipidus can be inherited, although this is rare. It occurs more commonly after head trauma and with brain neoplasms or infections. Individuals with central diabetes insipidus have a urine-concentrating defect that can be corrected by the administration of exogenous ADH.

The syndrome of inappropriate ADH secretion (SIADH) is a common clinical problem characterized by plasma ADH levels that are elevated above what would be expected on the basis of body fluid osmolality and blood volume and pressure—hence the term *inappropriate ADH secretion.* Individuals with SIADH retain water, and their body fluids become progressively hypoosmotic. In addition, their urine is more hyperosmotic than expected based on the low body-fluid osmolality. SIADH can be caused by infections and neoplasms of the brain, drugs (e.g., antitumor drugs), pulmonary diseases, and carcinoma of the lung.

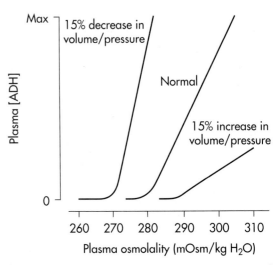

Figure 5-4 ■ Interaction between osmotic and hemodynamic stimuli for ADH secretion. With decreased blood volume and pressure, the osmotic set point is shifted to lower plasma osmolality values and the slope is increased. An increase in blood volume and pressure has the opposite effects.

Alterations in blood volume and pressure also affect the response to changes in body fluid osmolality (Figure 5-4). With a decrease in blood volume or pressure, the set point is shifted to lower osmolality values and the slope of the relationship is steeper. In terms of survival of the individual, this means that, faced with circulatory collapse, the kidneys will continue to conserve water, even though by doing so they reduce the osmolality of the body fluids. With an increase in blood volume or pressure the opposite occurs. The set point is shifted to higher osmolality values, and the slope is decreased.

ADH Actions on the Kidneys

The primary action of ADH on the kidneys is to increase the permeability of the collecting duct to water. In addition, ADH increases the permeability of the medullary portion of the collecting duct to urea.

The actions of ADH on water permeability of the collecting duct have been extensively studied. ADH binds to a receptor on the basolateral membrane of the cell. This receptor is termed the *V2 receptor* (i.e., *vasopressin 2 receptor*).[17] Binding to this receptor, which is coupled to adenylyl cyclase, increases the intracellular levels of cyclic adenosine monophosphate (cAMP).

---

17 A different ADH receptor (V1 receptor) is also present in blood vessels. This receptor mediates the vasoconstrictor response to ADH. It is this action of ADH that accounts for its alternative name, *vasopressin.*

The collecting ducts of some individuals do not respond normally to ADH. This lack of response can result from defects in the ADH receptor, lack of insertion of water channels into the apical membrane, or defective water channels. Regardless of the mechanism the urine of these individuals is not maximally concentrated. Consequently, they suffer from polyuria and polydipsia. This entity is termed *nephrogenic diabetes insipidus* to distinguish it from central diabetes insipidus. Although nephrogenic diabetes insipidus can be inherited, most causes are secondary to other factors, such as metabolic disorders (e.g., hypercalcemia) or certain drugs. For example, approximately 30%-40% of individuals taking lithium develop some degree of nephrogenic diabetes insipidus.

The rise in intracellular cAMP activates protein kinase A, which results in the insertion of vesicles containing water channels into the apical membrane of the cell. These water channels are preformed and reside in vesicles located beneath the cell's apical membrane. With the removal of ADH, these water channels are reinternalized into the cell, and the apical membrane is once again impermeable to water. This shuttling of water channels into and out of the apical membrane provides a rapid mechanism for controlling membrane water permeability. Because the basolateral membrane is freely permeable to water, any water that enters the cell through apical membrane water channels exits across the basolateral membrane, resulting in the net absorption of water from the tubule lumen.

ADH also increases the urea permeability of the distal portion of the inner medullary collecting duct. When ADH binds to its membrane receptor, cAMP levels rise within the inner medullary collecting duct cells. Ultimately, and by mechanisms not yet defined, this rise in intracellular cAMP activates specific urea transporters in the membrane, thereby increasing urea permeability.

■ THIRST

In addition to affecting the secretion of ADH, **changes in plasma osmolality and blood volume or pressure lead to alterations in the perception of thirst.** When body fluid osmolality is increased or the blood volume or pressure is reduced, the individual perceives thirst. Of these stimuli, hypertonicity is the more potent. An increase in plasma osmolality of only 2%-3% produces a strong desire to drink, whereas decreases in blood volume and pressure in the range of 10%-15% are required to produce the same response.

The neural centers involved in the thirst response have not been completely defined. It appears that osmoreceptors similar to, but distinct from, those involved in vasopressin release respond to changes in plasma osmolality. Like the vasopressin osmoreceptors, those involved in thirst respond only to effective osmoles. Even less is known about the pathways involved in the thirst response to decreased blood volume or pressure, but it is believed that the pathways may be the same as those involved in the vasopressin system.

The sensation of thirst is satisfied by the act of drinking even before sufficient water is absorbed from the gastrointestinal tract to correct the plasma osmolality. Oropharyngeal and upper gastrointestinal receptors appear to be involved in this response. However, relief of the thirst sensation via these receptors is short lived, and thirst is only completely satisfied when the plasma osmolality or blood volume or pressure is corrected.

It should be apparent that **the ADH and thirst systems work in concert to maintain water balance.** An increase in the plasma osmolality invokes drinking and, via ADH action on the kidneys, the conservation of water. Con-

With adequate access to water, the thirst mechanism can prevent the development of hyperosmolality. Indeed, it is this mechanism that is responsible for the polydipsia seen in response to the polyuria of both central and nephrogenic diabetes insipidus.

Water intake is also influenced by social and cultural factors. Thus, individuals will ingest water even in the absence of the thirst sensation. Normally the kidneys are able to excrete this excess water because they can excrete up to 18 L/day of urine. However, in some instances the volume of water ingested exceeds the capacity of the kidneys to excrete water. When this occurs, the body fluids become hypoosmotic.

versely, when the plasma osmolality is decreased, thirst is suppressed and, in the absence of ADH, renal water excretion is enhanced.

■ RENAL MECHANISMS FOR DILUTION AND CONCENTRATION OF THE URINE

Under normal circumstances the excretion of water is regulated separately from the excretion of solutes (e.g., NaCl). For this to occur the kidneys must be able to excrete urine that is either hypoosmotic or hyperosmotic with respect to the body fluids, which in turn requires that solute be separated from water at some point along the nephron. As discussed in Chapter 4, reabsorption of solute in the proximal tubule results in the reabsorption of a proportional amount of water; hence, there is no separation of solute and water in this portion of the nephron. Moreover, this is true regardless of whether the kidneys excrete dilute or concentrated urine. Henle's loop, and in particular **the thick ascending limb, is the major nephron site where this separation of solute and water occurs. Thus, the excretion of both di-**

lute and concentrated urine requires normal function of Henle's loop.

The production of hypoosmotic urine is conceptually easy to understand. The nephron must simply reabsorb solute from the tubular fluid and not allow water to follow. As just noted and as described in greater detail later, this occurs primarily in the thick ascending limb of Henle's loop. Under appropriate conditions (i.e., in the absence of ADH), the distal tubule and the collecting duct also contribute to this process.

The excretion of a hyperosmotic urine is conceptually more difficult to understand. This process requires the removal of water from the tubular fluid, which leaves solute behind. Because water can move only passively (driven by an osmotic gradient), the kidneys must be able to generate a hyperosmotic environment that can be used to remove water from the tubular fluid. Indeed, such an environment is generated in the interstitial fluid of the renal medulla. Henle's loop, especially the thick ascending limb, is critical for generating this hyperosmotic medullary environment. Once this hyperosmotic environment is established in the medullary interstitium, it can drive water reabsorption from the collecting duct.

Figure 5-5 summarizes the essential features of the mechanisms whereby the kidneys excrete either a dilute *(A)* or a concentrated *(B)* urine. First we will consider how the kidneys excrete a dilute urine (water diuresis) when ADH levels are low or zero. The following numbers refer to those encircled in Figure 5-5, *A*.

1. Fluid entering the descending thin limb of Henle's loop from the proximal tubule is isoosmotic with respect to plasma. This reflects the essentially isoosmotic nature of solute and water reabsorption in the proximal tubule (see Chapter 4).
2. The descending thin limb is highly permeable to water and much less so to solutes such as

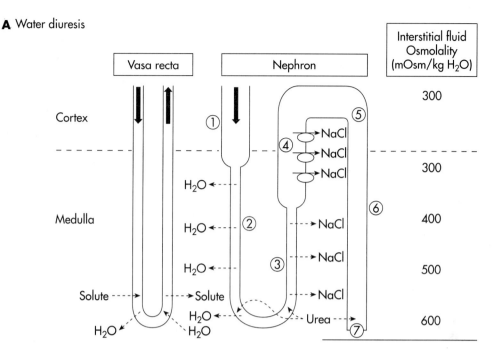

A Water diuresis

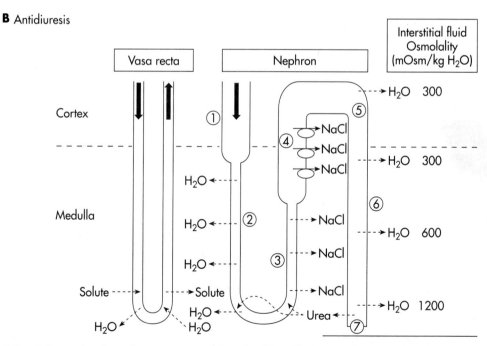

B Antidiuresis

Figure 5-5 ■ Schematic of nephron segments involved in dilution and concentration of the urine. Henle's loops of juxtamedullary nephrons are shown. A, Mechanism for the excretion of dilute urine (water diuresis). ADH is absent, and the collecting duct is essentially impermeable to water. Note also that during a water diuresis the osmolality of the medullary interstitium is reduced as a result of increased vasa recta blood flow and the entry of some urea into the medullary collecting duct. B, Mechanism for the excretion of a concentrated urine (antidiuresis). Plasma ADH levels are maximal, and the collecting duct is highly permeable to water. Under this condition the medullary interstitial gradient is maximal. See text for details.

NaCl and urea.[18] Consequently, as the fluid descends deeper into the hyperosmotic medulla, water is reabsorbed because of the osmotic gradient across the descending thin limb. By this process, fluid at the bend of the loop has an osmolality equal to that of the surrounding interstitial fluid. While the osmolalities of the tubular and interstitial fluids are similar at the bend of the loop, their compositions are markedly different. The tubular fluid [NaCl] is greater than that of the surrounding interstitial fluid. However, the [urea] of the tubular fluid is less than that of the interstitial fluid (see p. 88).

3. The ascending thin limb is impermeable to water but permeable to NaCl and urea. Consequently, as tubular fluid moves up the ascending limb, NaCl is passively reabsorbed (because luminal [NaCl] is greater than interstitial [NaCl]), whereas urea passively diffuses into the tubular fluid (because luminal [urea] is less than interstitial [urea]). The net effect is that the volume of the tubular fluid remains unchanged along the length of the thin ascending limb, but the [NaCl] decreases and the [urea] increases. Overall, the movement of NaCl out of the lumen of the thin ascending limb is greater than the movement of urea into the lumen, and dilution of the tubular fluid occurs.

4. The thick ascending limb of Henle's loop is impermeable to water and urea. This portion of the nephron actively reabsorbs NaCl and thereby dilutes the tubular fluid. Dilution occurs to such a degree that this segment is often referred to as the *diluting segment* of the kidney. Fluid leaving the thick ascending limb is hypoosmotic with respect to plasma (approximately 150 mOsm/kg H_2O).

5. The distal tubule and cortical portion of the collecting duct actively reabsorb NaCl and are impermeable to urea. In the absence of ADH the water permeability of these segments is low. Thus, when ADH is absent (i.e., decreased P_{osm}), the distal tubule and the cortical collecting duct are impermeable to water. Accordingly, the osmolality of tubule fluid in these segments is reduced further because NaCl is reabsorbed without water. Fluid entering the cortical portion of the collecting duct is hypoosmotic with respect to plasma (approximately 100 mOsm/kg H_2O).

6. The medullary collecting duct actively reabsorbs NaCl. Even in the absence of ADH this segment is slightly permeable to water and urea. Consequently, some urea enters the collecting duct from the medullary interstitium, and a small volume of water is reabsorbed.

7. The urine has an osmolality of approximately 50 mOsm/kg H_2O and contains low concentrations of NaCl and urea.

Next, we will consider how the kidneys excrete a concentrated urine (**antidiuresis**) when P_{osm} and plasma ADH levels are high. Numbers 1 through 7 refer to those encircled in Figure 5-5, *B*.

1-4. Steps 1 to 4 are similar when either a dilute or a concentrated urine is produced. It is important to recognize that although reabsorption of NaCl by the ascending thin and thick limbs of Henle's loop dilutes the tubular fluid, the reabsorbed NaCl accumulates in the medullary interstitium, raising its osmolality. **The accumulation of NaCl and urea in the medullary interstitium is critically important for the production of urine hyperosmotic to plasma because it provides the osmotic driving force for water reabsorption by the col-**

---

[18] Urea is an ineffective osmole for many cells within the body because it is freely permeable across the plasma membrane of these cells. However, in many portions of the nephron, urea permeability is quite low (see Table 5-3). In these regions of the nephron, urea can serve as an effective osmole.

lecting duct. The overall process by which Henle's loop, and in particular the thick ascending limb, generates the hyperosmotic medullary interstitial gradient is termed ***countercurrent multiplication.***[19]

5. Because of NaCl reabsorption by the thick ascending limb of Henle's loop, fluid reaching the distal tubule and collecting duct is hypoosmotic with respect to the surrounding interstitial fluid. Thus, there is an osmotic gradient across the distal tubule and collecting duct. In the presence of ADH, which increases the water permeability, water diffuses out of the tubule lumen and the tubule fluid osmolality increases. This begins the process of urine concentration. The maximum osmolality that the fluid in the cortical collecting duct can attain is approximately 300 mOsm/kg H_2O, which is the osmolality of the surrounding interstitial fluid and plasma. Although the fluid at this point has the same osmolality as that which entered the descending thin limb, its composition has been altered dramatically. Because of NaCl reabsorption by the preceding nephron segments, NaCl accounts for a much smaller por-

tion of the total tubular fluid osmolality. Instead, the tubule fluid osmolality reflects the presence of urea (filtered urea, plus urea added in the descending thin and ascending thin limbs of Henle's loop) and other nonreabsorbed solutes (e.g., creatinine).

6. The osmolality of the interstitial fluid in the medulla progressively increases from the corticomedullary junction, where it is approximately 300 mOsm/kg H_2O, to the papilla, where it is approximately 1200 mOsm/kg H_2O. Thus, an osmotic gradient exists between tubule fluid and the interstitial fluid along the entire medullary collecting duct. In the presence of ADH, which renders the medullary collecting duct permeable to water, the osmolality of tubule fluid increases. Because the initial portion of the collecting duct is impermeable to urea, it remains in the tubular fluid and its concentration increases as water is reabsorbed. In the presence of ADH, the urea permeability of the last portion of the medullary collecting duct is increased. Because the urea concentration of the tubular fluid has been increased by water reabsorption and its concentration in the tubular fluid is greater than its concentration in the interstitial fluid, some urea diffuses out of the tubule lumen and into the medullary interstitium. The maximal osmolality that the fluid in the medullary collecting duct can attain is equal to that of the surrounding interstitial fluid. The major components of the tubular fluid within the medullary collecting ducts are substances that have either escaped reabsorption or been secreted into the tubular fluid. Of these, urea is the most abundant.

7. The urine has an osmolality of 1200 mOsm/kg H_2O and contains high concentrations of urea and other nonreabsorbed solutes. Because urea in the tubular fluid tends to equilibrate with the interstitial urea, its concentration in the urine does not exceed that of the interstitium (approximately 600 mmole/L).

---

[19] The term *countercurrent multiplication* derives from both the form and function of Henle's loop. Henle's loop consists of two parallel limbs with tubular fluid flowing in opposite directions (countercurrent flow). Fluid flows into the medulla in the descending limb and out of the medulla in the ascending limb. The ascending limb is impermeable to water and reabsorbs solute from the tubular fluid. Thus, fluid within the ascending limb becomes diluted. This separation of solute and water by the ascending limb is termed the *single effect* of the countercurrent multiplication process. The solute removed from the ascending limb tubular fluid accumulates in the surrounding interstitial fluid and raises its osmolality. Because the descending limb is highly permeable to water, the increased osmolality of the medullary interstitium causes water to be absorbed and thereby concentrates the tubular fluid. The countercurrent flow within the descending and ascending limbs of Henle's loop magnifies, or "multiplies," the osmotic gradient between the tubule fluid in the descending and ascending limbs of Henle's loop.

Table 5-3 summarizes the transport and passive permeability properties of the nephron segments involved in the process of concentrating and diluting the urine.

Medullary Interstitial Fluid: Importance of Urea

As previously described, the generation of a hyperosmotic medullary interstitium, which is dependent on NaCl reabsorption by the ascending limb of Henle's loop, is critically important for the ability of the kidneys to excrete urine that is hyperosmotic with respect to plasma. Measurements of the composition of the medullary interstitial fluid have shown that its principal components are NaCl and urea and the distribution of these solutes is not uniform throughout the medulla. At the junction of the medulla and the cortex, the interstitial fluid has an osmolality of approximately 300 mOsm/kg H_2O, with virtually all osmoles attributable to NaCl. The concentrations of both NaCl and urea increase progressively with increasing depth into the medulla, and at the papilla the osmolality of the interstitial fluid is approximately 1200 mOsm/kg H_2O. Of this value, 600 mOsm/kg H_2O is attributed to NaCl and 600 mOsm/kg H_2O to urea.

The medullary gradient for NaCl results from the accumulation of NaCl reabsorbed by the nephron segments in the medulla by the process of countercurrent multiplication. The most important segment in this regard is the ascending limb (thick limb greater than thin limb) of Henle's loop.

Urea accumulation within the medullary interstitium is more complex and occurs most effectively when a hyperosmotic urine is excreted. Urea is generated by the liver as a result of protein metabolism and enters the tubular fluid by glomerular filtration. As indicated in Table 5-3, the permeability to urea of most nephron segments is relatively low, with the exception of the medullary collecting duct (especially in the presence of ADH). As fluid moves along the nephron, and especially as water is reabsorbed in the collecting duct, the urea concentration in the tubular fluid increases. When this urea-rich tubular fluid reaches the medullary collecting duct, where the

TABLE 5-3

Transport and permeability properties of nephron segments involved in urine concentration and dilution

Tubule segment	Active NaCl transport	Passive permeability*			Effect of ADH
		NaCl	Urea	H$_2$O	
Henle's loop					
Descending thin limb	0	+	+	+++	
Ascending thin limb	0	+++	+	0	
Thick ascending limb	+++	+	0	0	
Distal tubule	+	+	0	0	
Collecting duct					
Cortex	+	+	0	0	↑ H$_2$O permeability
Medulla	+	+	++	+	↑ H$_2$O and urea permeability

*Permeability is proportional to the number of + indicated: +, low permeability; +++, high permeability; 0, impermeable.

permeability to urea is not only high but increased by ADH, urea diffuses down its concentration gradient into the medullary interstitial fluid, where it accumulates. Some urea enters the descending thin and ascending thin limbs of Henle's loop and thereby causes the recycling of urea between the collecting duct and Henle's loop. This process of recycling also serves to trap urea in the medullary interstitium and thus facilitate its accumulation in the medulla.

As previously described, the hyperosmotic medullary interstitium is essential for concentrating the tubular fluid within the collecting duct. Because water reabsorption is a passive process driven by an osmotic gradient, **the maximal concentration that the urine can attain is equal to that of the medullary interstitium at the papilla** (approximately 1200 mOsm/kg H_2O). Because a hyperosmotic medullary interstitium is essential for urine concentration, any condition that reduces this gradient impairs the ability of the kidneys to concentrate the urine maximally.

Vasa Recta Function

The vasa recta, the capillary networks that supply blood to the medulla, are highly permeable to solute and water. As with Henle's loops, the vasa recta form a parallel set of hairpin loops within the medulla (see Figure 5-5 and Chapter 2). The vasa recta function not only to bring nutrients and oxygen to the tubules within the medulla but more importantly to remove excess water and solute, which is continuously added to the medullary interstitium by the nephron segments located in this region. **It should be emphasized that the ability of the vasa recta to maintain the medullary interstitial gradient is flow dependent.** A substantial increase in blood flow through the vasa recta ultimately dissipates the medullary gradient. Alternatively, if blood flow is reduced, the nephron segments within the medulla receive inadequate oxygen. Under this condition, tubular transport, especially by the thick ascending limb of Henle's loop, is impaired. As a result, the medullary interstitial osmotic gradient cannot be maintained.

Individuals on a protein-deficient diet can exhibit a defect in urine-concentrating ability. This inability to maximally concentrate the urine reflects decreased urea levels within the medullary interstitial fluid. When protein intake is inadequate, urea production in the body is decreased. Therefore the urea content and thus the osmolality of the medullary interstitium are reduced. This in turn reduces water reabsorption from the collecting duct and thereby reduces the concentrating ability of the kidneys. Ingestion of adequate amounts of protein corrects this defect.

The intake of large volumes of fluid results in the excretion of large volumes of urine (water diuresis). During a water diuresis, vasa recta blood flow increases and the gradient within the medullary interstitium is dissipated. If individuals who have drunk a large volume of water are abruptly deprived of water, they will not be able to maximally concentrate their urine (i.e., 1200 mOsm/kg H_2O). Normal concentrating ability will be restored once the medullary interstitial gradient is re-established. The time needed to reestablish the gradient is variable, depending on the magnitude and duration of the water diuresis.

Because water intake is not determined solely by thirst but influenced by social and behavioral factors, certain individuals drink large volumes of liquids over extended periods of time and thus undergo a prolonged water diuresis. Approximately 5% to 15% of patients with chronic psychiatric illness drink excessive quantities of water (psychogenic water drinkers) and thus demonstrate a concentrating defect if acutely challenged with water deprivation.

■ QUANTITATING RENAL DILUTING AND CONCENTRATING ABILITY

Assessment of the dilution and concentration processes involves measurements of urine osmolality and the volume of urine excreted. The range of urine osmolality is from 50 mOsm/kg H_2O to 1200 mOsm/kg H_2O. The corresponding range in urine volume is 18 L to as little as 0.5 L per day. It is important to recognize that these ranges are not fixed. They vary among individuals and are influenced importantly by the need for solute excretion (see p. 92).

A useful means to quantitate the handling of water by the kidneys is to measure the **free-water clearance.** As noted previously, the central process in the dilution or concentration of urine is the single effect of separating solute from water. Through this separation the kidneys, in a sense, generate a volume of water that is "free of all solute." When the urine is dilute, this **solute-free water** is excreted from the body. When the urine is concentrated, this solute-free water is returned to the systemic circulation. The concept of free-water clearance provides a means for quantitating the ability of the kidneys to generate solute-free water. This concept follows directly from renal clearance, as described in Chapter 3.

The clearance of total solute (i.e., osmoles) from plasma by the kidneys can be calculated as follows:

$$C_{osm} = \frac{U_{osm} \times \dot{V}}{P_{osm}} \qquad (5\text{-}1)$$

where: C_{osm} is termed the osmolar clearance; U_{osm} is the urine osmolality; $\dot{V}$ is the urine flow rate; and P_{osm} is the plasma osmolality. C_{osm} has units of volume/unit time. Free-water clearance (C_{H_2O}) is then calculated as follows:

$$C_{H_2O} = \dot{V} - C_{osm} \qquad (5\text{-}2)$$

Rearranging Equation 5-2 should make the following apparent:

$$\dot{V} = C_{H_2O} + C_{osm} \qquad (5\text{-}3)$$

In other words, it is possible to partition the total urine output ($\dot{V}$) into two hypothetical components. One component contains all the urine solutes and has an osmolality equal to that of plasma (i.e., $U_{osm} = P_{osm}$). This volume is defined by C_{osm} and represents a volume from which there has been no separation of solute and water. The second component is a volume of solute-free water (i.e., C_{H_2O}).

When dilute urine is produced, the value of C_{H_2O} is positive, indicating that solute-free water is excreted from the body. When concentrated urine is produced, the value of C_{H_2O} is negative, indicating that solute-free water is retained in the body. By convention, negative C_{H_2O} values are expressed as $T^C_{H_2O}$ **(tubular conservation of water).** The calculation of C_{H_2O} and $T^C_{H_2O}$ is illustrated in the following examples (see p. 91).

Two points regarding these examples require emphasis. First, changes in free-water excretion and reabsorption occur without changes in solute excretion (C_{osm} is unchanged). This underscores the fact that the control of water balance by the kidneys is independent of the control of excretion of solutes. Second, C_{H_2O} and $T^C_{H_2O}$ reflect net processes within the kidneys. For example, if C_{H_2O} is equal to zero, there is no net separation of solute and water by the kidneys. In actuality, solute and water were separated by the ascending limb of Henle's loop. However, this solute-free water was reabsorbed by the collecting duct (i.e., solute and water recombined) instead of being excreted (i.e., as dilute urine). The net effect is that C_{H_2O} is zero.

The determination of C_{H_2O} and $T^c_{H_2O}$ can provide important information about the function of those portions of the nephron involved in producing dilute and concentrated urine. Whether the kidneys excrete or reabsorb free water depends upon the presence of ADH. When no ADH is present or levels are low, solute-free water is

Consider a situation in which the kidneys must excrete 300 mOsm of solute. This occurs when urine is produced that is either isosmotic (U_{osm}/P_{osm} = 1), hypoosmotic (U_{osm}/P_{osm} <1), or hyperosmotic (U_{osm}/P_{osm} >1) with respect to plasma. We will examine each of these conditions separately. For simplicity of calculation we will assume P_{osm} = 300 mOsm/kg H_2O.

Example #1 - Isosmotic urine (U_{osm} = P_{osm}): If the urine flow rate under this condition is 2 L/day, C_{osm} is calculated as follows:

$$C_{osm} = \frac{300 \text{ mOsm/kg } H_2O \times 2L/day}{300 \text{ mOsm/kg } H_2O} = 2 \text{ L/day}$$

and C_{H_2O} is calculated as follows:

$$C_{H_2O} = 2 \text{ L/day} - 2 \text{ L/day} = 0 \text{ L/day}$$

Note that the urine flow rate ($\dot{V}$) is equal to C_{osm} and C_{H_2O} is zero. Therefore in this situation there is no excretion of solute-free water by the kidneys.

Example #2 - Dilute urine (U_{osm} < P_{osm}): In this situation the 300 mOsm of solute is excreted in twice the volume. Thus, U_{osm} = 150 mOsm/kg H_2O and $\dot{V}$ = 4 L/day. Accordingly, C_{osm} is calculated as follows:

$$C_{osm} = \frac{150 \text{ mOsm/kg } H_2O \times 4L/day}{300 \text{ mOsm/kg } H_2O} = 2 \text{ L/day}$$

and C_{H_2O} is calculated as follows:

$$C_{H_2O} = 4 \text{ L/day} - 2 \text{ L/day} = 2 \text{ L/day}$$

Note that C_{osm} is unchanged, and now solute-free water is excreted.

Example #3 - Concentrated urine (U_{osm} > P_{osm}): In this situation the 300 mOsm of solute is excreted in half the urine volume. Thus, U_{osm} = 600 mOsm/kg H_2O, and $\dot{V}$ = 1 L/day. C_{osm} is calculated as follows:

$$C_{osm} = \frac{600 \text{ mOsm/kg } H_2O \times 1L/day}{300 \text{ mOsm/kg } H_2O} = 2 \text{ L/day}$$

and C_{H_2O} is calculated as follows:

$$C_{H_2O} = 1 \text{ L/day} - 2 \text{ L/day} = -1 \text{ L/day } or \text{ } T^c_{H_2O} = 1 \text{ L/day.}$$

Note that C_{osm} is again unchanged. However, $\dot{V}$ is now less than C_{osm}. The difference between these parameters (1 L/day) represents the solute-free water reabsorbed by the kidneys and returned to systemic circulation.

excreted. When ADH levels are high, solute-free water is reabsorbed.

The following factors are necessary for the kidneys to excrete a maximum amount of solute-free water (C_{H_2O}):

1. ADH must be absent. This prevents water reabsorption by the collecting duct.
2. The tubular structures, which can separate solute from water (i.e., dilute the luminal fluid), must function normally. In the absence of ADH, the following nephron segments can dilute the luminal fluid:
   • Ascending thin limb of Henle's loop
   • Thick ascending limb of Henle's loop
   • Distal tubule
   • Collecting duct
   Because of its high transport rate, the thick ascending limb is quantitatively the most important of these segments involved in the separation of solute and water.
3. Adequate delivery of tubular fluid to the above nephron sites is required for maximal separation of solute and water. Factors that reduce delivery (e.g., decreased GFR or enhanced proximal tubule reabsorption) impair the ability of the kidneys to maximally excrete C_{H_2O}.

In the normal adult the maximum value of C_{H_2O} can be estimated at 10% of the glomerular filtration rate. Thus, if the GFR is 180 L/day, the maximum C_{H_2O} would be 18 L/day. The volume of urine excreted also depends on the amount of solute excreted. For example, if 600 mmoles of solute must be excreted to maintain steady-state balance, then the maximum volume of urine excreted at an osmolality of 50 mOsm/kg H_2O would be 12 L/day (i.e., 600 mosmoles/day ÷ 50 mOsm/kg H_2O = 12 L/day, with 1 kg of water equaling 1 L). Thus, to attain the maximum urine volume output of approximately 18 L/day, solute excretion would need to be 900 mosmoles/day. Diet determines the amount of solute that must be excreted each day by the kidneys.

Similar requirements also apply to the conservation of water by the kidneys ($T^c_{H_2O}$). For the kidneys to conserve water maximally, the following conditions must exist:

1. Adequate delivery of tubular fluid to those nephron segments in which separation of solute and water occurs: Most important in this regard is the thick ascending limb of Henle's loop. Delivery of tubular fluid to the loop of Henle is in turn dependent upon the GFR and proximal tubule reabsorption.
2. Normal reabsorption of NaCl by the nephron segments: Again, the most important segment is the thick ascending limb of Henle's loop.
3. Presence of a hyperosmotic medullary interstitium: The interstitial osmolality is maintained by NaCl reabsorption by Henle's loop (conditions 1 and 2) and by effective accumulation of urea. Urea accumulation in turn depends on adequate dietary protein intake.
4. Maximum levels of ADH and responsiveness of the collecting duct to ADH.

If these conditions are met, a small volume of hyperosmotic urine is excreted. The actual volume again depends on solute excretion. Thus, with a solute excretion of 600 mmoles/day and a maximum urine osmolality of 1200 mOsm/kg H_2O, the minimum urine volume is 0.5 L/day.

■ SUMMARY

1. The osmolality and volume of the body fluids are maintained within a narrow range, despite wide variation in water and solute intake. The kidneys play the central role in this regulatory process by virtue of their ability to vary the excretion of water and solutes.
2. Regulation of body fluid osmolality requires that water intake and loss from the body be equal. This involves the integrated interaction of the ADH secretory and thirst centers of the hypothalamus and the ability of the kidneys to excrete urine that is either hypoosmotic or hyperosmotic with respect to the body fluids.
3. When body fluid osmolality increases, ADH secretion and thirst are stimulated. ADH acts on the kidneys to increase the permeability of the collecting duct to water. Hence, water is reabsorbed from the lumen of the collecting duct, and a small volume of hyperosmotic urine is excreted. This renal conservation of water, together with increased water intake, restores body fluid osmolality to normal.
4. When body fluid osmolality decreases, ADH secretion and thirst are suppressed. In the absence of ADH the collecting duct is impermeable to water, and a large volume of hypoosmotic urine is excreted. With this increased excretion of water and a decreased intake of water caused by suppression of thirst, the osmolality of the body fluids is restored to normal.
5. Central to the process of concentrating and diluting the urine is Henle's loop. The transport of NaCl by Henle's loop allows the separation of solute and water, which is essential for the elaboration of hypoosmotic urine. By this same mechanism the interstitial fluid in the medullary portion of the kidney is ren-

dered hyperosmotic. This hyperosmotic medullary interstitial fluid in turn provides the osmotic driving force for the reabsorption of water from the lumen of the collecting duct when ADH is present.

6. Disorders of water balance result in alterations in body fluid osmolality. Changes in body fluid osmolality are manifested by a change in the plasma $[Na^+]$. Positive water balance (intake greater than excretion) results in a decrease in the body fluid osmolality and hyponatremia. Negative water balance (intake less than excretion) results in an increase in body fluid osmolality and hypernatremia.

7. The handling of water by the kidneys is quantitated by measuring the amount of solute-free water that is either excreted (C_{H_2O}) or reabsorbed ($T^c_{H_2O}$). Maximal excretion of solute-free water requires normal nephron function (especially the thick ascending limb of Henle's loop), adequate delivery of tubular fluid to the nephrons, and the absence of ADH. Maximal reabsorption of solute-free water requires normal nephron function (especially the thick ascending limb of Henle's loop), adequate delivery of tubular fluid to the nephrons, a hyperosmotic medullary interstitium, the presence of ADH, and responsiveness of the collecting duct to ADH.

■ KEY WORDS AND CONCEPTS

- Antidiuretic hormone (ADH)
- Diuresis/antidiuresis
- Supraoptic nuclei and paraventricular nuclei
- Neurohypophysis/posterior pituitary
- Osmotic and hemodynamic control of ADH secretion
- Osmoreceptors
- Effective and ineffective osmoles
- Set point for osmotic control of ADH secretion
- Baroreceptors
- Cellular events associated with ADH stimulation of collecting duct water permeability
- Polyuria
- Polydipsia
- Diabetes insipidus (central and nephrogenic)
- Syndrome of inappropriate secretion of ADH (SIADH)
- Thirst
- Countercurrent multiplication by Henle's loop
- Single effect of separating solute and water
- Diluting segment (thick ascending limb of Henle's loop)
- Medullary interstitial osmotic gradient
- Medullary accumulation of urea
- Solute-free water
- Free-water clearance (C_{H_2O})
- Free-water reabsorption/tubular conservation of water ($T^c_{H_2O}$)
- Osmolar clearance (C_{osm})

■ SELF-STUDY PROBLEMS

1. An individual's blood is drawn, and the following values are obtained (see Appendix B for normal values):

   Plasma $[Na^+]$ 135 mEq/L
   Serum [glucose]   100 mg/dL
   Serum [urea]   100 mg/dL
   Posm   310 mOsm/kg H_2O

   Would plasma ADH levels in this individual be elevated or suppressed?

2. In the table on p. 94, indicate the expected osmolality of tubular fluid in the absence and presence of ADH (assume that the plasma osmolality is 300 mOsm/kg H_2O and osmolality of the medullary interstitium is 1200 mOsm/kg H_2O at the papilla).

Nephron site	0-ADH	Max. ADH
Proximal tubule	————	————
Beginning of descending thin limb	————	————
Beginning of ascending thin limb	————	————
End of thick ascending limb	————	————
End of cortical collecting duct	————	————
Urine	————	————

3. Given the following data, calculate the free-water excreted by the kidneys.

   A. P_{osm} = 295 mOsm/kg H_2O
   U_{osm} = 70 mOsm/kg H_2O
   $\dot{V}$ = 3 ml/min

   B. P_{osm} = 295 mOsm/kg H_2O
   U_{osm} = 1100 mOsm/kg H_2O
   $\dot{V}$ = 0.4 ml/min

4. The ability of the kidneys to maximally concentrate the urine is impaired under each of the following conditions:

   a. Decreased renal perfusion (i.e., decreased GFR)

   b. Administration of a diuretic that inhibits active NaCl transport by the thick ascending limb of Henle's loop

   c. Nephrogenic diabetes insipidus
   What are the mechanisms responsible for the observed impairment in the kidneys' concentrating ability during each of these conditions?

5. An individual must excrete 800 mOsm of solute in a 24-hour period. What volume of urine is required if the individual can concentrate the urine to only 400 mOsm/kg H_2O? What volume of urine is required if this individual can concentrate the urine to 1200 mOsm/kg H_2O?

Regulation of Effective Circulating Volume and NaCl Balance

OBJECTIVES

Upon completion of this chapter the student should be able to answer the following questions:

1. Why do changes in Na^+ balance alter the volume of the extracellular fluid (ECF)?
2. What is the effective circulating volume, how is it influenced by changes in Na^+ balance, and how does it influence renal Na^+ excretion?
3. What are the mechanisms by which the body monitors the effective circulating volume?
4. What are the major signals acting on the kidneys to alter their excretion of Na^+?
5. How do changes in effective circulating volume alter Na^+ transport in each of the various portions of the nephron, and how do these changes in transport regulate renal Na^+ excretion?
6. What are the mechanisms involved in the formation of edema, and what role do the kidneys play in this process?

A s noted in Chapter 1, the major solute of the ECF is NaCl. Because NaCl is also the major determinant of ECF osmolality (see Chapter 5), alterations in Na^+ balance are often assumed to cause disturbances in ECF osmolality. However, under normal conditions this is not the case. Changes in Na^+ balance do not normally alter the ECF osmolality because the ADH and thirst systems maintain body fluid osmolality within a very narrow range (see Chapter 5). For example, addi- tion of NaCl to the ECF (without water) in- creases the $[Na^+]$ and osmolality of this com- partment (ICF osmolality also increases because of osmotic equilibration with the ECF). This in- crease in osmolality in turn stimulates thirst and the release of ADH from the posterior pituitary. The increased ingestion of water in response to thirst, together with the ADH-induced decrease in water excretion by the kidneys, quickly re- stores ECF osmolality to normal. However, the volume of the ECF is increased in proportion to the amount of water ingested, which in turn depends upon the amount of NaCl added to the ECF. Thus, in the new steady state, addition of NaCl to the ECF is equivalent to adding an isoosmotic solution. Conversely, a decrease in the NaCl content of the ECF results in a decrease in the volume of this compartment.

The kidneys are the major route for excretion of NaCl from the body. As such the kidneys play an important role in regulating the volume of the ECF. Under normal conditions the kidneys keep the volume of the ECF constant by adjusting the excretion of NaCl to match the amount ingested in the diet. If ingestion exceeds excretion, ECF volume increases above normal, whereas the opposite occurs if excretion exceeds ingestion. To defend itself against changes in ECF volume, the body relies on a system that monitors the volume of this compartment and sends signals to the kidneys to make appropriate adjustments in NaCl excretion.

This chapter reviews the physiology of the volume receptors and explains the various signals that act on the kidneys to regulate NaCl excretion, and thereby ECF volume, along with the responses of the various portions of the nephron to these signals. In addition, the pathophysiologic mechanisms involved in the formation of edema are presented, with emphasis on the role of NaCl handling by the kidneys.

■ CONCEPT OF EFFECTIVE
   CIRCULATING VOLUME

As already noted, the amount of NaCl in the ECF determines the volume of this body fluid compartment. To understand the role of renal Na^+ excretion in regulating the ECF volume, it is necessary to consider the concept of **effective circulating volume (ECV)**. ECV is not a measurable and distinct body fluid compartment; rather, it is related to the adequacy of tissue perfusion. Thus, it is related to the "fullness" of and "pressure" within the vascular tree. In the normal individual, ECV varies according to the volume of the ECF. However, this relationship is not maintained under some pathologic conditions.

The important point is that the kidneys alter their excretion of Na^+ in response to changes in ECV rather than ECF per se. When ECV is decreased, renal Na^+ excretion is reduced. This adaptive response restores the ECV to its normal

---

The typical diet contains approximately 140 mEq/day of Na^+ (~ 8 g of NaCl), and thus daily Na^+ excretion is also about 140 mEq. However, the excretion of Na^+ by the kidneys can vary over a wide range. Excretion rates as low as 10 mEq/day can be attained when individuals are placed on a low-salt diet. Conversely, the kidneys can increase their excretion rate to more than 1000 mEq/day when challenged by the ingestion of a high-salt diet. These changes in Na^+ excretion occur with only modest changes in the steady state Na^+ content of the body.

The response of the kidneys to abrupt changes in Na^+ intake typically takes from 3 to 5 days. During this transition period intake and excretion of Na^+ are not matched as they are in the steady state. Thus, the individual experiences either **positive Na^+ balance** (intake greater than excretion) or **negative Na^+ balance** (intake less than excretion). However, by the end of the transition period, intake once again equals excretion.

Provided the ADH and thirst systems are intact and normal, alterations in Na^+ balance result in changes in the volume of the ECF, not the serum $[Na^+]$ or plasma osmolality. Changes in ECF volume can be monitored by measuring body weight because 1 L of ECF equals 1 kg of body weight.

value and maintains adequate tissue perfusion. Conversely, an increase in the ECV results in enhanced renal Na+ excretion, termed **natriuresis.** Figure 6-1 illustrates the components of the ECV regulatory system, each of which is discussed in detail below.

Patients with congestive heart failure frequently have an increase in their ECF volume, which reflects the fact that reduced cardiac output, secondary to the heart disease, is sensed by the body as a decrease in the ECV. As a result the kidneys retain NaCl and water, and the volume of the ECF is expanded (manifested as tissue edema) in an attempt to increase the ECV. Thus, in congestive heart failure the ECF volume is increased, but the ECV is decreased.

For the normal individual the terms ECV and ECF can be, and quite often are, interchanged. However, it is the ECV, especially under certain pathologic conditions, that determines renal NaCl excretion. Consequently, to provide a framework for understanding the pathophysiologic basis of some clinically significant conditions, the remaining sections of this chapter will refer primarily to the ECV.

■ **ECV VOLUME SENSORS**

Table 6-1 lists the various ECV volume sensors in the body. The ECV volume sensors located in the vascular tree monitor its fullness and pressure. These appear to be the primary sensors for the ECV. Sensors related to the control of NaCl excretion by the kidneys are also presumed to exist within the brain and liver. Less is known about these latter two groups of receptors, and they are not considered further in this text. The sensors in the vascular system respond to stretch (**baroreceptors**) and are described in more detail below.

Vascular Low-Pressure Volume Sensors

Baroreceptors are located within the walls of the cardiac atria and pulmonary vessels and respond

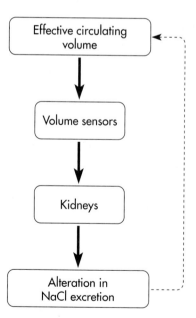

Figure 6-1 ■ General scheme for monitoring and controlling the effective circulating volume (ECV).

TABLE 6-1
ECV sensors

I. Vascular*
   A. Low pressure
      1. Cardiac atria
      2. Pulmonary vasculature
   B. High pressure
      1. Carotid sinus
      2. Aortic arch
      3. Juxtaglomerular apparatus of kidneys
II. Central nervous system
III. Hepatic

*Most sensitive sensors

to distension of these structures. Because of the low pressure within the atria and pulmonary vessels, these sensors respond primarily to the "fullness" of the vascular tree, sending signals to the brain's hypothalamic and medullary regions via afferent fibers in the vagus nerve. Activity of these sensors modulates both sympathetic nerve outflow and ADH secretion. For example, a decrease in filling of the pulmonary vessels and atria increases sympathetic nerve activity and stimulates ADH secretion. Conversely, distension of these structures decreases sympathetic nerve activity. In general, changes of 5% to 10% in blood volume and pressure are necessary to evoke a response.

The cardiac atria possess an additional mechanism related to control of renal NaCl excretion. The myocytes of the atria synthesize and store a peptide hormone. This hormone, termed *atrial natriuretic peptide (ANP)*, is released when the atria are distended (i.e., expansion of the ECV) and, by the mechanisms outlined in subsequent sections, reduces blood pressure and increases the excretion of NaCl and water by the kidneys.

Vascular High-Pressure Volume Sensors

Baroreceptors are also present in the arterial side of the vascular tree, located in the wall of the aortic arch, the carotid sinus, and the afferent arteriole of the kidneys. These baroreceptors respond primarily to blood pressure. The aortic arch and carotid baroreceptors, like the low-pressure baroreceptors, send input to the hypothalamic and medullary centers of the brain via the vagus and glossopharyngeal nerves. The response to this input also involves alterations in sympathetic outflow and ADH secretion. Thus, a decrease in blood pressure increases sympathetic nerve activity and ADH secretion. An increase in pressure tends to reduce sympathetic nerve activity. The sensitivity of the high-pressure baroreceptors is similar to those in the low-pressure side of the

---

Constriction of the renal artery (e.g., by an atherosclerotic plaque) reduces perfusion pressure to the kidney. The afferent arterioles sense this reduced perfusion pressure, resulting in the secretion of renin. The elevated renin levels cause increased production of angiotensin II, which in turn increases systemic blood pressure by its vasoconstrictive effect on arterioles throughout the vascular system. The afferent arterioles of the contralateral kidney (i.e., the kidney without stenosis of its renal artery) sense the increased systemic blood pressure, and renin secretion from that kidney is suppressed.

---

vascular system, with changes in pressure of 5% to 10% needed to evoke a response.

The **juxtaglomerular apparatus** (see Chapter 2), particularly the afferent arteriole, responds directly to changes in pressure. If perfusion pressure of the afferent arteriole is reduced, renin is released from the myocytes. Renin secretion is suppressed when perfusion pressure is increased. As described in subsequent sections, renin determines levels of angiotensin II and aldosterone, both of which play important roles in regulating renal Na^+ excretion (see Chapter 4).

■ VOLUME SENSOR SIGNALS

Once the various volume sensors have detected a change in the ECV, they send signals to the kidneys, which results in an appropriate adjustment in NaCl and water excretion. Accordingly, when the ECV is expanded, renal NaCl and water excretion is increased. Conversely, when the ECV is contracted, renal NaCl and water excretion is reduced. The signals involved in coupling the volume sensors to the kidney are both neural and hormonal. These are summarized in Table 6-2, as are their effects on renal NaCl and water excretion.

Signals involved in the control of renal NaCl and water excretion

Renal Sympathetic Nerves (↑ Activity: ↓ NaCl Excretion)
↓ Glomerular filtration rate
↑ Renin secretion
↑ Proximal tubule, thick ascending limb of Henle's loop, distal tubule, and collecting duct NaCl reabsorption

Renin-Angiotensin-Aldosterone (↑ Secretion: ↓ NaCl Excretion)
↑ Angiotensin II levels stimulate proximal tubule NaCl reabsorption
↑ Aldosterone levels stimulate thick ascending limb of Henle's loop and collecting duct NaCl reabsorption
↑ ADH secretion

Atrial Natriuretic Peptide (↑ Secretion: ↑ NaCl Excretion)
↑ Glomerular filtration rate
↓ Renin secretion
↓ Aldosterone secretion
↓ NaCl and water reabsorption by the collecting duct*
↓ ADH secretion and inhibition of ADH action on the collecting duct

ADH (↑ Secretion: ↓ H_2O Excretion)
↑ H_2O absorption by the collecting duct

*Urodilatin contributes to this effect.

Renal Sympathetic Nerves

As described in Chapter 2, **sympathetic nerve** fibers innervate the afferent and efferent arterioles of the glomerulus, as well as nephron cells. When ECV is decreased, a baroreceptor-mediated (low pressure and high pressure) increase occurs in renal sympathetic nerve activity. This has the following effects:

1. The afferent and efferent arterioles are constricted. This vasoconstriction (the effect appears to be greater on the afferent arteriole) decreases the hydrostatic pressure within the glomerular capillary lumen, and the glomerular filtration rate therefore falls. With this decrease in GFR the filtered load of Na^+ to the

nephrons is reduced (filtered load = GFR $\times$ plasma $[Na^+]$).

2. Renin secretion by the cells of the afferent and efferent arterioles is stimulated. As described below, renin ultimately increases circulating levels of angiotensin II and aldosterone.

3. NaCl reabsorption along the nephron is directly stimulated. Quantitatively the most important segment influenced by sympathetic nerve activity is the proximal tubule.

The combined effect of these actions contributes to an overall decrease in NaCl excretion, an adaptive response that works to restore ECV to its normal value. When the volume of ECV is increased, renal sympathetic nerve activity is reduced. This generally reverses the effects just described.

Renin-Angiotensin-Aldosterone System

Smooth muscle cells in the afferent and efferent arterioles are the site of synthesis, storage, and release of renin. Three factors play an important role in stimulating renin secretion:

1. Perfusion pressure: The afferent arteriole behaves as a high-pressure baroreceptor. When perfusion pressure to the kidneys is reduced, renin secretion is stimulated. Conversely, an increase in perfusion pressure inhibits renin release.
2. Sympathetic nerve activity: Activation of the sympathetic nerve fibers innervating the afferent and efferent arterioles results in increased renin secretion. Renin secretion decreases as renal sympathetic nerve activity decreases.
3. Delivery of NaCl to the macula densa: Delivery of NaCl to the macula densa regulates the GFR by a process termed *tubuloglomerular feedback* (see Chapter 3). By this feedback mechanism, increased NaCl delivery to the macula densa results in decreased GFR. Conversely, decreased NaCl delivery increases GFR. In addition, the macula densa plays a role in renin secretion. When NaCl delivery to the macula densa decreases, renin secretion is enhanced. Conversely, an increase in NaCl delivery inhibits renin secretion. This macula densa–mediated secretion of renin does not appear to be involved in the alterations in glomerular hemodynamics underlying the phenomenon of tubuloglomerular feedback.[20]

Figure 6-2 summarizes the essential components of the **renin-angiotensin-aldosterone system.** Renin alone does not have a physiologic function; it functions solely as a proteolytic enzyme. Its substrate is a circulating protein, **angiotensinogen,** which is produced by the liver. Angiotensinogen is cleaved by renin to yield a 10–amino-acid peptide, angiotensin I. Angiotensin I has no known physiologic function and is further cleaved to an 8–amino-acid peptide, angiotensin II, by a converting enzyme **(angiotensin-converting enzyme [ACE])** found on the surface of vascular endothelial cells (pulmonary and renal endothelial cells are important sites for the conversion of angiotensin I to angiotensin II). Angiotensin II has several important physiologic functions, including the following:

1. Stimulation of aldosterone secretion by the adrenal cortex
2. Arteriolar vasoconstriction, which increases blood pressure
3. Stimulation of ADH secretion and thirst
4. Enhancement of NaCl reabsorption by the proximal tubule

Angiotensin II is an important secretagogue for aldosterone (an increase in the plasma [K+] is the other important stimulus for aldosterone secretion), a steroid hormone produced by the glomerulosa cells of the adrenal cortex. Aldosterone acts in a number of ways on the kidneys (see also Chapters 4, 7, and 8). With regard to the regulation of the ECV, aldosterone reduces NaCl excretion by stimulating its reabsorption by the thick ascending limb of Henle's loop, the distal tubule, and the collecting duct.

---

20 It is thought that macula densa–mediated renin secretion may play a role in maintaining systemic arterial pressure under the condition of a reduced vascular volume. For example, when vascular volume is reduced, perfusion of the body tissues (including the kidneys) decreases. This in turn results in a decrease in the GFR and the filtered load of NaCl. The reduced delivery of NaCl to the macula densa then stimulates renin secretion, which through angiotensin II (a potent vasoconstrictor) acts to increase blood pressure and thereby maintain tissue perfusion.

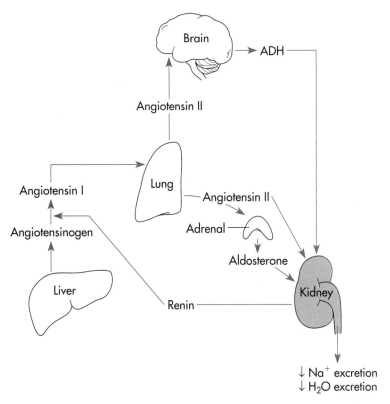

Figure 6-2 ■ Schematic representation of the essential components of the renin-angiotensin-aldosterone system. Activation of this system results in a decrease in the excretion of Na$^+$ and water by the kidneys. NOTE: Angiotensin I is converted to angiotensin II by an angiotensin-converting enzyme (ACE), which is present on all vascular endothelial cells. As shown, the endothelial cells within the lungs play a signficant role in this conversion process. See text for details.

The stimulation of Na$^+$ reabsorption by aldosterone in the late portion of the distal tubule and collecting duct has been studied extensively. Aldosterone enters the cell (principal cell) and binds to a cytoplasmic receptor. The hormone-receptor complex enters the nucleus and regulates transcription of messenger ribonucleic acid (mRNA), which encodes for a number of proteins important for Na$^+$ reabsorption by the cell. Although all the intracellular steps involved in the action of aldosterone have not been identified, the net effect on Na$^+$ reabsorption by the principal cell is to increase Na$^+$ entry into the cell across the apical membrane, as well as its exit from the cell across the basolateral membrane. The increase in apical membrane Na$^+$ entry occurs via Na$^+$-selective channels, and increased extrusion of Na$^+$ from the cell across the basolateral membrane occurs by the Na$^+$-K$^+$-ATPase. Because the transcellular reabsorption of Na$^+$ by the principal cell generates a lumen-negative transepithelial voltage (see Chapter 4), the enhanced Na$^+$ reabsorption from the luminal fluid increases the magnitude of this voltage. The passive movement of Cl$^-$ from the lumen to blood via the paracellular pathway is enhanced by the increase in the transepithelial voltage. Thus, aldosterone increases the reabsorption of NaCl from the tubular fluid. Reduced levels of aldosterone result in a decrease in the amount of NaCl reabsorbed by the principal cell.

Aldosterone also enhances NaCl reabsorption by cells of the thick ascending limb of Henle's loop. The precise cellular mechanisms involved in the action of aldosterone on the thick ascending limb cells have not yet been elucidated. However, it is likely that both Na^+ entry into the cell (perhaps via the apical membrane $1Na^+$-$1K^+$-$2Cl^-$ symporter) and its extrusion from the cell (via the basolateral membrane Na^+-K^+-ATPase) are stimulated.

As summarized in Table 6-2, activation of the renin-angiotensin-aldosterone system, as occurs with a decrease in the ECV, results in decreased excretion of NaCl by the kidneys. This system is suppressed when the ECV is expanded, and renal NaCl excretion is therefore enhanced.

Diseases of the adrenal cortex can alter aldosterone levels and thereby impair the ability of the kidneys to maintain an adequate ECV. With decreased secretion of aldosterone (hypoaldosteronism), there is reduced reabsorption of Na^+, primarily by the collecting duct, resulting in the loss of Na^+ in the urine. Because urinary Na^+ loss can exceed the amount ingested in the diet (negative Na^+ balance), the ECV decreases. In response to the decreased ECV, increased sympathetic tone and elevated levels of renin, angiotensin II, and ADH occur. With increased aldosterone secretion (hyperaldosteronism), the opposite effects are seen. Na^+ reabsorption by the collecting duct is enhanced, resulting in reduced excretion of Na^+. Consequently, the ECV is increased, sympathetic tone is decreased, and renin, angiotensin II, and ADH levels are decreased. As described below, atrial natriuretic peptide levels are also elevated in this setting.

Atrial Natriuretic Peptide

Atrial myocytes produce and store a peptide hormone called *atrial natriuretic peptide (ANP)* that relaxes vascular smooth muscle and promotes NaCl and water excretion by the kidney.[21] ANP is released with atrial stretch, as would occur with expansion of the ECV. The circulating form of ANP is 28 amino acids in length. In general, ANP actions as they relate to renal NaCl and water excretion antagonize those of the renin-angiotensin-aldosterone system. ANP actions include the following:

1. Vasodilatation of the afferent arterioles and vasoconstriction of the efferent arterioles of the glomerulus occur, increasing GFR and the filtered load of Na^+.
2. Renin secretion by the afferent and efferent arterioles is inhibited.
3. Aldosterone secretion by the glomerulosa cells of the adrenal cortex is inhibited. ANP reduces aldosterone secretion by two mechanisms: Angiotensin II–induced aldosterone secretion is reduced secondary to ANP inhibition of renin secretion, and ANP acts directly on the glomerulosa cells of the adrenal cortex to inhibit aldosterone secretion.
4. NaCl reabsorption by the collecting duct is inhibited. This is due in part to reduced levels of aldosterone; however, ANP also acts directly on the collecting duct cells. Through its second-messenger cyclic guanine monophosphate (cGMP), ANP inhibits Na^+ channels in the apical membrane of the cell and therefore NaCl reabsorption. This effect occurs predominantly in the medullary portion of the collecting duct.
5. ADH secretion by the posterior pituitary and ADH action on the collecting duct are inhib-

---

21 As noted in Chapter 4, urodilatin also acts on the collecting duct to decrease NaCl reabsorption.

ited, resulting in reduced water reabsorption by the collecting duct and increased excretion of water in the urine.

Taken together, these effects of ANP increase the excretion of NaCl and water by the kidneys. Hypothetically a reduction in circulating levels of ANP would be expected to decrease NaCl and water excretion, although no convincing evidence exists to support this.

Antidiuretic Hormone

When ECV is reduced by 5% to 10%, ADH secretion by the posterior pituitary is stimulated (see Chapter 5). The elevated levels of ADH cause decreased water excretion by the kidneys, which serves to help expand the ECV.

■ CONTROL OF Na⁺ EXCRETION WITH NORMAL ECV

The maintenance of a normal ECV, termed **euvolemia,** requires the precise balance between the amount of NaCl ingested and that excreted from the body[22]. Because the kidneys are the major route for NaCl excretion, the amount of NaCl in the urine reflects dietary intake. Thus, **in a euvolemic individual, daily urine NaCl excretion equals daily NaCl intake.**

The amount of NaCl excreted by the kidneys can vary widely. Under conditions of NaCl restriction (i.e., low NaCl diet), virtually no NaCl appears in the urine. Conversely, in individuals who ingest large quantities of NaCl, renal excretion can exceed 1000 mEq/day. The kidneys' response to variations in dietary NaCl usually takes several days. This is especially true when significant changes occur. During the transition period, excretion does not match intake, and the individual is in either **positive** (intake greater than

excretion) or **negative** (intake less than excretion) **NaCl balance.**

In the example shown in Figure 6-3, NaCl intake is abruptly increased. During the transition period required for the kidneys to increase NaCl excretion, a state of positive balance exists. The retained NaCl is added to the ECF, which increases in volume (water via the ADH system is also retained to keep plasma osmolality constant). The individual can detect this increase in the ECV (also the volume of the ECF) by a gain in body weight (1 L of ECF at 1 kg). Note that after several days, excretion again equals intake but at a higher level. When the intake is abruptly returned to its original level, a period of negative balance exists. However, after a few days, excretion again equals intake. Body weight also returns to its original level, reflecting the decrease in ECV.

Understanding the way renal NaCl excretion is regulated requires an understanding of the general features of Na⁺ handling along the nephron. Figure 6-4 summarizes the contribution of each nephron segment to the reabsorption of the filtered load of Na⁺ under euvolemic conditions. (The specific cellular mechanisms of Na⁺ transport are explained in Chapter 4.) The following discussion considers only the renal handling of Na⁺. Although not specifically addressed, Cl⁻ reabsorption is regulated similarly.

In a normal adult, the filtered load of Na⁺ can be calculated as follows:

$$\text{Filtered load of Na}^+ = \text{(GFR) (Plasma [Na}^+])\quad\text{(6-1)}$$
$$= \text{(180 L/day) (140 mEq/L)}$$
$$= \text{25,200 mEq/day}$$

With a typical diet, less then 1% of this filtered load is excreted in the urine (approximately 140 mEq/day). Because of the large filtered load of Na⁺, small changes in Na⁺ reabsorption by the nephron can have a large effect on Na⁺ balance and thus the ECV (and volume of the ECF). For example, an increase in Na⁺ excretion from 1%

---

[22] During euvolemia the ECV varies in direct proportion to the volume of the ECF. Thus, the two terms can be, and frequently are, interchanged.

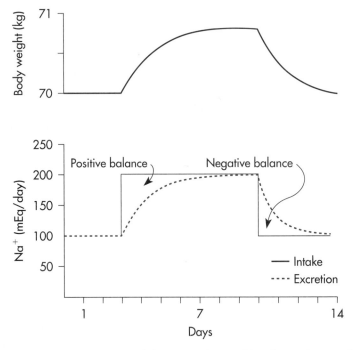

Figure 6-3 ■ **Response to step increases and decreases in NaCl intake. Na⁺ excretion by the kidneys** *(lower panel, dashed line)* **lags behind abrupt changes in Na⁺ intake** *(lower panel, solid line)*. **The change in ECF volume that occurs during the periods of positive and negative Na⁺ balance is reflected in alterations in body weight. See text for details.**

to 3% of the filtered load represents an additional loss of approximately 500 mEq/day. Because the ECF [Na⁺] is 140 mEq/L, Na⁺ loss of this magnitude would decrease ECF volume by more than 3 L (water excretion would be parallel to the loss of Na⁺ to maintain a constant body fluid osmolality; 500 mEq/day ÷ 140 mEq/L = −3.6 L/day).

During euvolemia the collecting duct is the main nephron segment where Na⁺ reabsorption is adjusted to maintain excretion at a level appropriate for dietary intake. This does not mean, however, that the other portions of the nephron are not important in this process. Because the reabsorptive capacity of the collecting duct is limited, these other portions of the nephron must reabsorb the bulk of the filtered load of Na⁺. Thus, during euvo-

lemia, Na⁺ handling by the nephron can be explained by two general processes:

1. **Na⁺ reabsorption by the proximal tubule, Henle's loop, and the distal tubule is regulated so that a relatively constant portion of the filtered load of Na⁺ is delivered to the collecting duct.** As indicated in Figure 6-4, the combined action of these nephron segments delivers 4% of the filtered load to the beginning of the collecting duct.

2. **Reabsorption of Na⁺ by the collecting duct is regulated so that the amount of Na⁺ excreted in the urine matches the amount ingested in the diet.** Thus, the collecting duct is the site where final adjust-

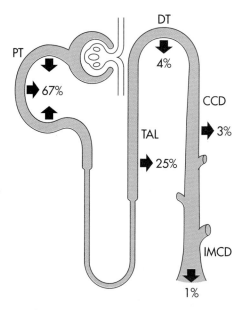

Figure 6-4 ■ **Segmental Na⁺ reabsorption. The percentage of the filtered load of Na⁺ reabsorbed by each nephron segment is indicated.** *PT,* **Proximal tubule;** *TAL,* **thick ascending limb;** *DT,* **distal tubule;** *CCD,* **cortical collecting duct;** *IMCD,* **inner medullary collecting duct.**

ments in Na⁺ excretion are made to maintain the euvolemic state.

Mechanisms for Keeping Constant the Rate of Na⁺ Delivery to the Collecting Duct

A number of mechanisms maintain delivery of a constant fraction of the filtered load of Na⁺ to the beginning of the collecting duct. These are autoregulation of GFR, and thus the filtered load of Na⁺, glomerulotubular balance, and load dependency of Na⁺ reabsorption by Henle's loop and the distal tubule.

Autoregulation of GFR (see Chapter 3) allows for the maintenance of a relatively constant filtration rate over a wide range of perfusion pressures. Because of this constant filtration rate, the filtered load of Na⁺ to the nephrons is also kept constant.

Despite the autoregulatory control of GFR, small variations occur. If an appropriate adjustment in Na⁺ reabsorption by the nephron did not compensate for these changes, marked changes in Na⁺ excretion would result. However, Na⁺ reabsorption in the euvolemic state, especially by the proximal tubule, does change in a way that is parallel to changes in GFR, a phenomenon termed **glomerulotubular balance (GT balance).** By this process, reabsorption of Na⁺, primarily by the proximal tubule, is adjusted to match the GFR. Thus, if GFR increases, the amount of Na⁺ reabsorbed by this nephron segment also increases. The opposite occurs if GFR decreases. (GT balance is further described in Chapter 4.)

The final mechanism that contributes to the constant delivery of Na⁺ to the beginning of the collecting duct relates to the ability of Henle's loop and the distal tubule to increase their Na⁺ reabsorptive rates in response to increased delivery. Of these two segments, Henle's loop, particularly the thick ascending limb, has the greater capacity to increase Na⁺ reabsorption in response to increased delivery. The mechanism by which the thick ascending limb is able to increase its Na⁺ reabsorptive rate in response to an increased delivered load is not completely understood.

Regulation of Collecting Duct Na⁺ Reabsorption

With a constant delivery of Na⁺, small adjustments in collecting duct reabsorption are sufficient to balance excretion and intake. (Recall that a 2% change in the fractional excretion of Na⁺ would produce more than a 3 L change in the volume of the ECF.) Aldosterone is the primary regulator of collecting duct Na⁺ reabsorption, and thus Na⁺ excretion, under this condition. When aldosterone levels are elevated, Na⁺ reabsorption by the principal cells of the collecting duct is increased (excretion decreased), and Na$^+$ reabsorption is decreased (excretion increased) when aldosterone levels are suppressed.

In addition to aldosterone, a number of other factors alter collecting-duct Na$^+$ reabsorption, including ANP, **urodilatin,** and sympathetic nerves. However, at present the relative roles of these other factors in the regulation of collecting-duct Na$^+$ reabsorption during euvolemia are not clear.

As long as variations in the dietary intake of NaCl are minor, the mechanisms described above can regulate renal Na$^+$ excretion appropriately, thereby maintaining the ECV at a normal level. However, significant changes in NaCl intake cannot be handled effectively by these mechanisms. When this occurs, ECV (and ECF volume) are altered. When ECV is altered, additional factors are called into play that act on the kidneys to adjust Na$^+$ reabsorption and reestablish the euvolemic state.

■ CONTROL OF Na$^+$ EXCRETION WITH INCREASED ECV

The volume sensors detect an increase in ECV, and signals are sent to the kidneys, resulting in the increased excretion of Na$^+$. The signals acting on the kidneys include the following:

1. Decreased activity of the renal sympathetic nerves
2. Release of ANP from atrial myocytes and urodilatin from distal tubular cells
3. Inhibition of ADH secretion from the posterior pituitary
4. Decreased renin secretion and thus decreased production of angiotensin II
5. Decreased secretion of aldosterone caused by reduced angiotensin II levels and elevated ANP levels.

Figure 6-5 illustrates the integrated response of the nephron to these signals. **The important difference between increased ECV and the euvolemic state is that in the former situation the renal response is not limited to the collecting duct; rather, it involves the entire nephron.**

Three general responses to an increase in the ECV occur (see Figure 6-5). The numbers correlate to those encircled in the figure.

1. GFR increases: GFR increases primarily as a result of the decrease in sympathetic nerve activity. Sympathetic fibers innervate the afferent and efferent arterioles of the glomerulus and control their diameter. Decreased sympathetic nerve activity, as occurs in this setting, leads to their dilatation. Because the effect appears to be greater on the afferent arteriole, the hydrostatic pressure within the glomerular capillary is increased and GFR increases. ANP has also been shown to increase GFR by dilating the afferent arterioles and constricting the efferent arterioles. Thus, the increased ANP levels found with this condition are also likely to contribute to this response. With the increase in GFR, the filtered load of Na$^+$ increases.

2. Reabsorption of Na$^+$ decreases in the proximal tubule: Several mechanisms appear to be involved in reducing Na$^+$ reabsorption by the proximal tubule, but the precise role of each is controversial. Because activation of the sympathetic nerve fibers innervating this nephron segment stimulates Na$^+$ reabsorption, the decreased sympathetic nerve activity resulting from increased ECV may contribute to the decreased Na$^+$ reabsorption that occurs. In addition, angiotensin II directly stimulates Na$^+$ reabsorption by the proximal tubule. Because angiotensin II levels are also reduced under this condition, it is possible that proximal tubule Na$^+$ reabsorption is decreased as a result. The increased hydrostatic pressure within the glomerular capillaries also leads to an increase in the hydrostatic pressure within the peritubular capillaries. This alteration in

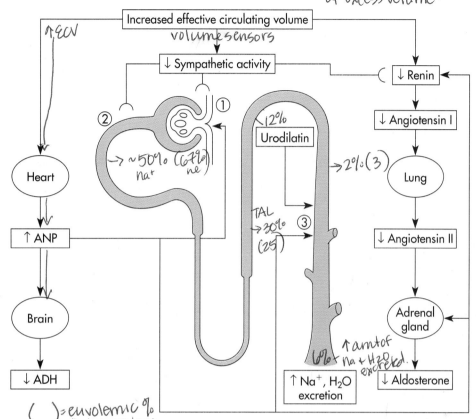

(Handwritten annotations on figure:)

↑ECV

volume sensors

2 → ~50% (67%)
Na⁺ (ne)

|2%

→2%(3)

TAL
→30%
(25)

↑ amt of
6% Na + H₂O excreted.

( ) = euvolemic % Na⁺ excretion

Figure 6-5 ■ **Integrated response to expansion of the effective circulating volume (ECV). Numbers re-fer to description of the response in the text.** Amt of Na⁺ reabsorption in TAL is load dependent

the capillary **Starling forces** reduces the absorption of solute (e.g., NaCl) and water from the lateral intercellular space, thus reducing tubular reabsorption (see Chapter 4 for mechanism).

3. Na⁺ reabsorption decreases in the collecting duct: Both the increase in the filtered load and the decrease in proximal tubule NaCl reabsorption result in the delivery of large amounts of NaCl to Henle's loop and the distal tubule. Because increased activity of sympathetic nerves and aldosterone both stimulate NaCl reabsorption by Henle's loop, the reduced nerve activity and low aldosterone levels seen with an expanded ECV could in theory reduce NaCl reabsorption by this nephron segment. However, because reabsorption by the thick ascending limb is load dependent, these effects are offset and the fraction of the filtered load of Na⁺ reabsorbed by Henle's loop is actually increased. Nevertheless, the amount of Na⁺ delivered to the beginning of the collecting duct is increased compared to the euvolemic state (see Figure 6-6).

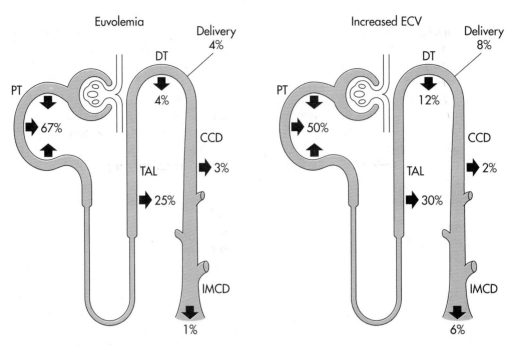

Figure 6-6 ■ **Segmental Na⁺ reabsorption during euvolemia and after expansion of the effective circulating volume (ECV). Note that with expansion of the ECV, delivery of Na⁺ to the collecting duct is increased from 4% to 8%. With inhibition of Na⁺ reabsorption by the collecting duct, Na⁺ excretion is increased from 1% to 6%.** *PT,* **Proximal tubule;** *TAL,* **thick ascending limb;** *DT,* **distal tubule;** *CCD,* **cortical collecting duct;** *IMCD,* **inner medullary collecting duct.**

The amount of Na⁺ delivered to the beginning of the collecting duct varies in proportion to the degree of ECV expansion. This increased load of Na⁺ overwhelms the reabsorptive capacity of the collecting duct, which is reduced even further by the actions of ANP and urodilatin and the decrease in the circulating levels of aldosterone.

The final component in the response to ECV expansion is the excretion of water. As Na⁺ excretion increases, plasma osmolality begins to fall. This results in decreased secretion of ADH. ADH secretion is also decreased in response to the elevated levels of ANP. In addition, ANP and urodilatin inhibit the action of ADH on the collecting duct. Together, these effects decrease water reabsorption by the collecting duct, thereby

increasing water excretion by the kidneys. Thus, the excretion of Na⁺ and water occurs in concert; ECV is restored toward normal, and body fluid osmolality remains constant. The time course of this response (hours to days) and the degree to which the ECV is returned toward its normal level depend upon the magnitude and duration of the increase in ECV. Thus, if the increase in the ECV is small and of limited duration (e.g., the result of a single ingestion of a Na⁺ load), the mechanisms just described generally return the ECV to its normal level within 24 hours. However, if the increase in the ECV is large and prolonged, the response will take several days. Moreover, the ECV may not be completely restored to its normal level.

In summary, the nephron's response to ECV expansion involves the integrated action of all its component parts. The filtered load is increased, proximal tubule reabsorption is reduced (**GFR is increased, and proximal reabsorption is decreased; thus, GT balance does not occur under this condition**), and the delivery of NaCl to the beginning of the collecting duct is increased. This increased delivery, with inhibition of collecting duct reabsorption, results in the excretion of a larger fraction of the filtered load of Na^+.

■ **CONTROL OF Na^+ EXCRETION WITH DECREASED ECV**

Volume sensors detect a decrease in ECV. Signals are sent to the kidneys, and Na^+ and water excretion are reduced. The signals involved are essentially the opposite of those involved with the response to ECV expansion and include the following:

1. Increased renal sympathetic nerve activity
2. Increased secretion of renin, which results in increased angiotensin II levels and thus increased secretion of aldosterone by the adrenal cortex
3. Inhibition of ANP secretion by the atrial myocytes and urodilatin by the distal tubule
4. Stimulation of ADH secretion by the posterior pituitary

The integrated response of the nephron to these signals is illustrated in Figure 6-7.

The nephron's response to ECV contraction involves all nephron segments. The general response is as follows (the numbers correlate to those encircled in the figure):

1. GFR decreases: Afferent and efferent arteriolar constriction occurs as a result of increased renal sympathetic nerve activity. The effect appears to be greater on the afferent arteriole, causing the hydrostatic pressure in the glomerular capillary to fall and thereby decreasing the GFR. This in turn reduces the filtered load of Na^+.

2. Na^+ reabsorption by the proximal tubule is increased: Several mechanisms appear to be involved in augmenting Na^+ reabsorption in this segment. For example, increased sympathetic nerve activity and angiotensin II directly stimulate Na^+ reabsorption by the proximal tubule. The decreased hydrostatic pressure within the glomerular capillaries also leads to a decrease in the hydrostatic pressure within the peritubular capillaries. This alteration in the capillary Starling forces facilitates the movement of fluid from the lateral intercellular space into the capillary, thereby stimulating reabsorption of solute and water by the proximal tubule (see Chapter 4 for mechanism).

3. Na^+ reabsorption by the collecting duct is enhanced: The reduced filtered load and enhanced proximal tubule reabsorption result in decreased delivery of Na^+ to Henle's loop and the distal tubule. Increased sympathetic nerve activity and aldosterone stimulate Na^+ reabsorption by the thick ascending limb and distal tubule. Because sympathetic nerve activity is increased and aldosterone levels are elevated with a decreased ECV, the potential for increased Na^+ reabsorption by these segments exists. However, Na^+ transport by the thick ascending limb and distal tubule is load dependent. This offsets the stimulatory effects of increased sympathetic nerve activity and aldosterone, and the fraction of the filtered load of Na^+ reabsorbed by these segments is actually less than that seen in the euvolemic state. Nevertheless, the net result is that less Na^+ is delivered to the beginning of the collecting duct. This is illustrated in Figure 6-8.

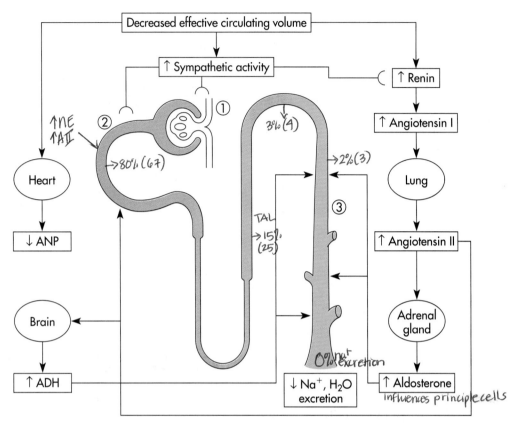

Figure 6-7 ■ Integrated response to a decrease in the effective circulating volume. Numbers refer to description of the response in text. Urodilatin levels are also decreased (and not depicted).

The small amount of Na^+ delivered to the collecting duct is virtually all reabsorbed because transport in this segment is enhanced. This stimulation of collecting-duct Na^+ reabsorption is primarily due to increased aldosterone levels. Additionally, ANP and urodilatin, which inhibit collecting duct reabsorption, are not present.

Finally, water reabsorption by the collecting duct is enhanced by ADH, the levels of which are elevated because of the activation of the low-pressure and high-pressure vascular baroreceptors. As a result, water excretion is reduced, and together with the Na^+ retained by the kidneys the ECV is returned toward normal, and body

fluid osmolality remains constant. The time course of this reexpansion (hours to days) and the degree to which the ECV is returned toward normal depend upon the magnitude of the decrease in ECV, as well as the dietary intake of Na^+. Thus, the kidneys can reduce Na^+ excretion, but the ECV will be restored to its normal level only if adequate amounts of Na^+ are ingested.

In summary, the nephron's response to a reduction in the ECV involves the integrated action of all its nephron segments. The filtered load of Na^+ is decreased, proximal tubule reabsorption is enhanced (GFR is decreased, while proximal reabsorption is increased; thus, GT-balance does

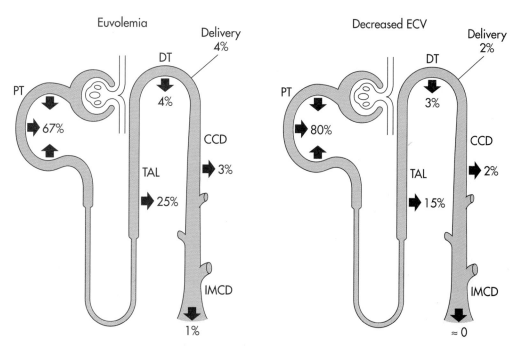

Figure 6-8 ■ Segmental Na⁺ reabsorption during euvolemia and after a decrease in the effective circulating volume (ECV). Note that with contraction of the ECV, delivery of Na⁺ to the collecting duct is reduced from 4% to 2%. The collecting duct reabsorbs virtually all of the Na⁺ it receives, and Na⁺ excretion is reduced to near zero. *PT,* Proximal tubule; *TAL,* thick ascending limb; *DT,* distal tubule; *CCD,* cortical collecting duct; *IMCD,* inner medullary collecting duct.

not occur under this condition), and the delivery of Na⁺ to the beginning of the collecting duct is reduced. This decreased delivery, together with enhanced Na⁺ reabsorption by the collecting duct, results in the virtual elimination of Na⁺ from the urine.

■ EDEMA AND THE ROLE OF THE KIDNEYS

Edema is the accumulation of excess fluid within the interstitial space. The Starling forces across the capillaries determine the movement of fluid into and out of the vascular compartment and the interstitial space (see Chapter 1). Alterations of these forces under pathologic conditions can lead to increased movement of fluid from the vascular space into the interstitium, re-

sulting in edema formation. However, for edema to be detected clinically (e.g., swelling of ankles), NaCl and water must be retained by the kidneys.

The role of the kidneys in the formation of edema can be appreciated by recognizing that the interstitial compartment must contain 2 to 3 L of excess fluid before edema is detectable. The source of this fluid is the vascular compartment (i.e., plasma), which has a volume of 3 to 4 L in the normal individual. Thus, the movement of 2 to 3 L out of the plasma compartment into the interstitial compartment would result in a marked decrease in blood pressure. As described below, this would prevent further movement of fluid from the vascular compartment into the interstitial compartment. However, retention of NaCl and water by the kidneys replenishes the plasma volume, thereby maintaining the blood pressure. As a result, accumulation of fluid in the interstitial compartment continues, and edema develops.

Alterations in Starling Forces

In Chapter 1 the Starling forces and their determination of fluid movement across the capillary wall were explained. Edema results from a change in the Starling forces that alters these fluid dynamics.

Capillary Hydrostatic Pressure (P_c) Increasing the P_c favors the movement of fluid out of the capillary or retards its movement into the capillary, thereby promoting edema formation. Normally the resistance of the precapillary arteriole is well regulated, such that changes in systemic blood pressure do not result in marked alterations in P_c. However, postcapillary resistance is not regulated to the same degree. Therefore alterations in the pressure within the venous side of the circulation do have significant effects on P_c. Consequently, an increase in the venous pressure elevates P_c. This reduces the amount of fluid reabsorbed from the interstitium back into the capillary lumen, resulting in the accumulation of edema fluid.

Plasma Oncotic Pressure (π_c) A decrease in π_c favors movement of fluid out of the capillary lumen and inhibits its reabsorption from the interstitium. Because albumin is the most abundant plasma protein, alterations in π_c result primarily from changes in the plasma [albumin].

Lymphatic Obstruction Obstruction of the lymphatics increases interstitial hydrostatic pressure (P_i) and thereby interferes with and reduces the volume of interstitial fluid that is returned to the circulation via this route. As a result, edema can form.

With renal diseases that produce the nephrotic syndrome, the permeability of the glomerular capillary is abnormally high, causing large quantities of albumin to be filtered and lost in the urine (i.e., proteinuria). If the rate of loss exceeds the rate at which albumin is synthesized by the liver, plasma [albumin] falls. The resultant change in π_c contributes to the formation of edema seen in this situation.

Because the liver synthesizes many of the plasma proteins including albumin, hypoalbuminemia is often seen in individuals with liver failure. The reduced plasma [protein] contributes to the formation of edema and ascites (i.e., accumulation of fluid in the peritoneal cavity) in these individuals.

Heart failure (i.e., decreased ability of the heart to pump blood) is one of the common conditions producing an increase in P_c. Because of poor cardiac performance, the pressure in the venous circulation is elevated. P_c can also be elevated secondary to venous thrombosis. With heart failure, pressures within all capillary beds throughout the body are increased, and generalized edema results. In contrast, edema resulting from venous thrombosis is localized to the tissues drained by the affected vein.

The most common cause of lymphatic obstruction is malignancy. When malignant cells spread to lymph nodes, obstruction can occur. Edema in this situation is confined regionally to the structures drained by the obstructed lymphatic vessels.

Capillary Permeability An increase in capillary permeability favors increased movement of fluid across the capillary wall, aiding capillary-to-interstitium movement at the arteriolar end and interstitium-to-capillary movement at the venous end. Because permeability is increased, albumin can accumulate in the interstitium. The oncotic pressure of this albumin contributes to the accumulation of excess fluid in the interstitial compartment, and edema forms.

The venom of many stinging and biting insects contains substances that increase the permeability of capillaries (i.e., increased K_f). This increased permeability can result in the accumulation of excess interstitial fluid. The accumulation of fluid and the associated swelling are usually limited to a small region around the site of the insect sting/bite. Insect stings and bites do not produce generalized edema (i.e., accumulation of excess interstitial fluid throughout the body) unless a systemic allergic reaction occurs.

The Role of the Kidneys

In each of the conditions described above, excess fluid accumulates in the interstitium at the expense of the plasma volume. If the plasma volume is not maintained near a normal level, this fluid accumulation is self-limiting. Consider the situation that exists with heart failure. Because of decreased cardiac performance, venous pressure is elevated. This raises capillary hydrostatic pressure, and fluid accumulates in the interstitium. Because the source of this fluid is the plasma, and assuming plasma volume is not maintained by some mechanism (as described later), plasma volume decreases. This in turn decreases venous and capillary hydrostatic pressures, and movement of fluid into the interstitium ceases.

Figure 6-9 illustrates what occurs when an alteration in the capillary Starling forces causes fluid accumulation in the interstitium. As fluid moves from the vascular compartment into the interstitium, vascular volume is decreased. The volume sensors detect this decrease in ECV and send signals to the kidneys, resulting in a decrease in the excretion of NaCl and water. This retention of NaCl and water serves to restore the vascular volume (i.e., plasma volume). With restoration of plasma volume, and assuming the condition altering the Starling forces still exists (e.g., untreated heart failure), additional fluid moves into the interstitium and edema forms. This cycle continues until a new steady state is reached at the capillary level, such that the amount of fluid moving out of the capillary lumen into the interstitium is again balanced by the amount moving in the opposite direction. This steady state can be attained even when the underlying cause is uncorrected. As edema fluid accumulates in the interstitial compartment, the hydrostatic pressure in this compartment increases. This pressure increase occurs as a result of the limited compliance of the surrounding tissue (e.g., skin).[23] Eventually the hydrostatic pressure within the interstitium rises to a level at which net accumulation in the interstitial compartment ceases.

The importance of NaCl retention by the kidneys in edema formation provides two approaches for treatment. The first involves dietary manipulation. The ultimate source of NaCl is the diet. Thus, if dietary intake of NaCl is restricted, the amount that can be retained by the kidneys is reduced and edema formation is limited. The second approach is to inhibit the kidneys' ability to retain NaCl. This is accomplished by the use of diuretics, which, as described in Chapter 10,

---

[23] The situation is analogous to the pressure increase that occurs as a balloon is inflated. Initially the volume of the balloon increases without a large increase in pressure. However, as the balloon reaches its limit of distensibility, the pressure increases.

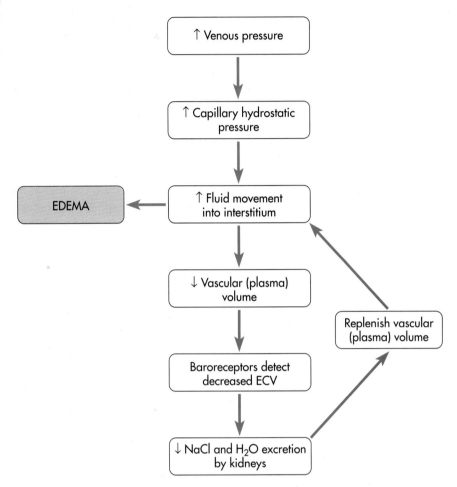

Figure 6-9 ■ **Steps involved in the development of edema resulting from an increase in venous pressure (e.g., during heart failure). Retention of NaCl and water by the kidneys maintains plasma volume, allowing the accumulation of fluid in the interstitium. See text for details.**

inhibit Na^+ transport mechanisms in the nephron. Thus, NaCl excretion is increased and NaCl retention blunted.

■ SUMMARY

1. The volume of the ECF and ECV is determined by Na^+ balance. When intake of Na^+ exceeds excretion, the ECF and ECV increase (positive Na^+ balance). Conversely, when excretion of Na^+ exceeds intake, the ECF and ECV decrease (negative Na^+ balance). The kidneys are the primary route for Na^+ excretion.

2. The coordination of Na^+ intake and excretion, and thus the maintenance of a normal ECV, requires the integrated action of the kidneys with the cardiovascular and sympathetic nervous systems. Cardiovascular volume receptors detect changes in the ECV, and by sympathetic and hormonal signals effect appro-

priate adjustments in Na^+ excretion by the kidneys.

3. Under normal conditions (euvolemia), Na^+ excretion by the kidneys is matched to the amount of Na^+ ingested in the diet. The kidneys accomplish this by reabsorbing virtually all of the filtered load of Na^+ (typically less than 1% of the filtered load is excreted). During euvolemia the collecting duct is responsible for making small adjustments in urinary Na^+ excretion to effect Na^+ balance. The major factor regulating collecting duct Na^+ reabsorption is aldosterone, which acts to stimulate Na^+ reabsorption.

4. When the ECV is increased, low- and high-pressure volume sensors initiate a response that ultimately leads to increased excretion of Na^+ by the kidneys and the return of the ECV to normal. The components of this response include a decrease in sympathetic outflow to the kidney, a suppression of the renin-angiotensin-aldosterone system, and release from the cardiac atria of atrial natriuretic peptide. By the actions of these effectors, glomerular filtration rate is enhanced, which increases the filtered load of Na^+, and Na^+ reabsorption by the proximal tubule and collecting duct is reduced. Together these changes in renal Na^+ handling enhance Na^+ excretion.

5. When the ECV is decreased, the above sequence of events is reversed (increased sympathetic outflow to the kidney, activation of the renin-angiotensin-aldosterone system, and suppression of atrial natriuretic peptide secretion). This decreases the glomerular filtration rate, enhances reabsorption of Na^+ by the proximal tubule and collecting duct, and thus reduces Na^+ excretion.

6. The development of generalized edema requires both an alteration in the Starling forces across capillary walls favoring the accumulation of fluid in the interstitium and retention of NaCl and water by the kidneys.

■ KEY WORDS AND CONCEPTS

- Effective circulating volume (ECV)
- Natriuresis
- ECV volume sensors
- Baroreceptors
- Sympathetic nerves
- Atrial natriuretic peptide (ANP)
- Urodilatin
- Juxtaglomerular apparatus
- Renin-angiotensin-aldosterone system
- Angiotensinogen
- Angiotensin-converting enzyme
- Antidiuretic hormone (ADH)
- Euvolemia
- Positive and negative Na^+ balance
- Glomerulotubular balance (GT balance)
- Starling forces
- Expansion of ECV
- Contraction of ECV
- Edema

■ SELF-STUDY PROBLEMS

1. An individual experiences an acute episode of vomiting and diarrhea and loses 3 kg in body weight over a 24-hour period. A blood sample shows that the plasma $[Na^+]$ is normal at 145 mEq/L. Indicate whether the following parameters would be increased, decreased, or unchanged from what they were before this illness (i.e., normal values).

Plasma osmolality	_____
ECV	_____
Plasma ADH levels	_____
Urine osmolality	_____
Sensation of thirst	_____

2. An individual is euvolemic and ingests a diet that contains 200 mEq/day of Na^+ on average. What would the Na^+ excretion rate of this individual be over a 24-hour period?

Regulatory signals	Increased ECV	Decreased ECV
Renal sympathetic nerves	_____	_____
ANP	_____	_____
Renin-angiotensin	_____	_____
Aldosterone	_____	_____
Vasopressin	_____	_____

3. Indicate on the above table whether the signals listed are increased or decreased by the indicated change in ECV.

4. A patient with heart failure has developed edema with swelling of the ankles and fluid in the lungs. During the past 2 weeks, the individual's weight has increased by 4 kg. Assuming that the entire weight gain is the result of the accumulation of fluid, calculate the following:

Volume of accumulated fluid: _____ L
Amount of Na$^+$ retained by
   the kidneys: _____ mEq

5. As illustrated below, administration of high doses of aldosterone to a normal individual leads to a transient retention of Na$^+$ by the kidneys (i.e., positive Na$^+$ balance). However, after several days, Na$^+$ excretion increases to the level it at which it was before hormone administration. When the hormone is stopped, Na$^+$ excretion transiently increases (i.e., negative Na$^+$ balance) but returns to its initial level over several days. Delineate the mechanisms involved in these transient changes in Na$^+$ excretion.

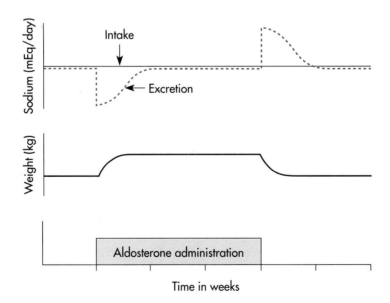

7

Regulation of
Potassium Balance

Upon completion of this chapter the student should be able to answer the following questions:

1. How does the body maintain K^+ homeostasis?
2. What is the distribution of K^+ within the body compartments? Why is this distribution important?
3. What are the hormones and factors that regulate plasma K^+ levels? Why is this regulation important?
4. How do the various segments of the nephron transport K^+, and how does the mechanism of K^+ transport by these segments determine how much K^+ is excreted in the urine?
5. Why are the distal tubule and collecting duct so important in regulating K^+ excretion?
6. How do plasma K^+ levels, aldosterone, ADH, tubular fluid flow rate, and acid-base balance influence K^+ excretion?

P otassium (K^+) is one of the most abundant cations in the body. It is critical for many cell functions, and its concentration in cells and extracellular fluid remains constant despite wide fluctuations in dietary K^+ intake. Two sets of regulatory mechanisms safeguard K^+ homeostasis.

First, several mechanisms regulate the potassium $[K^+]$ in the extracellular fluid.[24] Second, another set of mechanisms maintains a constant amount of K^+ in the body by adjusting renal K^+ excretion to match dietary K^+ intake. The kidneys regulate K^+ excretion. This chapter focuses on the hormones and factors that influence the $[K^+]$ in the extracellular fluid compartments and the hormones and factors that regulate the amount of K^+ excreted in the urine.

---

24 The $[K^+]$ in the ECF is monitored in the clinical setting by measuring the plasma $[K^+]$. For simplicity in this book, we use plasma $[K^+]$ interchangebly with ECF $[K^+]$.

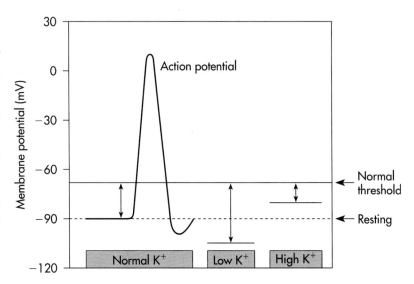

Figure 7-1 ■ The effects of variations in plasma [K⁺] on the resting membrane potential of skeletal muscle. Hyperkalemia causes the membrane potential to become less negative and decreases the excitability by inactivating fast Na⁺ channels. Hypokalemia hyperpolarizes the membrane potential and thereby reduces excitability.

The importance of K⁺ balance is evident in the clinical setting, where cardiac arrhythmias are produced by both hypokalemia and hyperkalemia. Figure 7-2 illustrates several electrocardiograms (ECGs) from patients with various levels of plasma [K⁺]. The first sign of hyperkalemia is the appearance of tall, thin T waves. Further increases in plasma [K⁺] prolong the P-R interval, depress the S-T segment, and lengthen the QRS interval. Finally, as plasma [K⁺] approaches 10 mEq/L, the P wave disappears, the QRS interval broadens, the ECG appears as a sine wave, and the ventricles fibrillate (i.e., muscles contract in a rapid, uncoordinated manner). Hypokalemia prolongs the Q-T interval, inverts the T wave, and lowers the S-T segment. The ECG is a fast and easy way to determine whether changes in plasma [K⁺] influence the heart and other excitable cells. In contrast, measurements of plasma [K⁺] by the clinical laboratory require a blood sample, and values are often not immediately available.

■ OVERVIEW OF K⁺ HOMEOSTASIS

Total body K⁺ is 50 mEq/kg of body weight, or 3500 mEq for a 70 kg individual. Ninety-eight percent of the K⁺ in the body is within cells, where its average concentration is 150 mEq/L. A high intracellular concentration of K⁺ is required for many cell functions, including cell growth and division and volume regulation. Only 2% of total body K⁺ is located in the ECF, where its normal concentration is approximately 4 mEq/L (see Appendix B). When the [K⁺] of the ECF exceeds 5 mEq/L, **hyperkalemia** exists. Conversely, **hypokalemia** exists when the [K⁺] of the ECF is less than 3.5 mEq/L.

The large concentration difference of K⁺ across cell membranes (approximately 146 mEq/L) is maintained by the operation of the Na⁺-K⁺-ATPase. This K⁺ gradient is important in maintaining the potential difference across cell membranes. Thus, K⁺ is critical for the excitability of nerve and muscle cells, as well as for the contractility of cardiac, skeletal, and smooth muscle cells (Figure 7-1).

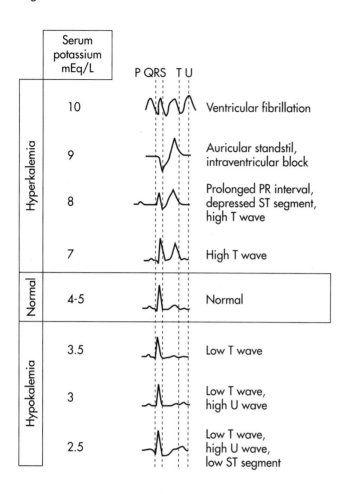

Serum potassium mEq/L		
Hyperkalemia		
	10	Ventricular fibrillation
	9	Auricular standstil, intraventricular block
	8	Prolonged PR interval, depressed ST segment, high T wave
	7	High T wave
Normal	4-5	Normal
Hypokalemia		
	3.5	Low T wave
	3	Low T wave, high U wave
	2.5	Low T wave, high U wave, low ST segment

Figure 7-2 ■ **Electrocardiographs (ECGs) from individuals with varying plasma [K⁺]. Hyperkalemia increases the height of the T wave, and hypokalemia inverts the T wave. See the text for details. (Modified from Barker L, Burton J, Zieve P: *Principles of ambulatory medicine*, Baltimore, 1982, Williams & Wilkins.)**

■ INTERNAL K⁺ DISTRIBUTION

Within minutes after a meal the K^+ absorbed by the gastrointestinal tract enters the ECF (Figure 7-3). If the K^+ ingested during a normal meal (~33 mEq) were to remain in the ECF compartment, plasma [K^+] would increase by a potentially lethal 2.4 mEq/L (33 mEq added to 14 L of ECF):

$$\frac{33 \text{ mEq}}{14 \text{ L}} = \Delta\ 2.4 \text{ mEq/L}$$

The rapid uptake of K^+ into cells prevents this rise in plasma [K^+]. **Because the excretion of K^+ by the kidneys after a meal is relatively slow (hours), the buffering of K^+ by cells is essential to prevent life-threatening hyperkalemia.** To maintain a constant level of total body K^+, all of the K^+ absorbed by the gastrointestinal tract must eventually be excreted by the kidneys. This K^+ is slowly excreted so that after 6 hours it is eliminated from the body, and the amount of K^+ therefore remains constant.

Several hormones promote the uptake of K^+ into cells after a rise in plasma [K^+] and thereby prevent dangerous hyperkalemia. As illustrated in Figure 7-3 and summarized in the box on p. 121, these hormones include epinephrine, insulin, and aldosterone. They all increase K^+ up-

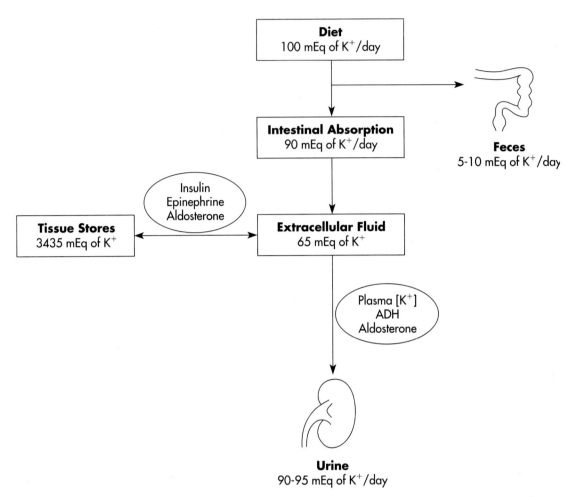

Figure 7-3 ■ **Overview of potassium (K⁺) homeostasis.** An increase in plasma insulin, epinephrine, and aldosterone stimulates K⁺ movement into cells and decreases plasma [K⁺], whereas a fall in the plasma concentration of these hormones increases plasma [K⁺]. The amount of K⁺ in the body is determined by the kidneys. An individual is in K⁺ balance when dietary intake and urinary output (plus output by the gastrointestinal tract) are equal. The excretion of K⁺ by the kidneys is regulated by plasma [K⁺], aldosterone, and ADH (antidiuretic hormone).

take into skeletal muscle, liver, bone, and red blood cells by stimulating the Na⁺-K⁺-ATPase pump. Acute stimulation of K⁺ uptake, which occurs within minutes, is mediated by an increased turnover rate of existing Na⁺-K⁺-ATPase, whereas the chronic increase in K⁺ uptake, which takes hours to days, is mediated by an increase in the number of Na⁺-K⁺-ATPase pumps. A rise in plasma [K⁺] subsequent to K⁺ absorption by the gastrointestinal tract stimulates insulin secretion from the pancreas, aldosterone release from the adrenal cortex, and epinephrine secretion from

> ## *Major Factors and Hormones Influencing the Distribution of K+ between the ICF and the ECF*
>
> **Physiologic: Keep Plasma [K+] Constant**
>
> Epinephrine
> Insulin
> Aldosterone
>
> **Pathophysiologic: Displace Plasma [K+] from Normal**
>
> Acid-base balance
> Plasma osmolality
> Cell lysis
> Exercise

> α-Adrenoceptor activation is important in preventing hypokalemia after exercise. The importance of β_2 receptors is illustrated by two observations. First, the rise in plasma [K+] after a K+-rich meal is greater if the subject has been pretreated with propranolol, a β-adrenergic blocker. Second, the release of epinephrine during stress (e.g., coronary ischemia) can rapidly lower plasma [K+].

the adrenal medulla. In contrast, a decrease in plasma [K+] inhibits release of these hormones. Whereas insulin and epinephrine act within a few minutes, aldosterone requires about 1 hour to stimulate K+ uptake into cells.

Epinephrine

Catecholamines affect the distribution of K+ across cell membranes by activating α and β_2-adrenergic receptors. Stimulation of α receptor releases K+ from cells, especially in the liver, whereas stimulation of β_2 receptors causes K+ uptake by cells.

Insulin

Insulin also stimulates K+ uptake into cells. The importance of insulin is illustrated by two observations. First, the rise in plasma [K+] after a K+-rich meal is greater in patients with diabetes mellitus (i.e., insulin deficiency) than in normal people. Second, infusion of insulin (and glucose to prevent insulin-induced hypoglycemia) constitutes acute therapy for hyperkalemia. **Insulin is the most important hormone that shifts K+ into cells after ingestion of K+ in a meal.**

Aldosterone

Like catecholamines and insulin, aldosterone also promotes K+ uptake into cells. A rise in aldosterone levels (e.g., primary aldosteronism) causes hypokalemia, and a fall in aldosterone levels (e.g., Addison's disease) causes hyperkalemia. As discussed later, aldosterone also stimulates urinary K+ excretion. Thus, aldosterone alters plasma [K+] by acting on K+ uptake into cells and altering urinary K+ excretion.

Thus far the discussion has focused on hormones that maintain the distribution of K+ across cell membranes constant. Other factors, however, influence K+ movement across the cell membrane, but they are not homeostatic mechanisms because they displace plasma [K+] from normal levels.

Acid-Base Balance

In general, metabolic acidosis increases plasma [K+], and metabolic alkalosis decreases it. In contrast, respiratory acid-base disorders have little or no effect on plasma [K+]. A metabolic acidosis produced by the addition of inorganic acids (e.g., HCl, H_2SO_4) increases plasma [K+] to a much greater extent than does a similar acidosis produced by the accumulation of organic acids (e.g., lactic acid, acetic acid, keto acids). The reduced pH promotes movement of H+ into cells and the reciprocal movement of K+ out of cells. Metabolic alkalosis has the opposite effect:

plasma [K$^+$] decreases as K$^+$ moves into cells and H$^+$ leaves cells. The mechanism responsible for this shift is not fully understood. Some researchers suggest that the movement of H$^+$ occurs as the cells' buffer changes in the [H$^+$] of the extracellular fluid. As H$^+$ moves across the cell membranes, K$^+$ moves in the opposite direction, and thus cations are neither gained nor lost across the cell membranes. Although organic acids produce a metabolic acidosis, they do not cause a significant degree of hyperkalemia. Two possible explanations have been suggested for the reduced effect of organic acids to cause hyperkalemia. First, the organic anion may enter the cell with H$^+$, thereby eliminating the need for K$^+$-H$^+$ exchange across the membrane. Second, organic anions may stimulate insulin secretion, which moves K$^+$ into cells, counteracting the direct effect of the acidosis, which moves K$^+$ out of cells.

Plasma Osmolality

Plasma osmolality also influences the distribution of K$^+$ across cell membranes. An increase in the osmolality of the extracellular fluid enhances K$^+$ release by cells and thus increases extracellular [K$^+$]. The plasma K$^+$ level may increase by 0.4 to 0.8 mEq/L for a 10 mOsm/kg H$_2$O elevation in plasma osmolality. Hypoosmolality has the opposite action. The changes in plasma [K$^+$] associated with alterations in osmolality are related to changes in cell volume. For example, as plasma osmolality increases, water leaves cells because of the osmotic gradient across the plasma membrane. Water leaves cells until the intracellular osmolality becomes equal to the extracellular osmolality. This loss of water shrinks the cells and causes the cell [K$^+$] to rise. The rise in intracellular [K$^+$] provides a driving force for K$^+$ efflux from the cells. This sequence increases the plasma [K$^+$]. A fall in plasma osmolality has the opposite effect.

Cell Lysis

Cell lysis causes hyperkalemia, which results from the addition of intracellular K$^+$ to the extracellular fluid.

Exercise

During exercise more K$^+$ is released from skeletal muscle cells than during rest. Release of K$^+$ during the recovery phase of the action potential and the ensuing hyperkalemia depend on the degree of exercise. Plasma [K$^+$] increases by 0.3 mEq/L with slow walking and may increase by up to 2 mEq/L or more above normal with exercise.

Acid-base balance, plasma osmolality, cell lysis, and exercise do not maintain plasma [K$^+$] at a normal value and therefore do not contribute to K$^+$ homeostasis. The extent to which these pathophysiologic states alter plasma [K$^+$] depends on the integrity of the homeostatic mechanisms that regulate plasma [K$^+$] (e.g., secretion of epinephrine, insulin, and aldosterone).

■ K$^+$ EXCRETION BY THE KIDNEYS

The kidneys play the major role in maintaining K$^+$ balance. As illustrated in Figure 7-3 the kidneys excrete 90%-95% of the K$^+$ ingested in the diet. Excretion equals intake even when intake increases by as much as tenfold. This equality between urinary excretion and dietary intake underscores the importance of the kidneys in main-

Severe trauma (e.g., burns) and some diseases such as tumor lysis syndrome and rhabdomyolysis (i.e., destruction of skeletal muscle) cause cell destruction and release of K$^+$ (and other cell solutes) into the extracellular fluid. In addition, gastric ulcers may cause seepage of red blood cells into the gastrointestinal tract. The blood cells are digested, and the K$^+$ released from the cells is absorbed and can cause hyperkalemia.

Exercise-induced changes in plasma [K$^+$] usually do not produce symptoms and are reversed after several minutes of rest. However, in individuals (1) who have certain endocrine disorders that affect the release of insulin, epinephrine, or aldosterone; (2) whose ability to excrete K$^+$ is impaired (e.g., renal failure); or (3) who are on certain medications, such as β-adrenergic blockers, exercise can lead to potentially life-threatening hyperkalemia. For example, during exercise plasma [K$^+$] may increase by 2 to 4 mEq/L or more in individuals taking β-adrenergic blockers for hypertension.

In individuals with advanced renal disease the kidneys are unable to eliminate K$^+$ from the body, and plasma [K$^+$] rises. The resulting hyperkalemia reduces the resting membrane potential (i.e., the voltage becomes less negative) and decreases the excitability of neurons, cardiac cells, and muscle cells by inactivating fast Na$^+$ channels in the membrane. Severe, rapid increases in plasma [K$^+$] can lead to cardiac arrest and death. In contrast, in patients taking diuretic drugs for hypertension, urinary K$^+$ excretion often exceeds dietary K$^+$ intake. Accordingly, negative K$^+$ balance exists and hypokalemia develops. This decline in extracellular [K$^+$] hyperpolarizes the resting cell membrane potential (i.e., the voltage becomes more negative) and reduces the excitability of neurons, cardiac cells, and muscle cells. Severe hypokalemia can lead to paralysis, cardiac arrhythmia, and death. Hypokalemia can also impair the ability of the kidneys to concentrate the urine and can stimulate renal production of NH$_4^+$. Therefore maintenance of a high intracellular [K$^+$], a low extracellular [K$^+$], as well as a high K$^+$ concentration gradient across cell membranes is essential for a number of cellular functions.

taining K$^+$ homeostasis. Although small amounts of K$^+$ are lost each day in the stool and sweat (approximately 5%-10% of the K$^+$ ingested in the diet), this amount is essentially constant, not regulated, and therefore relatively much less important than the K$^+$ excreted by the kidneys.[25] **The primary event in determining urinary K$^+$ excretion is K$^+$ secretion from the blood into the tubular fluid by the cells of the distal tubule and collecting duct system.** The transport pattern of K$^+$ by the major nephron segments is illustrated in Figure 7-4.

Because K$^+$ is not bound to plasma proteins, it is freely filtered by the glomerulus. Normally, when individuals ingest an average diet, urinary K$^+$ excretion is 15% of the amount filtered. Accordingly, K$^+$ must be reabsorbed along the nephron. When dietary K$^+$ intake is augmented, however, K$^+$ excretion can exceed the amount filtered, indicating that K$^+$ can also be secreted.

The proximal tubule reabsorbs 67% of the filtered K$^+$ under most conditions. Approximately 20% of the filtered K$^+$ is reabsorbed by Henle's loop, and, as with the proximal tubule, reabsorp-

tion is a constant fraction of the amount filtered. In contrast to these segments, which are capable of only reabsorbing K$^+$, the distal tubule and the collecting duct have the capacity to either reabsorb or secrete K$^+$. The rate of K$^+$ reabsorption or secretion by the distal tubule and the collecting duct depends on a variety of hormones and factors. When K$^+$ intake is normal (100 mEq/day), K$^+$ is secreted. A rise in dietary K$^+$ intake increases K$^+$ secretion so that the amount of K$^+$ appearing in the urine may approach 80% of the amount filtered (Figure 7-4). In contrast, a low-potassium diet activates K$^+$ reabsorption along the distal tubule and collecting duct so that urinary excretion falls to 1% of the K$^+$ filtered by

---

25 Loss of K$^+$ in the feces can become significant during periods of diarrhea and chronic renal failure.

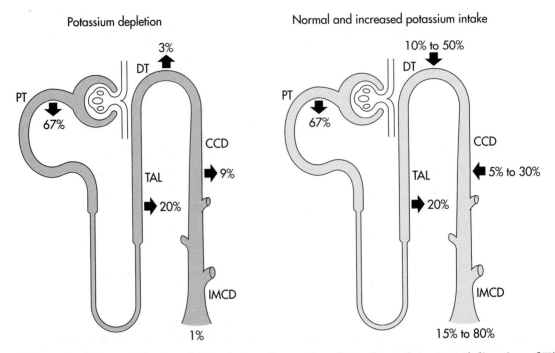

Potassium depletion

Normal and increased potassium intake

Figure 7-4 ■ **K$^+$ transport along the nephron. K$^+$ excretion depends on the rate and direction of K$^+$ transport by the distal tubule and the collecting duct. Percentages refer to the amount of filtered K$^+$ reabsorbed or secreted by each nephron segment. Left panel, Dietary K$^+$ depletion. An amount of K$^+$ equal to 1% of the filtered load of K$^+$ is excreted. Right panel, Normal and increased dietary K$^+$ intake. An amount of K$^+$ equal to 15% to 80% of the filtered load is excreted. *PT*, Proximal tubule; *TAL*, thick ascending limb; *DT*, distal tubule; *CCD*, cortical collecting duct; *IMCD*, inner medullary collecting duct.**

the glomerulus (Figure 7-4). The kidneys are not able to reduce K$^+$ excretion to the same low levels that they can for Na$^+$ (0.2%). Therefore hypokalemia can develop in individuals placed on a K$^+$-deficient diet.

Because the magnitude and direction of K$^+$ transport by the distal tubule and collecting duct are variable, the overall rate of urinary K$^+$ excretion is determined by these tubular segments.

■ **CELLULAR MECHANISMS OF K$^+$ TRANSPORT BY THE DISTAL TUBULE AND COLLECTING DUCT**

Figure 7-5 illustrates the cellular mechanism of K$^+$ secretion by principal cells in the distal tubule and collecting duct. Secretion from blood

into tubular fluid is a two-step process involving the following: (1) K$^+$ uptake across the basolateral membrane by Na$^+$-K$^+$-ATPase and (2) diffusion of K$^+$ from the cell into the tubular fluid. The operation of the Na$^+$-K$^+$-ATPase creates a high intracellular [K$^+$], which provides the chemical driving force for K$^+$ exit across the apical membrane through K$^+$ channels. Although K$^+$ channels are also present in the basolateral membrane, K$^+$ preferentially leaves the cell across the apical membrane and enters the tubular fluid for two reasons. First, the electrochemical gradient of K$^+$ across the apical membrane favors the downhill movement into the tubular fluid. Second, K$^+$ is able to cross the apical membrane more readily than the basolateral mem-

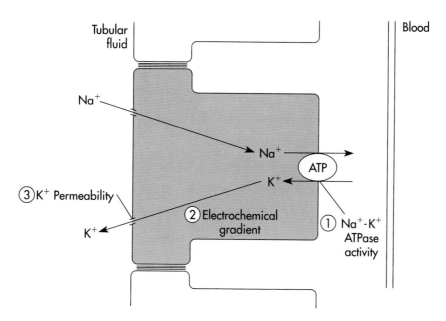

Figure 7-5 ■ Cellular mechanism of K⁺ secretion by the principal cell in the distal tubule and collecting duct. The numbers indicate the sites where K⁺ secretion is regulated: *1,* Na⁺-K⁺-ATPase; *2,* Electrochemical gradient of K⁺ across the apical membrane; and *3,* the K⁺ permeability of the apical membrane.

brane. Therefore K⁺ preferentially diffuses across the apical membrane into the tubular fluid. The three major factors that control the rate of K⁺ secretion by the distal tubule and the collecting duct are as follows (see Figure 7-5):

1. The activity of the Na⁺-K⁺-ATPase
2. The driving force (electrochemical gradient) for K⁺ movement across the apical membrane
3. The ability of K⁺ to cross the apical membrane

Every change in K⁺ secretion results from an alteration in one or more of these factors.

In contrast, the cellular pathways and mechanisms of K⁺ reabsorption in the distal tubule and collecting duct are not completely understood. Intercalated cells may reabsorb K⁺ by an H⁺-K⁺-ATPase transport mechanism located in the apical membrane. This transporter mediates K⁺ uptake in exchange for H⁺. However, the pathway of K⁺ exit from intercalated cells into the blood is unknown. Reabsorption of K⁺ is activated by a diet low in K⁺.

■ REGULATION OF K⁺ SECRETION BY THE DISTAL TUBULE AND COLLECTING DUCT

Regulation of K⁺ excretion is achieved mainly by alterations in K⁺ secretion by principal cells of the distal tubule and collecting duct. Plasma [K⁺] and aldosterone are the major physiologic regulators of K⁺ secretion. ADH also stimulates K⁺ secretion; however, it is less important than plasma [K⁺] and aldosterone. Other factors, including the flow rate of tubular fluid and acid-base balance, influence K⁺ secretion by the distal tubule and collecting duct. However, they are not homeostatic mechanisms because they disturb K⁺ balance.

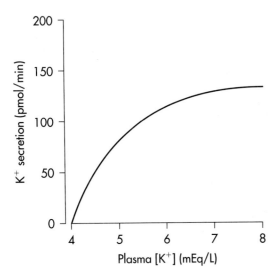

Figure 7-6 ■ The relationship between plasma [K⁺] and K⁺ secretion by the distal tubule and the cortical collecting duct.

Chronic **hypokalemia,** a plasma [K⁺] less than 3.5 mEq/L, occurs most often in individuals who receive diuretics for hypertension. Hypokalemia also occurs in individuals who vomit, abuse laxatives, or have nasogastric suction, diarrhea, or hyperaldosteronism. Hypokalemia occurs because the excretion of K⁺ by the kidneys exceeds dietary intake of K⁺. Vomiting, nasogastric suction, diuretics, and diarrhea all can decrease the effective circulating volume (ECV), which in turn stimulates aldosterone secretion. Because aldosterone stimulates K⁺ excretion by the kidneys, its action contributes to the development of hypokalemia.

Chronic **hyperkalemia,** a plasma [K⁺] greater than 5 mEq/L, occurs most frequently in individuals with a reduced urine flow or a low plasma aldosterone level or in individuals with renal disease whose GFR falls to less than 20% of normal. In these individuals hyperkalemia occurs because the excretion of K⁺ by the kidneys is less than dietary intake of K⁺. Less common causes for hyperkalemia occur with deficiencies of insulin, epinephrine, or aldosterone secretion or with metabolic acidosis caused by inorganic acids.

Major Factors and Hormones Influencing K⁺ Excretion

Physiologic: Keep K⁺ Balance Constant

Plasma [K⁺]
Aldosterone
ADH

Pathophysiologic: Displace K⁺ Balance

Flow rate of tubular fluid
Acid-base balance

Hormones and Factors That Regulate Urinary K⁺ Excretion

Plasma [K⁺] Plasma [K⁺] is an important determinant of K⁺ secretion by the distal tubule and collecting duct (Figure 7-6). Hyperkalemia (e.g., resulting from a high-K⁺ diet or rhabdomyolysis), stimulates secretion within minutes. Several mechanisms are involved. First, hyperkalemia stimulates the Na⁺-K⁺-ATPase pump and thereby increases K⁺ uptake across the basolateral membrane. This raises intracellular [K⁺] and increases the electrochemical driving force for K⁺ exit across the apical membrane. Second, hyperkalemia also increases the ability of K⁺ to cross the apical membrane. Third, hyperkalemia stimulates aldosterone secretion by the adrenal cortex, which, as discussed later, acts synergistically with plasma [K⁺] to stimulate K⁺ secretion. Fourth, hyperkalemia also increases the flow rate of tubular fluid by inhibiting NaCl and water reabsorption across the proximal tubule, which stimulates K⁺ secretion by the distal tubule and collecting duct.

Hypokalemia (e.g., caused by a low-K⁺ diet or diarrhea) decreases K⁺ secretion by actions opposite to those described for hyperkalemia. Hence, hypokalemia inhibits the Na⁺-K⁺-ATPase pump, decreases the electrochemical driving force for K⁺ efflux across the apical membrane, reduces the ability of K⁺ to cross the apical membrane, and causes a reduction in plasma aldosterone levels.

Aldosterone A chronic (i.e., 24 hours or longer) elevation in plasma aldosterone concentration enhances K^+ secretion across the distal tubule and collecting duct by increasing the amount of Na^+-K^+-ATPase in principal cells (Figure 7-7). This elevates cell $[K^+]$. Aldosterone also increases the driving force for K^+ exit across the apical membrane and increases the ability of K^+ to cross the apical membrane. Aldosterone secretion is increased by hyperkalemia and angiotensin II (following activation of the renin-angiotensin system), and secretion is decreased by hypokalemia and atrial natriuretic peptide.

An acute increase in aldosterone (i.e., over hours) enhances the activity of the Na^+-K^+-ATPase, but K^+ excretion does not increase. The reason for this relates to the effect of aldosterone on Na^+ reabsorption and tubular flow. Aldosterone stimulates Na^+ reabsorption and thereby decreases tubular flow by stimulating water reabsorption. The decrease in flow decreases K^+ secretion (discussed in more detail later). However, chronic stimulation of Na^+ reabsorption expands the ECF and thereby returns flow to normal, which allows the direct stimulatory effect of aldosterone on the distal tubule and collecting duct to increase K^+ excretion.

Glucocorticoids also stimulate K^+ excretion. However, this effect is indirect and mediated by an increase in the GFR that increases tubular flow.

Antidiuretic Hormone Antidiuretic hormone (ADH) increases the electrochemical driving force for K^+ exit across the apical membrane of principal cells by stimulating Na^+ uptake across the apical membrane, which depolarizes

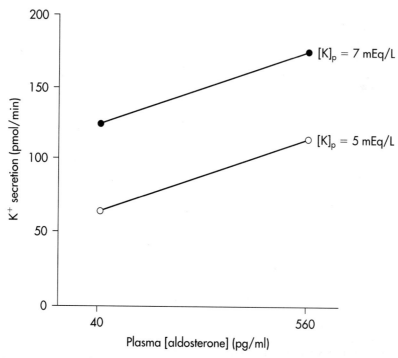

Figure 7-7 ■ The relationship between plasma aldosterone and K^+ secretion by the distal tubule and the cortical collecting duct. Note that K^+ secretion is increased further when the plasma $[K^+]$ ($[K]_p$) is increased.

(i.e., reduces) the electrical potential difference across the apical membrane. Despite this effect, ADH does not change K^+ secretion by these nephron segments. The reason for this relates to the effect of ADH on tubular fluid flow. ADH decreases tubular fluid flow by stimulating water reabsorption. The decrease in tubular flow decreases K^+ secretion (discussed in more detail later). As illustrated in Figure 7-8, changes in ADH levels do not alter K^+ secretion by the distal tubule and collecting duct or urinary K^+ excretion because the stimulatory effect of ADH on the electrochemical driving force for K^+ exit across the apical membrane is offset by the inhibitory effect of decreased tubular fluid flow. If ADH did not increase the electrochemical gradient favoring K^+ secretion, urinary K^+ excretion would fall as ADH levels increase (decreasing

urine flow) and K^+ balance would change in response to alterations in water balance. Thus, these effects of ADH on tubular flow and the electrochemical driving force for K^+ exit across the apical membrane enable urinary K^+ excretion to be maintained at a constant rate despite wide fluctuations in water excretion.

Factors That Perturb K^+ Excretion

Flow of Tubular Fluid A rise in the flow of tubular fluid (e.g., diuretic treatment, extracellular fluid volume expansion) stimulates K^+ secretion within minutes, whereas a fall in flow (e.g., extracellular fluid volume contraction caused by hemorrhage, severe vomiting, or diarrhea) reduces K^+ secretion by the distal tubule and collecting duct (Figure 7-9). Increments in tubular fluid flow are more effective in stimulating K^+

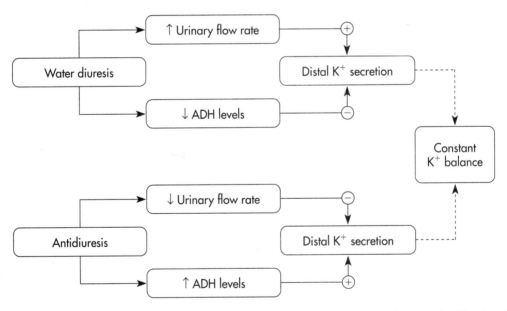

Figure 7-8 ■ **Opposing effects of ADH on K^+ secretion by the distal tubule and cortical collecting duct. Secretion is stimulated by an increase in the electrochemical gradient for K^+ across the apical membrane and perhaps by an increase in the K^+ permeability of the apical membrane. In contrast, secretion is reduced by a fall in the flow rate of tubular fluid. Because these effects oppose each other, net K^+ secretion is not affected by ADH.**

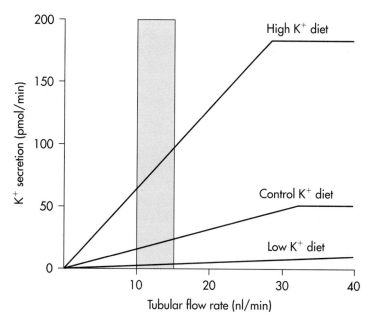

Figure 7-9 ■ **Relationship between tubular flow rate and K⁺ secretion by the distal tubule and cortical collecting duct. A diet high in K⁺ increases the slope of the relationship between flow rate and secretion and increases the maximum rate of secretion. A diet low in K⁺ has the opposite effects. The shaded bar indicates the flow rate under most physiologic conditions.**

secretion as dietary K⁺ intake is increased from a diet low in K⁺ to one high in K⁺. Alterations in tubular fluid flow influence K⁺ secretion by changing the driving force for K⁺ exit across the apical membrane. As K⁺ is secreted into the tubular fluid, the [K⁺] of the fluid increases. This reduces the electrochemical driving force for K⁺ exit across the apical membrane and thereby reduces the rate of secretion. An increase in tubular fluid flow minimizes the rise in tubular fluid [K⁺] as the secreted K⁺ is washed downstream. A second mechanism responsible for flow-dependent stimulation of K⁺ secretion is related to Na⁺ reabsorption. A rise in flow increases the amount of Na⁺ entering the distal tubule and collecting duct, which in turn enhances Na⁺ reabsorption. The increase in Na⁺ reabsorption stimulates K⁺ uptake across the basolateral membrane by in-

creasing the activity of the Na⁺-K⁺-ATPase, which promotes K⁺ secretion.

Because diuretic drugs increase the flow of tubular fluid through the distal tubule and collecting duct, they also enhance urinary K⁺ excretion. In contrast, a decline in tubular fluid flow inhibits K⁺ secretion. A decline in the tubular fluid flow facilitates the rise in tubular fluid [K⁺] and thereby reduces secretion.

Acid-Base Balance Another factor that modulates K⁺ secretion is the [H⁺] of the extracellular fluid (Figure 7-10). Acute alterations (over a period of minutes to hours) in the pH of the plasma influence K⁺ secretion by the distal tubule and collecting duct. Alkalosis (i.e., a plasma pH above normal) increases H⁺ secretion, whereas acidosis (i.e., a plasma pH below normal) decreases K⁺ secretion. Acute acidosis re-

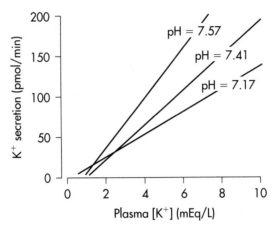

Figure 7-10 ■ **Effect of plasma pH on the relationship between plasma [K⁺] and K⁺ secretion by the distal tubule and collecting duct.**

duces K⁺ secretion by two mechanisms: (1) it inhibits the Na⁺-K⁺-ATPase pump and thereby reduces cell [K⁺] and the electrochemical driving force for K⁺ exit across the apical membrane, and (2) it reduces the ability of K⁺ to cross the apical membrane. Alkalosis has the opposite effects.

The effect of metabolic acidosis on K⁺ excretion is time dependent. When a metabolic acidosis is prolonged for several days, urinary K⁺ excretion is stimulated (Figure 7-11). This occurs because chronic metabolic acidosis decreases water and NaCl reabsorption by the proximal tubule by inhibiting the Na⁺-K⁺-ATPase. Hence, the flow of tubular fluid is augmented through the distal tubule and collecting duct. The inhibition of proximal tubular water and NaCl reabsorption also causes a decrease in ECV and thereby stimulates aldosterone secretion. In addition, chronic acidosis, caused by inorganic acids, increases plasma [K⁺], which stimulates aldosterone secretion. The rise in tubular fluid flow, plasma [K⁺], and aldosterone offsets the effects of acidosis on cell [K⁺] and apical membrane permeability so that K⁺ secretion rises. Thus, metabolic acidosis may either inhibit or stimulate potassium excretion, depend-

ing on the natural duration of the disturbance.

The acid-base balance and the flow of tubular fluid do not maintain K⁺ balance at a normal value and therefore do not contribute to K⁺ homeostasis. The extent to which changes in flow and acid-base balance alter K⁺ balance and plasma [K⁺] depends on the integrity of the homeostatic mechanisms that regulate K⁺ balance and plasma [K⁺].

Interaction Among Hormones and Factors That Influence K⁺ Secretion by the Distal Tubule and Collecting Duct

As discussed previously, the rate of urinary K⁺ excretion is frequently determined by simultaneous changes in hormone levels, acid-base balance, or flow (Table 7-1). Frequently the powerful effect of flow often enhances or opposes the response of the distal tubule and collecting duct to hormones and changes in acid-base balance. This interaction can be beneficial, as with hyperkalemia, in which the change in flow enhances K⁺ excretion and thereby restores K⁺ homeostasis, or detrimental, as with alkalosis, in which changes in flow and acid-base status perturb K⁺ homeostasis.

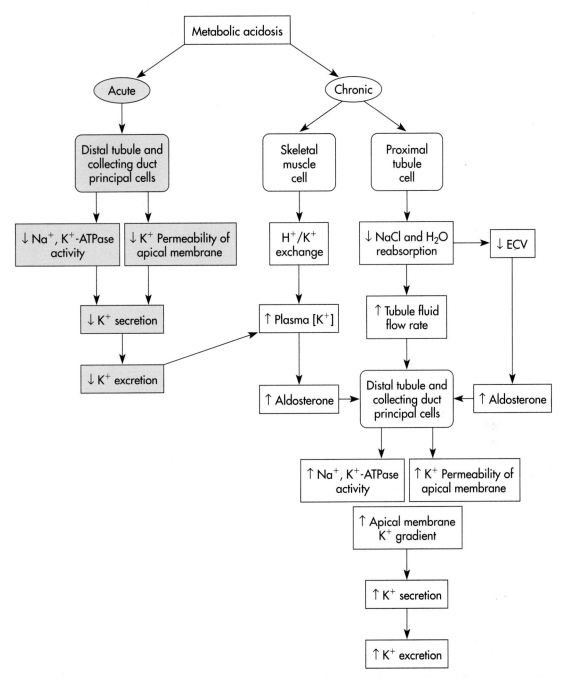

Figure 7-11 ■ **Acute versus chronic effect of metabolic acidosis on K⁺ excretion. See text for details.**

Interaction between the direct/indirect effects of hormones and factors on K$^+$ secretion by the distal tubule and collecting duct and flow of tubular fluid

	Direct or indirect	Tubular fluid flow	Urinary excretion
Hyperkalemia	↑	↑	↑↑
Alodsterone			
Acute	↑	↓	NC
Chronic	↑	NC	↑
Glucocorticoids	NC	↑	↑
ADH	↑	↓	NC
Acidosis			
Acute	↓	NC	↓
Chronic	↓	↑↑	↑
Alkalosis	↑	↑	↑↑

NC, No change. (Modified from Field MJ, Berliner RW, Giebisch GH: *Regulation of renal potassium metabolism.* In Narins R, editor: *Textbook of nephrology: clinical disorders of fluid and electrolyte metabolism,* ed 5, New York, 1994, McGraw Hill.)

■ **SUMMARY**

1. One of the most abundant cations in the body, K$^+$ is crucial for many cellular functions, including cell growth and division and the excitability of nerve and muscle.

2. K$^+$ homeostasis is maintained by hormones that regulate plasma [K$^+$] and by the kidneys, which adjust K$^+$ excretion to match dietary K$^+$ intake. Plasma [K$^+$] is maintained by insulin, epinephrine, and aldosterone. In contrast, cell lysis and exercise and changes in acid-base balance and plasma osmolality perturb plasma [K$^+$].

3. K$^+$ excretion by the kidneys is determined by the rate of K$^+$ secretion by the distal tubule and collecting duct. K$^+$ secretion by these tubular segments is regulated by plasma [K$^+$], aldosterone, and ADH. In contrast, changes in tubular fluid flow and acid-base disturbance perturb K$^+$ excretion by the kidneys.

■ **KEY WORDS AND CONCEPTS**

- Hyperkalemia
- Hypokalemia
- Internal K$^+$ balance
- Insulin
- Epinephrine
- Plasma osmolality
- Acid-base balance
- External K$^+$ balance
- Cellular mechanisms of K$^+$ secretion by the distal tubule and collecting duct
- Hormones and factors regulating K$^+$ excretion
- Aldosterone
- ADH
- Plasma [K$^+$]
- Tubular fluid flow rate

■ SELF-STUDY PROBLEMS

1. What would happen to the rise in plasma [K$^+$] following an intravenous K$^+$ load if the subject had a combination of sympathetic blockade and insulin deficiency?

2. What effect would aldosterone deficiency have on urinary K$^+$ excretion? What would happen to plasma [K$^+$], and what effect would this have on K$^+$ excretion?

3. Describe the homeostatic mechanisms involved in maintaining the plasma [K$^+$] following ingestion of a meal rich in K$^+$.

4. If the GFR declined by 50% (e.g., because of a loss of one kidney) and the filtered load of K$^+$ also declined by 50%, would the remaining kidney be able to maintain K$^+$ balance? If so, how would this occur? If not, would the subject become hyperkalemic?

Regulation of
Acid-Base Balance

OBJECTIVES

Upon completion of this chapter the student should be able to answer the following questions:

1. How does the CO_2/HCO_3^- system operate as a buffer, and why is it an important buffer of the extracellular fluid (ECF)?
2. How does metabolism of food produce acid and alkali, and what effect does the composition of the diet have on systemic acid-base balance?
3. What is the difference between volatile and nonvolatile acids?
4. How do the kidneys contribute to systemic acid-base balance?
5. Why are urinary buffers necessary for the excretion of acid by the kidneys?
6. What are the mechanisms for H^+ transport in the various segments of the nephron, and how are these mechanisms regulated?
7. How do the various segments of the nephron contribute to the process of reabsorbing the filtered HCO_3^-?
8. How do the kidneys form new HCO_3^-?
9. How is ammonium produced by the kidneys, and why is it considered a urinary buffer?
10. What are the major mechanisms by which the body defends itself against changes in acid-base balance?
11. What is the difference between simple metabolic and respiratory acid-base disorders, and how are they differentiated by blood gas measurements?

The concentration of H^+ in the body fluids is low compared with that of other ions. For example, Na^+ is present at a concentration some three million times greater than that of H^+ ($[Na^+]$ = 140 mEq/L; $[H^+]$ = 40 nEq/L). Because of the low $[H^+]$ of the body fluids, it is commonly expressed as the negative logarithm, or pH. Table 8-1 lists $[H^+]$ and corresponding pH over the physiologic range.

The coordinated functions of the liver, lungs, and kidneys create acid-base balance. Acid or alkali[26] addition to or production by the body must be matched by excretion from the body for the maintenance of acid-base balance. Through metabolism the liver adds various acid and alkali equivalents to the ECF (other cells, such as skeletal muscle, can also add acid to the body via metabolism, especially under anaerobic conditions). In a normal adult, acid or alkali is added to the body fluids by metabolism, and the amount of acid or alkali added is determined primarily by the diet.

With a normal diet the body produces approximately 15 to 20 moles of acid per day. Virtually all of this acid is derived from CO_2 (CO_2 + $H_2O \leftrightarrow H_2CO_3$) and is therefore called *volatile acid.* The lungs handle this potential acid load by excreting CO_2. In addition, the metabolism of food produces acid and alkali that cannot be excreted by the lungs. In people on a typical meat-containing diet, acid production exceeds alkali production. This acid, termed *nonvolatile acid,* is produced at a small fraction of the rate of volatile acid production (50 to 100 mmoles/day versus 15 to 20 moles/day). The kidneys, together with various buffers, play an important role in the handling of nonvolatile acid and thereby minimize its effect on body fluid pH.

---

26 Acids are defined as substances that add H^+ to the body fluids, whereas alkalis remove H^+ from the body fluids.

TABLE 8 - 1	
Relationship between pH and [H⁺]	
pH	**[H⁺], nEq/L**
7.8	16
7.7	20
7.6	26
7.5	32
7.4	40
7.3	50
7.2	63
7.1	80
7.0	100
6.9	125
6.8	160

Many of the body's metabolic functions are exquisitely sensitive to pH, and normal function can occur only within a very narrow range. The pH range of the ECF that is generally compatible with life is 6.8 to 7.8 (160 to 16 nEq/L of H^+). Normally the ECF pH is maintained between 7.35 and 7.45. This chapter examines the mechanisms the body uses to maintain the pH of the body fluids within this normal range, with special emphasis on the role of the kidneys.

■ THE CO_2/HCO_3^- BUFFER SYSTEM

Bicarbonate (HCO_3^-) is an important buffer of the extracellular fluid (ECF). Given a plasma $[HCO_3^-]$ of 23 to 25 mEq/L and a volume of 14 L, the ECF can potentially buffer 350 mEq of H^+. The CO_2/HCO_3^- buffer system differs from the other buffer systems of the body (e.g., phosphate) because it is regulated by both the lungs and the kidneys. This is best appreciated by considering the following reaction:

$$CO_2 + H_2O \overset{CA}{\leftrightarrow} H_2CO_3 \leftrightarrow H^+ + HCO_3^- \qquad (8\text{-}1)$$

The first reaction (hydration/dehydration of CO_2) is the rate-limiting step. This normally slow reaction is greatly accelerated in the presence of the enzyme **carbonic anhydrase (CA).** The second reaction, the ionization of H_2CO_3 to H^+ and HCO_3^-, is virtually instantaneous.

To quantitate these reactions, it is convenient and simpler to consider H^+ and HCO_3^- as products and CO_2 and H_2CO_3 as reactants. Thus:

$$K' = \frac{[H^+][HCO_3^-]}{[CO_2][H_2CO_3]} \quad (8\text{-}2)$$

Because this simplification combines the dissociation reaction ($H_2CO_3 \leftrightarrow H^+ + HCO_3^-$) with the hydration/dehydration reaction ($CO_2 + H_2O \leftrightarrow H_2CO_3$), K' is not a true dissociation constant. Instead, it is termed an *apparent dissociation constant.* The value of K' depends on temperature and solution composition. For plasma at $37°$ C, K' has a value of $10^{-6.1}$ ($pK' = 6.1$).

The terms in the denominator of Equation 8-2 represent the total amount of CO_2 dissolved in solution. Most of this CO_2 is in the gas form, with only 0.3% being H_2CO_3. Because the amount of CO_2 in solution depends on its partial pressure (P_{CO_2}) and its solubility (α), Equation 8-2 can be rewritten as follows[27]:

$$K' = \frac{[H^+][HCO_3^-]}{\alpha P_{CO_2}} \quad (8\text{-}3)$$

For plasma at $37°$ C, $\alpha = 0.03$.

A more useful form of this equation is obtained by solving for $[H^+]$:

$$[H^+] = \frac{K'\, \alpha P_{CO_2}}{[HCO_3^-]} \quad (8\text{-}4)$$

Taking the negative logarithm of both sides of the equation yields the following:

$$-\log[H^+] = \frac{-\log[K'] + -\log\alpha P_{CO_2}}{-\log[HCO_3^-]} \quad (8\text{-}5)$$

$$pH = pK' + \log \frac{[HCO_3^-]}{\alpha P_{CO_2}}$$

or

$$pH = 6.1 + \log \frac{[HCO_3^-]}{0.03 P_{CO_2}} \quad (8\text{-}6)$$

Equation 8-6 is the **Henderson-Hasselbalch equation.** Inspection of it shows that the pH of the ECF varies when either $[HCO_3^-]$ or P_{CO_2} is altered. Disturbances of acid-base balance that result from a change in the ECF $[HCO_3^-]$ are termed *metabolic acid-base disorders,* whereas those resulting from a change in the P_{CO_2} are termed *respiratory acid-base disorders.* These disorders are considered in more detail in a subsequent section. The kidneys are primarily responsible for regulating the $[HCO_3^-]$, whereas the lungs control the P_{CO_2}.

■ METABOLIC PRODUCTION OF ACID AND ALKALI

In the normal individual the metabolism of dietary foodstuffs produces a number of substances that can have an impact on acid-base status. When insulin is present and the tissues are adequately perfused, cellular metabolism of carbohydrates and fats produces large quantities of CO_2 (approximately 15 to 20 mol/day).[28] This CO_2, which is a potential acid in the body fluids (as H_2CO_3), is termed *volatile acid* and is excreted from the body by the lungs. In addition, the normal diet contains a number of constituents whose metabolism produces acids other than CO_2. These are termed *nonvolatile* acids.

---

27 α is not strictly a gas solubility constant; rather it is a constant that relates the P_{CO_2} to the total concentration of H_2CO_3 and the dissolved CO_2.

28 In the absence of insulin, or when tissue hypoxia exists, carbohydrates and fats are incompletely metabolized. When this occurs, large quantities of nonvolatile acids are produced (e.g., lactic acid and β-hydroxybutyric acid).

Metabolites of amino acids constitute a major portion of nonvolatile acid production. The sulfur-containing amino acids cysteine and methionine yield sulfuric acid when metabolized, whereas hydrochloric acid results from the metabolism of the cationic amino acids lysine, arginine, and histidine. This acid production is partially offset by the metabolism of the anionic amino acids aspartate and glutamate, which results in the production of HCO_3^-.

The diet also contains a number of other substances that can have an impact on acid-base balance. For example, ingested phosphate (as $H_2PO_4^-$) constitutes another nonvolatile acid load to the body. A number of organic anions (e.g., citrate) produce HCO_3^- when metabolized. Finally, during the process of digestion and absorption of gastrointestinal fluid, some HCO_3^- is normally lost in the feces. This HCO_3^- loss is equivalent to the addition of nonvolatile acid to the body. On a typical diet, dietary intake, cellular metabolism, and fecal HCO_3^- loss result in the net addition of approximately 1 mEq/kg body weight of nonvolatile acid to the body each day (50 to 100 mEq/day for most adults). It should be emphasized that the production of nonvolatile acids is highly dependent on the diet. For example, a vegetarian diet can result in lessened acid production.

The nonvolatile acids produced during metabolism do not circulate as free acids but are immediately buffered.

$$H_2SO_4 + 2NaHCO_3 \leftrightarrow Na_2SO_4 + 2CO_2 + 2H_2O \quad \text{(8-7)}$$

$$HCl + NaHCO_3 \leftrightarrow NaCl + CO_2 + H_2O \quad \text{(8-8)}$$

This buffering process yields the Na^+ salts of the strong acids and removes HCO_3^- from ECF. Buffering of strong acids by HCO_3^- minimizes the effect of the strong acids on lowering the pH of the ECF. **In order to maintain acid-base balance, the kidneys must excrete these Na^+ salts and replenish the HCO_3^- lost by titration.**

■ OVERVIEW OF RENAL ACID EXCRETION

To maintain acid-base balance, the kidneys must excrete an amount of acid equal to nonvolatile acid production. In addition, they must prevent the loss of HCO_3^- in the urine. The latter task is quantitatively more important because the filtered load of HCO_3^- is approximately 4320 mEq/day (24 mEq/L × 180 L/day = 4320 mEq/day), compared with only 50 to 100 mEq/day of nonvolatile acid.

Both the reabsorption of filtered HCO_3^- and the excretion of acid are accomplished through the process of H^+ secretion by the nephrons. Thus, in a single day the nephrons must secrete approximately 4390 mEq of H^+ into the tubular fluid. Most of the H^+ does not leave the body in the urine but serves to reabsorb the filtered HCO_3^-. Only 50 to 100 mEq are excreted. As a result of this acid excretion the urine is normally acidic.

Theoretically the kidneys could excrete the nonvolatile acids and replenish the HCO_3^- lost during titration by reversing the reactions shown in Equations 8-7 and 8-8. However, because the pKs of these acids are so low, this process would require a urine pH of 1.0, and the minimum urine pH attainable by the kidneys is only 4.0 to 4.5. Consequently, the kidneys cannot excrete the free acids but must excrete their salts while excreting H^+ with other urinary buffers. The two major urinary buffers are **ammonia** (NH_3/NH_4^+) and phosphate ($HPO_4^=/H_2PO_4^-$). Urinary phosphate and, to a lesser degree, other buffer species (e.g., creatinine) are collectively termed ***titratable acid.***[29]

---

[29] The term *titratable acid* is derived from the method by which these buffers are quantitated in the laboratory. Typically, alkali (OH^-) is added to a urine sample to titrate its pH to that of plasma (i.e., 7.4). The amount of alkali added is equal to the H^+ titrated by these urine buffers and is termed *titratable acid.*

The overall process of **net acid excretion (NAE)** by the kidneys can be quantitated as follows:

$$NAE = [(U_{NH_4^+} \times \dot{V}) + (U_{TA} \times \dot{V})] \\ - (U_{HCO_3^-} \times \dot{V})$$ (8-9)

where: $U_{NH_4^+} \times \dot{V}$ and $U_{TA} \times \dot{V}$ are the rates of H^+ excretion (mEq/day) as NH_4^+ and titratable acid (TA); and $U_{HCO_3^-} \times \dot{V}$ is the amount of HCO_3^- lost in the urine (equivalent to adding H^+ to the body). **To maintain acid-base balance, net acid excretion must equal nonvolatile acid production.**

■ HCO_3^- REABSORPTION ALONG THE NEPHRON

Glomerular filtration delivers 4320 mEq/day of HCO_3^- to the nephron. Figure 8-1 illustrates the contribution of the various nephron segments to the reabsorption of this HCO_3^-. The reabsorption of HCO_3^- is critically important for the prevention of its loss in the urine. Under normal conditions, virtually all of the filtered HCO_3^- is reabsorbed and none appears in the urine.

Approximately 80% of the filtered load of HCO_3^- is reabsorbed in the proximal tubule. The cellular mechanisms involved in reabsorption are illustrated in Figure 8-2. The apical membrane of the proximal tubular cell contains a Na^+-H^+ antiporter that secretes H^+ into the tubular fluid, using the energy in the lumen-to-cell Na^+ gradient. Recent evidence indicates that a portion of H^+ secretion is also mediated by an H^+-ATPase. Within the cell, H^+ and HCO_3^- are produced in a reaction catalyzed by carbonic anhydrase (see Equation 8-1). The H^+ is secreted into the tubular fluid, whereas the HCO_3^- exits the cell across the basolateral membrane and returns to the peritubular blood.

Although the electrochemical gradient for HCO_3^- favors its passive movement out of the cell across the basolateral membrane, simple diffusion does not appear to occur to a significant

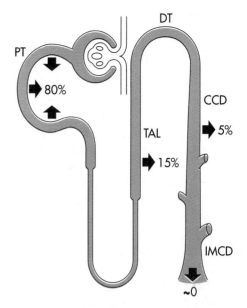

Figure 8-1 ■ Segmental reabsorption of HCO_3^-. The fraction of the filtered load of HCO_3^- reabsorbed by the various segments of the nephron is shown. Normally the entire filtered load of HCO_3^- is reabsorbed. *PT*, Proximal tubule; *TAL*, thick ascending limb; *DT*, distal tubule; *CCD*, cortical collecting duct; *IMCD*, inner medullary collecting duct.

degree; instead HCO_3^- movement out of the cell across the basolateral membrane is coupled to other ions. The majority of HCO_3^- exits via a symporter that couples the efflux of 1 Na^+ with 3 HCO_3^-. Additionally, some of the HCO_3^- exits in exchange for Cl^- (Cl^-- HCO_3^- antiporter).

Within the tubular fluid the secreted H^+ combines with the filtered HCO_3^- to form H_2CO_3. This is rapidly converted to CO_2 and H_2O. Carbonic anhydrase present in the apical membrane and exposed to the tubular fluid contents facilitates the conversion of H_2CO_3 to H_2O and CO_2. Because both CO_2 and H_2O can readily penetrate the tubule, they are rapidly reabsorbed. The net effect of this process is that for each HCO_3^- removed from the tubular fluid, one HCO_3^- appears in the peritubular blood.

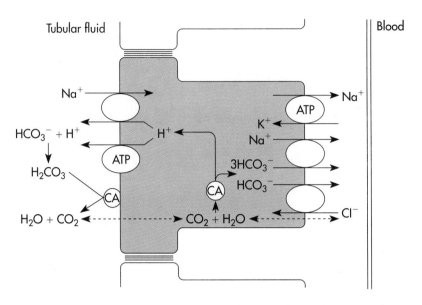

Figure 8-2 ■ Cellular mechanism for reabsorption of filtered HCO$_3^-$ by cells of the proximal tubule. *CA*, Carbonic anhydrase.

An additional 15% of the filtered load of HCO$_3^-$ is reabsorbed by Henle's loop. The majority of this HCO$_3^-$ is reabsorbed by the cells of the thick ascending limb. The mechanism for HCO$_3^-$ reabsorption by the cells of the thick ascending limb appears to be similar to that described for the proximal tubule. H$^+$ is secreted into the tubular fluid by an apical membrane Na$^+$-H$^+$ antiporter. HCO$_3^-$ exits the cell across the basolateral membrane coupled to Na$^+$ (Na$^+$-3HCO$_3^-$ symporter) and is returned to the peritubular blood.

The distal tubule and collecting duct reabsorb the small amount of HCO$_3^-$ that escapes reabsorption by the proximal tubule and Henle's loop (5% of the filtered load). The mechanism by which this occurs does not depend on Na$^+$ (i.e., apical membrane Na$^+$-H$^+$ antiporter), as is the case in the earlier nephron segments. Figure 8-3 shows the mechanism of HCO$_3^-$ reabsorption by the collecting duct. Here, H$^+$ secretion occurs via the intercalated cell (see Chapter 2). Within

the cell, H$^+$ and HCO$_3^-$ are produced by the hydration of CO$_2$, a reaction that is catalyzed by carbonic anhydrase. The H$^+$ is secreted into the tubular fluid by two mechanisms. The first involves an apical membrane H$^+$-ATPase. The second couples the secretion of H$^+$ with the reabsorption of K$^+$ via an H$^+$-K$^+$-ATPase similar to that of the stomach. The HCO$_3^-$ exits the cell across the basolateral membrane in exchange for Cl$^-$ (Cl$^-$-HCO$_3^-$ antiporter) and enters the peritubular capillary blood.

A second population of intercalated cells exists within the collecting duct; these cells secrete HCO$_3^-$ rather than H$^+$ into the tubular fluid and appear to have the H$^+$-ATPase located in the basolateral membrane and a Cl$^-$/HCO$_3^-$ antiporter in the apical membrane (see Figure 8-3). Their activity can be increased during metabolic alkalosis when the kidneys must excrete excess HCO$_3^-$. However, under normal conditions H$^+$ secretion predominates in the collecting duct.

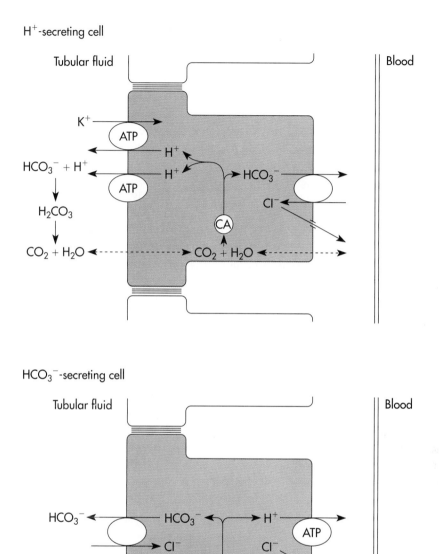

Figure 8-3 ■ **Cellular mechanisms for reabsorption and secretion of HCO_3^- by intercalated cells of the collecting duct.** *CA,* **Carbonic anhydrase.**

H$^+$ does not readily cross the apical membrane of the cells of the collecting duct, and the pH of the tubular fluid can be rendered quite acidic. Indeed, the most acidic tubular fluid along the nephron (pH = 4.0 to 4.5) is produced here. By comparison, the permeability of the proximal tubule to H$^+$ and HCO$_3^-$ is much higher, and the tubular fluid pH falls to only 6.5 in this segment. The ability of the collecting duct to lower the pH of the tubular fluid is critically important for the excretion of urinary buffers.

■ REGULATION OF HCO$_3^-$ REABSORPTION

HCO$_3^-$ reabsorption (i.e., H$^+$ secretion) is regulated by several factors (Table 8-2). The primary sites for regulation of HCO$_3^-$ reabsorption are the proximal tubule and collecting duct.

Because of glomerulotubular balance, any change in the filtered load of HCO$_3^-$ that results from alterations in the glomerular filtration rate (GFR) is matched by an appropriate change in HCO$_3^-$ reabsorption by the proximal tubule. Thus, proximal tubular HCO$_3^-$ reabsorption increases when the filtered load is increased and decreases when the filtered load is reduced.

The major fraction of proximal tubular HCO$_3^-$ reabsorption occurs as a result of H$^+$ secretion by the Na$^+$-H$^+$ antiporter located in the apical membrane of the cells. Consequently, factors that regulate Na$^+$ homeostasis (see Chapter 6) alter HCO$_3^-$ reabsorption secondarily. Thus, expansion of the ECF, which inhibits proximal tubular Na$^+$ reabsorption, also decreases the reabsorption of HCO$_3^-$. Conversely, HCO$_3^-$ reabsorption is enhanced when ECF is decreased.

TABLE 8-2

Factors regulating HCO$_3^-$ reabsorption (H$^+$ secretion) by the nephron

Factor	Nephron site of action
Increasing H$^+$ Secretion	
Increase in filtered load of HCO$_3^-$	Proximal tubule
Decrease in ECF volume	Proximal tubule
Decrease in plasma [HCO$_3^-$] ($\downarrow$ pH)	Proximal tubule, thick ascending limb of Henle's loop, and collecting duct
Increase in blood Pco$_2$	Proximal tubule, thick ascending limb of Henle's loop, and collecting duct
Increase in aldosterone	Collecting duct
Decreasing H$^+$ Secretion	
Decrease in filtered load of HCO$_3^-$	Proximal tubule
Increase in ECF volume	Proximal tubule
Increase in plasma [HCO$_3^-$] ($\uparrow$ pH)	Proximal tubule, thick ascending limb of Henle's loop, and collecting duct
Decrease in blood Pco$_2$	Proximal tubule, thick ascending limb of Henle's loop, and collecting duct
Decrease in aldosterone	Collecting duct

As might be expected, changes in systemic acid-base balance also affect HCO_3^- reabsorption. Systemic acidosis, whether produced by a decrease in the plasma $[HCO_3^-]$ (metabolic) or by an increase in the Pco_2 (respiratory), stimulates HCO_3^- reabsorption all along the nephron (i.e., proximal tubule, Henle's loop, and the collecting duct). This stimulation is believed to occur as a result of acidification of the intracellular fluid, which in turn produces a more favorable cell-to-lumen H^+ gradient and enhances H^+ secretion across the apical membrane of the cell. There is also evidence that acidification of the intracellular fluid results in the insertion of more transporters into the membranes of the cells. The insertion of H^+-ATPase into the apical membrane of collecting duct intercalated cells is an important component of the response to systemic acidosis. It is likely that insertion of acid-base–related transporters into the apical and perhaps also the basolateral membrane occurs in other nephron segments as well and constitutes an important mechanism for regulating transport in response to systemic acid-base disorders (or other regulatory factors). Metabolic and respiratory alkalosis inhibit HCO_3^- reabsorption along the nephron. The mechanisms involved are thought to be the opposite of those involved in stimulation of HCO_3^- reabsorption with acidosis.

Aldosterone is an important regulatory factor for HCO_3^- reabsorption, especially in the collecting duct. Aldosterone stimulates H^+ secretion by the intercalated cells of the collecting duct. This effect reflects both the direct action of the hormone on the intercalated cell and an indirect effect via aldosterone stimulation of Na^+ reabsorption by the principal cell. With regard to aldosterone's indirect effect (see Chapters 4 and 6), Na^+ reabsorption by the principal cells of the collecting duct produces a lumen-negative transepithelial voltage. When Na^+ reabsorption is stimulated by aldosterone, the magnitude of the lumen-negative voltage is increased. This in turn

favors intercalated cell H^+ secretion by reducing the electrochemical gradient against which the apical membrane H^+-ATPase must pump (the H^+-ATPase is affected by a change in voltage).[30] The cellular mechanism by which aldosterone directly stimulates intercalated cell H^+ secretion is not yet fully understood. However, it probably involves the synthesis of additional transporters and their insertion into the cell membranes. As would be expected, collecting duct H^+ secretion is decreased when aldosterone levels are reduced.

Other factors influence renal H^+/HCO_3^- transport but are not primarily involved in regulating acid-base balance. For example, parathyroid hormone (PTH) inhibits HCO_3^- reabsorption by the proximal tubule. PTH is primarily involved in the maintenance of Ca^{++} and Pi balance (see Chapter 9). However, when PTH acts on proximal tubular cells, it also inhibits the Na^+-H^+ antiporter in the apical membrane. Angiotensin II stimulates proximal tubule HCO_3^- reabsorption. This action is related to stimulation of Na^+ reabsorption (see Chapter 6) and is mediated by increased activity of the Na^+-H^+ antiporter. Finally, hypokalemia can stimulate proximal tubular HCO_3^- reabsorption. The mechanism for this stimulation is not completely understood but may reflect hypokalemia-induced acidification of the intracellular fluid (see Chapter 7).

■ FORMATION OF NEW HCO_3^-: THE ROLE OF AMMONIUM

As previously discussed, the reabsorption of HCO_3^- is important for the maintenance of acid-base balance. HCO_3^- loss in the urine would decrease the plasma $[HCO_3^-]$ and would be equivalent to the addition of H^+ to the body. However,

---

30 Because the H^+-K^+-ATPase of intercalated cells is electroneutral, indirect stimulation of this transporter by the lumen-negative voltage would not occur.

HCO_3^- reabsorption alone does not replenish the HCO_3^- lost during the titration of the nonvolatile acids produced by metabolism. To maintain acid-base balance, the kidneys must replace this lost HCO_3^- with new HCO_3^-. The production of new HCO_3^- is critically dependent on the availability of urinary buffers. Figure 8-4 illustrates how the titration of these buffers results in the **formation of new HCO_3^-**. When tubular fluid is free of HCO_3^- in the collecting duct because of HCO_3^- reabsorption in upstream tubular segments, H^+ secreted into tubular fluid combines with a urinary buffer. Thus, H^+ secretion results in the excretion of the H^+ with a buffer, and the HCO_3^- produced in the cell from the hydration of CO_2 is added back to the blood.

As previously noted, the two major urinary buffers are ammonium (NH_3/NH_4^+) and phosphate ($HPO_4^=/H_2PO_4^-$). Phosphate is derived solely from the diet. The amount excreted in the urine as titratable acid therefore depends on the filtered load minus the amount reabsorbed by the nephron. **Ammonium is produced by the kidneys, and its synthesis and subsequent excretion can be regulated in response to the acid-base requirements of the body. Because of this, ammonia is the more important urinary buffer.**

Ammonium is produced in the kidneys by the metabolism of glutamine. The kidneys receive the glutamine (primarily from the liver) and the Na^+ salts of the nonvolatile acids (e.g., Na_2SO_4) in the renal arterial plasma. The kidneys metabolize the glutamine, excrete NH_4^+ with the acid salts, and return $NaHCO_3$ to the body in the renal vein plasma. It is important to recognize that the formation of new HCO_3^- by this process depends on the kidneys' ability to excrete the NH_4^+ in the urine. If NH_4^+ is not excreted in the urine but instead enters the systemic circulation, it will

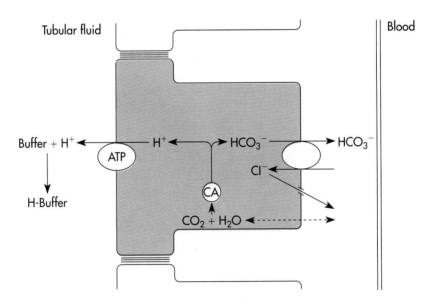

Figure 8-4 ■ General scheme for the excretion of H^+ with non-HCO_3^- urinary buffers. The primary urinary buffers are NH_3 and $HPO_4^=$ (titratable acid). For simplicity, only the H^+-ATPase is shown. H^+ secretion by the H^+-K^+-ATPase also titrates luminal buffers. *CA*, Carbonic anhydrase.

titrate plasma HCO_3^-, thus negating the process of new HCO_3^- generation.[31] The process by which the kidneys excrete NH_4^+ is complex. Figure 8-5 illustrates the essential features of this process.

Ammonium is produced in proximal tubular cells from glutamine. Each glutamine molecule produces two molecules of NH_4^+ and a divalent anion. Metabolism of this anion ultimately provides two molecules of HCO_3^-.

$$(8\text{-}10)$$
$$\text{Glutamine} \leftrightarrow 2NH_4^+ + Anion^{-2} \leftrightarrow 2HCO_3^- + 2NH_4^+$$

The HCO_3^- exits the cell across the basolateral membrane and enters the peritubular blood as new HCO_3^-. NH_4^+ exits the cell across the apical membrane and enters the tubular fluid. A major mechanism for the secretion of NH_4^+ into the tubular fluid involves the Na^+-H^+ antiporter, with NH_4^+ substituting for H^+. In addition, NH_3 can diffuse out of the cell into the tubular lumen, where it is protonated to NH_4^+. A significant portion of the NH_4^+ secreted by the proximal tubule is reabsorbed by Henle's loop. The thick ascending limb is the primary site of this NH_4^+ reabsorption. NH_4^+ substitutes for K^+ on the $1Na^+$-$1K^+$-$2Cl^-$ symporter. In addition, the lumen-positive transepithelial voltage in this segment drives paracellular reabsorption of NH_4^+. The reabsorbed NH_4^+ accumulates in the medullary interstitium, where it exists in chemical equilibrium with NH_3.[32] It then reenters the tubular fluid of the collecting duct. The mechanism by which this occurs involves the processes of **nonionic diffusion** and **diffusion trapping.** The collecting duct does

not have a specific transport mechanism for the secretion of NH_4^+, nor do the cells have a significant permeability to NH_4^+. However, NH_3 is able to penetrate the cells of the collecting duct and diffuse from the medullary interstitium into the lumen of the collecting duct. As described previously, H^+ secretion by the intercalated cells of the collecting duct results in acidification of the luminal fluid. (Luminal fluid pH as low as 4.0 to 4.5 can be achieved.) Consequently, NH_3 diffusing from the medullary interstitium into the collecting duct lumen (nonionic diffusion) is protonated to NH_4^+ by the acidic tubular fluid. Because NH_4^+ is less able to penetrate the collecting duct than is NH_3, NH_4^+ is trapped in the tubular lumen (diffusion trapping) and eliminated from the body in the urine.

H^+ secretion by the collecting duct is critical for the excretion of NH_4^+. If collecting duct H^+ secretion is inhibited, the NH_4^+ reabsorbed by the thick ascending limb is not excreted in the urine. Instead it is returned to systemic circulation, where it will titrate HCO_3^-. If this occurs, net acid excretion by the kidneys is reduced, and insufficient quantities of new HCO_3^- are added to systemic circulation to replenish what was titrated by the buffering of nonvolatile acids.

An important feature of the NH_4^+ system is that it can be regulated. Alterations in ECF pH cause changes in NH_4^+ production, presumably by affecting intracellular pH. During systemic acidosis the enzymes in the proximal tubular cell, which are responsible for the metabolism of glutamine, are stimulated. This involves the synthesis of new enzyme and requires several days for complete adaptation. With increased levels of this enzyme, NH_4^+ production is increased, thus allowing more H^+ excretion and enhanced production of new HCO_3^-. Conversely, NH_4^+ production is reduced with alkalosis.

Plasma $[K^+]$ also alters NH_4^+ production. Hyperkalemia inhibits NH_4^+ production, whereas hypokalemia stimulates production. Although

---

31 The mechanism by which NH_4^+ titrates HCO_3^- is indirect and occurs as a result of the synthesis of urea from NH_4^+ by the liver (i.e., the urea cycle). When urea is synthesized from NH_4^+, H^+ are generated. These H^+ are rapidly buffered by HCO_3^-.

32 Ammonia is a weak base that is present as both NH_4^+ and NH_3, with the relative amounts of each species determined by the pKa (pKa = 9.0).

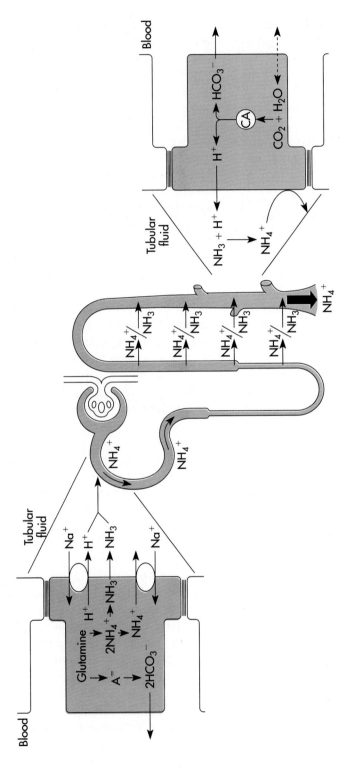

Figure 8-5 ■ Production, transport, and excretion of ammonia by the nephron. Glutamine is metabolized to NH_4^+ and HCO_3^- in the proximal tubule. The NH_4^+ is secreted into the lumen, and the HCO_3^- enters the blood. The secreted NH_4^+ is reabsorbed in Henle's loop primarily by the thick ascending limb and accumulates in the medullary interstitium, where it exists as both NH_4^+ and NH_3. NH_3 diffuses into the tubular fluid of the collecting duct, and H^+ secretion by the collecting duct leads to accumulation of NH_4^+ in the lumen by the processes of nonionic diffusion and diffusion trapping. Traditionally, NH_3 has been termed a *urinary buffer;* and this designation has been used here. However, as illustrated by this scheme, it is more appropriate to view NH_4^+ excretion as a "marker" of glutamine metabolism in the proximal tubule. Accordingly, for each molecule of NH_4^+ excreted, a molecule of HCO_3^- has to be added back to the ECF.

the mechanism by which plasma K^+ alters NH_4^+ production is not fully understood, alterations in plasma $[K^+]$ are believed to cause changes in intracellular $[H^+]$ by exchanging H^+ for K^+ (see Chapter 7); this change in intracellular pH is thought to then control NH_4^+ production. By this mechanism, exchange of extracellular K^+ for intracellular H^+ during hyperkalemia would raise intracellular pH and thereby inhibit NH_4^+ production. The opposite would occur during hypokalemia.

■ RESPONSE TO ACID-BASE DISORDERS

The pH of the ECF is maintained within a very narrow range (7.35 to 7.45).[33] **Acidosis** occurs

---

[33] For simplicity, the value of 7.40 will be used as normal, and deviations from this single value are deemed abnormal. Similarly, the normal range for Pco_2 is 33 to 44 mm Hg. However, a Pco_2 of 40 mm Hg is used as the normal reference value. Finally, a value of 24 mEq/L is considered a normal ECF $[HCO_3^-]$, even though the normal range is 22 to 28 mEq/L.

when the blood pH falls below this range, whereas **alkalosis** exists when the blood pH exceeds this range. When the acid-base disorder results from a primary change in the $[HCO_3^-]$, it is termed a *metabolic* disorder. When the primary disturbance is an alteration in the blood Pco_2, it is termed a *respiratory* disorder.

When an acid-base disturbance develops, the body employs a series of mechanisms to defend itself against the change in the pH of the ECF. It is important to recognize that these defense mechanisms do not correct the acid-base disturbance but merely minimize the change in pH imposed by the disturbance. Restoration of the blood pH to its normal value requires correction of the underlying process or processes that produced the acid-base disorder. For example, metabolism of fats in the absence of insulin leads to the accumulation of keto acids (i.e., nonvolatile acid) in the blood and the development of metabolic acidosis. The acid-base defense mechanisms mini-

---

Renal tubular acidosis (RTA) refers to conditions in which urine acidification is impaired. Under these conditions the kidneys are unable to excrete a sufficient amount of net acid to balance nonvolatile acid production, and metabolic acidosis results. RTA can occur by a defect either in proximal tubular H^+ secretion/HCO_3^- reabsorption (proximal RTA) or in distal tubular H^+ secretion (distal RTA).

Proximal RTA can be caused by a variety of hereditary and acquired conditions (e.g., cystinosis, Fanconi syndrome, administration of carbonic anhydrase inhibitors). H^+ secretion by proximal tubular cells is impaired and results in a decrease in the reabsorption of the filtered load of HCO_3^-. Consequently, HCO_3^- is lost in the urine, plasma $[HCO_3^-]$ decreases, and metabolic acidosis ensues.

Distal RTA also occurs in a number of hereditary and acquired conditions (e.g., medullary sponge kidney, the use of drugs such as amphotericin B, and secondary to urinary obstruction).

Depending on the cause, secretion of H^+ by intercalated cells of the collecting duct is impaired or the ability of H^+ to penetrate the collecting duct is increased. In either case the ability to acidify the tubular fluid is impaired. Consequently, trapping of NH_4^+ is reduced. This in turn decreases net acid excretion, with the subsequent development of metabolic acidosis.

Failure to produce sufficient quantities of urinary ammonium can also reduce the amount of net acid excreted by the kidneys. In this situation, proximal tubular HCO_3^- reabsorption is normal, as is H^+ secretion by the distal tubule and collecting duct, and the urine pH is maximally acidic. However, because of the lack of sufficient quantities of NH_4^+, net acid excretion is less than net acid production, and metabolic acidosis develops.

If the metabolic acidosis resulting from any of these forms of RTA is severe, individuals must ingest alkali (e.g., $NaHCO_3$) to maintain acid-base balance.

mize the fall in pH that occurs in this condition, but normal acid-base balance is not restored until insulin is administered and keto-acid production ceases.

The body has three general defenses against changes in body fluid pH produced by acid-base disturbances. These mechanisms are as follows:

1. Extracellular and intracellular buffering
2. Adjustments in blood P_{CO_2} by alterations in the ventilatory rate of the lungs
3. Adjustments in renal acid excretion

Extracellular and Intracellular Buffering

The first line of defense against acid-base disorders is extracellular and intracellular buffering. The response of the extracellular buffers is virtually instantaneous, whereas cellular buffering is somewhat slower and can take several minutes to complete.

Metabolic disorders that result from the addition of nonvolatile acids or alkali to the body fluids are buffered in both the extracellular and intracellular fluids. The CO_2/HCO_3^- buffer system is the principal ECF buffer. Buffering of acid and alkali by this system involves the following reaction:

$$H^+ + HCO_3^- \leftrightarrow H_2CO_3 \leftrightarrow H_2O + CO_2 \qquad (8\text{-}11)$$

When nonvolatile acid is added to the body fluids or alkali is lost from the body, the reaction of Equation 8-11 is driven to the right, HCO_3^- is consumed during the process of buffering the acid load, and the plasma $[HCO_3^-]$ is reduced. Conversely, when nonvolatile alkali is added to the body fluids or acid is lost from the body, the reaction is driven to the left. H^+ is consumed, causing more HCO_3^- to be produced from the dissociation of H_2CO_3. As a consequence, $[HCO_3^-]$ increases.

Although the CO_2/HCO_3^- buffer system is the principal ECF buffer, phosphate and plasma protein provide additional extracellular buffering.

$$H^+ + HPO_4^= \leftrightarrow H_2PO_4^- \qquad (8\text{-}12)$$
$$H^+ + Protein^- \leftrightarrow H\text{-}Protein$$

The combined action of the CO_2/HCO_3^-, phosphate, and plasma protein buffering processes accounts for approximately 50% of the buffering of a nonvolatile acid load and 70% of a nonvolatile alkali load. The remainder of the buffering under these two conditions occurs intracellularly. Intracellular buffering involves the movement of H^+ into cells (during buffering of nonvolatile acid) or the movement of H^+ out of cells (during buffering of nonvolatile alkali). H^+ is titrated inside the cell by HCO_3^-, phosphate, and the histidine groups on protein.

Bone represents an additional source of extracellular buffer ($NaHCO_3$, $KHCO_3$, $CaCO_3$, $CaHPO_4$). With chronic acidosis, buffering by bone results in demineralization (i.e., Ca^{++} is released from bone as Ca^{++}-containing buffers bind H^+ in exchange for Ca^{++}).

With respiratory acid-base disorders, body fluid pH changes as a result of alterations in $[H_2CO_3]$, which is determined directly by the P_{CO_2} (see Equation 8-1). Virtually all buffering in respiratory acid-base disorders occurs intracellularly. When P_{CO_2} rises (respiratory acidosis), CO_2 moves into the cell, where it combines with H_2O to form H_2CO_3. This dissociates to H^+ and HCO_3^-. The H^+ is buffered by cellular proteins, and HCO_3^- exits the cell and raises the plasma $[HCO_3^-]$.

This process is reversed when P_{CO_2} is reduced (respiratory alkalosis). Under this condition the hydration reaction ($H_2O + CO_2 \leftrightarrow H_2CO_3$) is shifted to the left by the decrease in P_{CO_2}. This in turn shifts the dissociation reaction ($H_2CO_3 \leftrightarrow H^+ + HCO_3^-$) to the left, thereby reducing the plasma $[HCO_3^-]$.

Respiratory Defense

The lungs are the second line of defense to acid-base disorders. As indicated by the Henderson-

Hasselbalch equation (see Equation 8-6), changes in the P_{CO_2} alter the blood pH: an increase in P_{CO_2} decreases pH, and a decrease in P_{CO_2} increases pH.

The ventilatory rate determines the P_{CO_2}. Increased ventilation decreases P_{CO_2}, whereas P_{CO_2} increases with decreased ventilation. The blood P_{CO_2} and pH are important regulators of the ventilatory rate. **Chemoreceptors** located in the brain (ventral surface of medulla) and periphery (carotid and aortic bodies) sense changes in P_{CO_2} and [H^+] and alter the ventilatory rate. With metabolic acidosis an increase in [H^+] (decrease in pH) increases the ventilatory rate. Conversely, during metabolic alkalosis a decrease in [H^+] (increase in pH) leads to a decrease in the ventilatory rate.[34] The respiratory response to metabolic acid-base disturbances may take place in several minutes or require several hours to complete.

Renal Defense

The third and final line of defense against acid-base disorders is the kidneys. In response to an alteration in the plasma pH and P_{CO_2} the kidneys make appropriate adjustments in the excretion of HCO_3^- and net acid. The renal response requires several days to complete, reflecting the time needed to increase the synthesis and activity of the enzymes involved in NH_4^+ production.

In the case of acidosis (increase in [H^+] or P_{CO_2}), secretion of H^+ by the nephron is stimulated and the entire filtered load of HCO_3^- is reabsorbed. The production and excretion of NH_4^+ are also stimulated, thus increasing net acid excretion by the kidneys (see Equation 8-9). The new HCO_3^- generated during the process of net acid excretion is returned to the body, and the plasma [HCO_3^-] increases.

---

34 With maximal hyperventilation, P_{CO_2} can be reduced to approximately 10 mm Hg. Because hypoxia, which is a potent stimulator of ventilation, also develops with hypoventilation, the degree to which P_{CO_2} can be increased is limited. In an otherwise normal individual, hypoventilation cannot raise the P_{CO_2} above 60 mm Hg.

Insulin-dependent diabetics can develop a metabolic acidosis (secondary to the production of keto acids) if insulin dosages are not adequate. As a compensatory response to this acidosis, deep and rapid breathing develops. This breathing pattern is termed *Kussmaul's respiration*. With prolonged Kussmaul's respiration the muscles involved can become fatigued. When this happens, respiratory compensation is impaired and the acidosis can become more severe.

Loss of gastric contents from the body (i.e., vomiting, nasogastric suction) produces a metabolic alkalosis secondary to the loss of HCl. If the volume of gastric fluid loss is significant, the effective circulating volume (ECV) is also decreased. Under this condition the kidneys cannot excrete sufficient quantities of HCO_3^- to compensate for the metabolic alkalosis. HCO_3^- excretion does not occur, because the decreased ECV results in enhanced proximal tubular Na^+ reabsorption and increased levels of aldosterone (see Chapter 6). These responses in turn limit HCO_3^- excretion because Na^+ reabsorption in the proximal tubule is coupled to H^+ secretion via the Na^+-H^+-antiporter. In addition, the elevated aldosterone levels stimulate H^+ secretion by the collecting duct. Thus, this condition is characterized by a metabolic alkalosis and a paradoxically acidic urine. Correction of the alkalosis only occurs when the ECV is restored to its normal value. With restoration of the ECV, HCO_3^- reabsorption by the proximal tubule decreases, as does H^+ secretion by the collecting duct. As a result, HCO_3^- excretion increases and the plasma [HCO_3^-] returns to normal.

With alkalosis (decrease in [H^+] or P_{CO_2}), secretion of H^+ by the nephron is inhibited, and as a result net acid excretion and HCO_3^- reabsorption are reduced. HCO_3^- appears in the urine, thereby reducing the plasma [HCO_3^-].

■ SIMPLE ACID-BASE DISORDERS

Table 8-3 summarizes the primary alterations and the subsequent defense mechanisms associated with the various simple acid-base disorders. The respiratory and renal defense mechanisms are commonly referred to as *compensatory responses* in discussions of these disorders. Accordingly, **the lungs compensate for metabolic disorders, and the kidneys compensate for respiratory disorders.** Note again that these **compensatory mechanisms do not correct the underlying disorder but simply reduce the magnitude of the change in blood pH. Complete recovery from the acid-base disorder requires correction of the underlying cause.**

Metabolic Acidosis

Metabolic acidosis is characterized by a low plasma [HCO_3^-] and a low plasma pH. This condition can develop by the addition of nonvolatile acid to the body (e.g., diabetic ketoacidosis), the loss of nonvolatile alkali (e.g., with diarrhea), or the failure of the kidneys to excrete sufficient net acid to replenish the HCO_3^- used to titrate nonvolatile acids (e.g., renal tubular aci-

dosis or renal failure). As described above, buffering of H^+ occurs in both the extracellular and intracellular fluids. With a fall in pH the respiratory centers are stimulated, and the ventilatory rate is increased **(respiratory compensation).** This reduces P_{CO_2}, which further minimizes the fall in plasma pH. In general, there is a 1.2 mm Hg decrease in the P_{CO_2} for every 1 mEq/L fall in plasma [HCO_3^-]. Thus, if plasma [HCO_3^-] were reduced to 14 mEq/L from a normal value of 24 mEq/L, the expected decrease in P_{CO_2} would be 12 mm Hg and the measured P_{CO_2} would be 28 mm Hg (normal P_{CO_2} = 40 mm Hg).

Finally, renal excretion of net acid is increased. This occurs by eliminating all HCO_3^- from the urine (enhanced reabsorption of filtered HCO_3^-) and increasing ammonium excretion (enhanced production of new HCO_3^-). If the process that initiated the acid-base disturbance is corrected, the enhanced excretion of acid by the kidneys ultimately returns the pH and [HCO_3^-] to normal. With correction of the pH the ventilatory rate also returns to normal.

Metabolic Alkalosis

Metabolic alkalosis is characterized by an elevated plasma [HCO_3^-] and pH. This can occur by the addition of nonvolatile alkali to the body (e.g., ingestion of antacids), as a result of a decreased ECV (e.g., hemorrhage), or, more commonly, from loss of nonvolatile acid (e.g., loss of

TABLE 8-3

Characteristics of simple acid-base disorders

Disorder	Plasma pH	Primary alteration	Defense mechanisms
Metabolic acidosis	↓	↓ Plasma [HCO_3^-]	ICF and ECF buffers; Hyperventilation (↓ P_{CO_2})
Metabolic alkalosis	↑	↑ Plasma [HCO_3^-]	ICF and ECF buffers; Hypoventilation (↑ P_{CO_2})
Respiratory acidosis	↓	↑ P_{CO_2}	ICF buffers; ↑ Renal NAE excretion
Respiratory alkalosis	↑	↓ P_{CO_2}	ICF buffers; ↓ Renal NAE excretion

When nonvolatile acid is added to the body fluids, the [H$^+$] increases (pH decreases) and the [HCO$_3$$^-$] decreases. In addition, the concentration of the anion, which is associated with the nonvolatile acid, increases. This change in the [anion] provides a convenient way to analyze and help determine the cause of a metabolic acidosis by calculating what is termed the **anion gap.** The anion gap represents the difference between the concentration of the major plasma cation (Na$^+$) and the major plasma anions (Cl$^-$ and HCO$_3$$^-$).

$$\text{Anion gap} = [\text{Na}^+] - ([\text{Cl}^-] + [\text{HCO}_3{}^-]) \tag{8-13}$$

Under normal conditions the anion gap is in the range of 8 to 16 mEq/L.[35] If the anion of the nonvolatile acid is Cl$^-$, the anion gap will be normal (i.e., the decrease in [HCO$_3$$^-$] is matched by an increase in [Cl$^-$]). The metabolic acidosis associated with diarrhea or renal tubular acidosis has a normal anion gap. In contrast, if the anion of the nonvolatile acid is not Cl$^-$ (e.g., lactate, β-hydroxybutyrate), the anion gap will increase (i.e., the decrease in [HCO$_3$$^-$] is not matched by an increase in the [Cl$^-$] but rather by an increase in the [unmeasured anion]). The anion gap is increased in the metabolic acidosis associated with renal failure, diabetes (ketoacidosis), lactic acidosis, and the ingestion of large quantities of aspirin. Thus, calculation of the anion gap is a useful way to identify the etiology of a metabolic acidosis.

gastric HCl with vomiting). Buffering occurs in the extracellular and intracellular fluid compartments. The increase in pH inhibits the respiratory centers, reduces the ventilatory rate, and thus elevates Pco$_2$ (**respiratory compensa-**

tion). With appropriate respiratory compensation, a 0.7 mm Hg increase in Pco$_2$ occurs for every 1 mEq/L rise in plasma [HCO$_3$$^-$].

The renal compensatory response to metabolic alkalosis is to increase the excretion of HCO$_3$$^-$ by reducing its reabsorption along the nephron. Normally this occurs quite rapidly and effectively. However, as already noted, when the alkalosis occurs in the setting of decreased ECV (e.g., vomiting in which fluid loss occurs with H$^+$ loss), HCO$_3$$^-$ excretion does not occur, and enhanced renal excretion of HCO$_3$$^-$ and correction of the alkalosis occur only with restoration of a normal ECV. Enhanced renal excretion of HCO$_3$$^-$ eventually returns the pH and [HCO$_3$$^-$] to normal, provided that the underlying cause of the initial acid-base disturbance is corrected. With correction of the pH the ventilatory rate is also returned to normal.

Respiratory Acidosis

Respiratory acidosis is characterized by elevated Pco$_2$ and reduced plasma pH. It results from decreased gas exchange across the alveoli, as a result of either inadequate ventilation (e.g., drug-induced depression of the respiratory centers) or impaired gas diffusion (e.g., pulmonary edema, as may occur in cardiovascular disease). In contrast to the metabolic disorders, buffering during respiratory acidosis occurs almost entirely in the intracellular compartment. The increase in Pco$_2$ and the decrease in pH stimulate both HCO$_3$$^-$ reabsorption by the nephron and ammonium excretion (**renal compensation**). Together, these responses increase net acid excretion and generate new HCO$_3$$^-$.

The renal compensatory response takes several days to occur. Consequently, respiratory acid-base disorders are commonly divided into acute and chronic phases. In the acute phase, there has not been sufficient time for the renal compensatory response to occur, and the body relies on intracellular buffering to minimize the change in

---

[35] An anion gap (i.e., a difference between the concentration of cations and anions) does not actually exist. All cations are balanced by anions. The gap simply reflects the parameters that are measured. In reality:

$$[\text{Na}^+] + [\text{unmeasured cations}] =$$
$$[\text{Cl}^-] + [\text{HCO}_3{}^-] + [\text{unmeasured anions}]$$

pH. During this phase, and because of the buffering, there is a 1 mEq/L increase in plasma $[HCO_3^-]$ for every 10 mm Hg rise in P_{CO_2}. In the chronic phase, renal compensation occurs, and there is a 3.5 mEq/L increase in plasma $[HCO_3^-]$ for each 10 mm Hg rise in P_{CO_2}. Correction of the underlying disorder returns the P_{CO_2} to normal, and the renal excretion of acid decreases to its initial level.

Respiratory Alkalosis

Respiratory alkalosis is characterized by reduced P_{CO_2} and elevated plasma pH. It results from increased gas exchange in the lungs, usually due to increased ventilation from stimulation of the respiratory centers (e.g., by drugs or CNS disorders). Hyperventilation can also occur as a response to anxiety or fear. As noted, buffering is primarily intracellular. In the acute phase of respiratory alkalosis, plasma $[HCO_3^-]$ decreases 2 mEq/L for every 10 mm Hg fall in P_{CO_2}. The elevated pH and reduced P_{CO_2} inhibit HCO_3^- reabsorption by the nephron and reduce ammonium excretion (renal compensation). As a result of these two effects, net acid excretion is reduced. The response takes several days and results in a 5 mEq/L decrease in plasma $[HCO_3^-]$ for every 10 mm Hg reduction in P_{CO_2}. Correction of the underlying disorder returns P_{CO_2} to normal, and renal excretion of acid increases to its initial level.

■ ANALYSIS OF ACID-BASE DISORDERS

Analysis of an acid-base disorder is directed at identifying the underlying cause so that appropriate therapy can be initiated. The patient's medical history and associated physical findings often provide valuable clues about the nature and origin of an acid-base disorder. Additionally, analysis of an arterial blood sample is frequently required. Such an analysis is straightforward if approached in a systematic fashion. For example, consider the following data:

$$pH = 7.35 \quad [HCO_3^-] = 16 \text{ mEq/L} \quad P_{CO_2} = 30 \text{ mm Hg}$$

The acid-base disorder represented by these values or any other set of values can be determined by the following three-step approach (Figure 8-6).

1. Examination of the pH: After an initial consideration of the plasma pH, the underlying disorder can be classified as either an acidosis or an alkalosis. Note that the defense mechanisms of the body cannot by themselves correct an acid-base disorder. Thus, even if the defense mechanisms are completely operative, the pH still indicates the origin of the initial disorder. In the preceding example the pH of 7.35 indicates an acidosis.

2. Determination of metabolic versus respiratory disorder: Simple acid-base disorders are either metabolic or respiratory. The $[HCO_3^-]$ and P_{CO_2} must next be examined to determine which disorder is present. As indicated by the Henderson-Hasselbalch equation (see Equation 8-6), acidosis could be the result of a decrease in the $[HCO_3^-]$ (metabolic) or an increase in the P_{CO_2} (respiratory). Alternatively, alkalosis could result from an increase in the $[HCO_3^-]$ (metabolic) or a decrease in the P_{CO_2} (respiratory). For the preceding example the $[HCO_3^-]$ is reduced from normal (normal = 23 to 25 mEq/L), as is the P_{CO_2} (normal = 40 mm Hg). The disorder must therefore be a metabolic acidosis; it cannot be a respiratory acidosis because the P_{CO_2} is reduced.

3. Analysis of compensatory response: Metabolic disorders lead to compensatory changes in ventilation and thus in P_{CO_2}, whereas respiratory disorders cause compensatory changes in renal acid excretion and thus in plasma $[HCO_3^-]$. P_{CO_2} is decreased in an appropriately compensated metabolic acidosis, whereas it is elevated with a compensated meta-

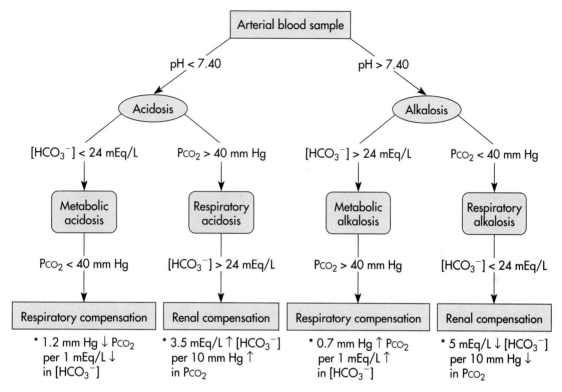

Figure 8-6 ■ **Approach for the analysis of simple acid-base disorders.**

bolic alkalosis. With respiratory acidosis, complete compensation results in an elevation of $[HCO_3^-]$. Conversely, $[HCO_3^-]$ is reduced in response to respiratory alkalosis. In the preceding example P_{CO_2} is reduced from normal, and the magnitude of this reduction (10 mm Hg decrease in P_{CO_2} for an 8 mEq/L increase in $[HCO_3^-]$) is as expected. Therefore the acid-base disorder is a simple metabolic acidosis with appropriate respiratory compensation.

If the appropriate compensatory response is not present, a **mixed acid-base disorder** should be suspected. A mixed disorder reflects the presence of two or more underlying causes

for the acid-base disturbance. A mixed disorder should be suspected when analysis of the arterial blood gas indicates that appropriate compensation has not occurred. For example, consider the following data:

$$pH = 6.96 \quad [HCO_3^-] = 12 \text{ mEq/L} \quad P_{CO_2} = 55 \text{ mm Hg}$$

Following the three-step approach outlined above reveals that the disturbance is an acidosis that has both a metabolic component ($[HCO_3^-]$ < 24 mEq/L) and a respiratory component (P_{CO_2} > 40 mm Hg). Thus, this disorder is mixed. An example of such a disorder is an individual with a history of chronic pulmonary disease, such as emphysema (i.e., chronic respiratory acidosis), who develops an acute gastrointestinal illness with diarrhea. Diarrhea results in the development of a metabolic acidosis because diarrhea fluid depletes large quantities of HCO_3^- from the body.

A mixed acid-base disorder is also indicated when a patient has abnormal P_{CO_2} and plasma $[HCO_3^-]$ but normal plasma pH. Such a situation occurs with the ingestion of a large quantity of aspirin. The salicylic acid (active ingredient in aspirin) produces a metabolic acidosis and at the same time stimulates the respiratory centers, causing hyperventilation and a respiratory alkalosis. Thus, the patient has reduced plasma $[HCO_3^-]$ and P_{CO_2}.

■ SUMMARY

1. The pH of the body fluids is maintained within a narrow range by the coordinated function of the lungs and kidneys. Volatile (CO_2-derived) and nonvolatile acids, together with any acid or alkali ingested in the diet, must be excreted for acid-base balance to be maintained.

2. The lungs are the excretory route for the volatile acid, whereas the kidneys are the route for excretion of the nonvolatile acid.

3. The body uses buffer systems to minimize changes in body fluid pH; the CO_2/HCO_3^- buffer system of the ECF is the most important because it is regulated by both the lungs and the kidneys.

4. The kidneys maintain acid-base balance by the excretion of an amount of acid equal to the amount of nonvolatile acid produced by cellular metabolism and metabolism of food ingested in the diet. The kidneys also prevent the loss of HCO_3^- in the urine by reabsorbing virtually all the HCO_3^- that is filtered at the glomerulus. Both the reabsorption of filtered HCO_3^- and the excretion of acid are accomplished by secretion of H^+ by the nephrons.

5. Urinary buffers are necessary for effective excretion of acid because the minimum pH of the urine is only 4.0 to 4.5. Phosphate (titratable acid) is a urinary buffer. Ammonium excretion results in new HCO_3 formation. Renal ammonium production and excretion are regulated in response to acid-base disturbances.

6. Respiratory acid-base disorders result from primary alterations in the blood P_{CO_2}. Elevation of P_{CO_2} produces acidosis, and the kidneys respond by increasing the excretion of acid. Conversely, reduction of P_{CO_2} produces alkalosis, and renal acid excretion is reduced. The kidneys respond to respiratory acid-base disorders over several hours to days.

7. Metabolic acid-base disorders result from primary alterations in the plasma $[HCO_3^-]$, which in turn result from addition of acid to, or loss of alkali from, the body. In response to metabolic acidosis, pulmonary ventilation is increased, which decreases the P_{CO_2}. An increase in the $[HCO_3^-]$ causes alkalosis. This decreases pulmonary ventilation, which elevates the P_{CO_2}. The pulmonary response to metabolic acid-base disorders occurs in a matter of minutes.

■ KEY WORDS AND CONCEPTS

- CO_2/HCO_3^- buffer system
- Carbonic anhydrase (CA)
- Henderson-Hasselbalch equation
- Volatile and nonvolatile acids
- Net acid excretion (NEA)
- Titratable acid
- Ammonia/ammonium
- Reabsorption of filtered HCO_3^-
- Formation of new HCO_3^-
- Nonionic diffusion and diffusion trapping of ammonia
- Acidosis (metabolic and respiratory)

- Alkalosis (metabolic and respiratory)
- Anion gap
- Chemoreceptors and control of respiration
- Acid-base defense mechanisms
- Respiratory compensation
- Renal compensation
- Simple acid-base disorders
- Mixed acid-base disorders
- Extracellular and intracellular chemical buffers

■ SELF-STUDY PROBLEMS

1. If there were no urinary buffers, how much urine (L/day) would the kidneys have to produce in order to excrete net acid equal to the amount of nonvolatile acid produced from metabolism? Assume that nonvolatile acid production is 70 mEq/day and the minimum urine pH is 4.0.
2. In the following table, indicate the simple acid-base disorder that exists for the laboratory data given. Use the following as normal values: pH = 7.40; $[HCO_3^-]$ = 24 mEq/L; P_{CO_2} = 40 mm Hg.
3. A previously healthy individual develops a gastrointestinal illness with nausea and vomiting. The following laboratory data are obtained after 12 hours of this illness:

Body weight:	70 kg
Blood pressure:	120/80 mm Hg
Plasma pH:	7.48
P_{CO_2}:	44 mm Hg
Plasma $[HCO_3^-]$:	32 mEq/L
Urine pH:	7.5

a. What is the acid-base disorder of this individual? What was its origin?

The illness continues, and 48 hours later the following laboratory data are obtained.

Body weight:	68 kg
Blood pressure:	80/40 mm Hg
Plasma pH:	7.50
P_{CO_2}:	48 mm Hg
Plasma $[HCO_3^-]$:	36 mEq/L
Urine pH:	6.0

b. Has the acid-base disturbance changed? How do you explain the paradoxical decrease in urine pH?

4. What effect would administration of a drug that inhibits carbonic anhydrase be expected to have on urine HCO_3^- excretion, and by what mechanism? What type of acid-base disorder could result from the use of this drug?

pH	$[HCO_3^-]$ mEq/L	P_{CO_2} mm Hg	Disorder	Compensation
7.34	15	29	_____	_____
7.49	35	48	_____	_____
7.47	14	20	_____	_____
7.34	31	60	_____	_____
7.26	26	60	_____	_____
7.62	20	20	_____	_____
7.09	15	50	_____	_____
7.40	15	25	_____	_____

9

Regulation of Calcium and Phosphate Balance

Upon completion of this chapter the student should be able to answer the following questions:

1. What is the physiologic importance of calcium (Ca^{++}) and phosphate (Pi)?
2. How does the body maintain Ca^{++} and Pi homeostasis?
3. What is the relative importance of the kidneys versus the gastrointestinal tract and bone in maintaining plasma Ca^{++} and Pi levels?
4. What hormones and factors regulate plasma Ca^{++} and Pi levels?
5. What are the cellular mechanisms responsible for Ca^{++} and Pi reabsorption along the nephron?
6. What hormones regulate renal Ca^{++} and Pi excretion?

C a^{++} and inorganic phosphate (Pi)[36] are multivalent ions that subserve many complex and vital functions. In a normal adult the renal excretion of these ions is balanced by gastrointestinal absorption. If the plasma concentrations decline substantially, gastrointestinal absorption, bone resorption, and renal tubular reabsorption increase and return plasma concentrations of Ca^{++} and Pi to normal levels. During growth and pregnancy, intestinal absorption exceeds urinary excretion, and these ions accumulate in newly formed fetal tissue and bone. In contrast, bone disease (e.g., osteoporosis) or a decline in lean body mass increases urinary multivalent ion loss without a change in intestinal absorption. These conditions produce a net loss of Ca^{++} and Pi from the body.

This brief introduction reveals that **the kidneys, in conjunction with the gastrointestinal tract and bone, play a major role in maintaining plasma Ca^{++} and Pi levels.** Accordingly, this chapter will discuss Ca^{++} and Pi handling by the kidneys with an emphasis on the hormones and factors that regulate urinary excretion.

---

36 At physiologic pH, inorganic phosphate exists as $HPO_4^=$ and $H_2PO_4^-$ (pK = 6.8). For simplicity we collectively refer to these ion species as *Pi.*

■ CALCIUM

Calcium ions play a major role in many processes, including bone formation, cell division and growth, blood coagulation, hormone-response coupling, and electrical stimulus-response coupling (such as muscle contraction and neurotransmitter release). Ninety-nine percent of Ca^{++} is stored in bone, 1% is found in the intracellular fluid, and 0.1% is located in the extracellular fluid (ECF) (Table 9-1). The total $[Ca^{++}]$ in plasma is 10 mg/dl (2.5 mM or 5 mEq/L), and its concentration is normally maintained within very narrow limits. A low ionized plasma $[Ca^{++}]$, hypocalcemia, increases the excitability of nerve and muscle cells and can lead to hypocalcemic tetany, which is characterized by skeletal muscle spasms. An elevated ionized plasma $[Ca^{++}]$, **hypercalcemia,** may produce decreased neuromuscular excitability, cardiac arrhythmias, lethargy, disorientation, and even death.

Overview of Ca^{++} Homeostasis

The maintenance of Ca^{++} homeostasis depends on two factors:

1. The total amount of Ca^{++} in the body
2. The distribution of Ca^{++} between bone and ECF compartments

Total body Ca^{++} is determined by the relative amounts of Ca^{++} absorbed by the gastrointestinal tract and excreted by the kidneys (Figure 9-1). Ca^{++} absorption by the gastrointestinal tract occurs by an active, carrier-mediated transport mechanism that is stimulated by **calcitriol,** a metabolite of **vitamin D3.**[37] Net Ca^{++} absorption is normally 200 mg/day, but it can increase to 600 mg/day when calcitriol levels rise. In adults, Ca^{++} excretion by the kidneys is equal to the amount absorbed by the gastrointestinal tract (200 mg/day), and it changes in accordance with the reabsorption of Ca^{++} by the gastrointestinal tract. Thus, in adults, Ca^{++} balance is maintained because the amount of Ca^{++} ingested in an average diet (1000 mg/day) is equal to the amount lost in the feces (800 mg/day: the amount that escapes absorption by the gastrointestinal tract) plus the amount excreted in the urine (200 mg/day).

The second factor that controls Ca^{++} homeostasis is the distribution of Ca^{++} between bone and the ECF. Three hormones, parathyroid hormone (PTH), calcitriol, and calcitonin, are the most important hormones that regulate the distribution of Ca^{++} between bone and the ECF and thereby regulate plasma $[Ca^{++}]$. PTH is secreted by the parathyroid glands, and its secretion is

---

[37] Vitamin D_3 is ingested in the diet and can be synthesized in the skin in the presence of UV light. Vitamin D_3 is converted in the liver to calcifediol and then in the kidney, primarily in the proximal tubule, to the active metabolite calcitriol.

T A B L E   9 - 1

Body content and distribution of Ca^{++} and Pi

Ion	Body content	Bone	Compartment	
			Intracellular	Extracellular
Ca^{++}	1300 g	99%	1%	0.10%
Pi	700 g	86%	14%	0.03%

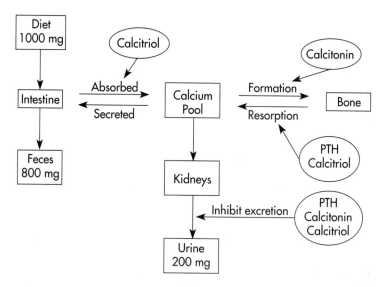

Figure 9-1 ■ **Overview of Ca^{++} homeostasis. See text for details.**

stimulated by a decline in plasma [Ca^{++}] (i.e., **hypocalcemia**). PTH increases plasma [Ca^{++}] in the following ways:

1. By stimulating bone resorption
2. By increasing Ca^{++} reabsorption by the kidneys
3. By stimulating the production of calcitriol, which in turn increases Ca^{++} absorption by the gastrointestinal tract and stimulates bone resorption

Hypercalcemia reduces PTH secretion, which leads to actions opposite to those described above. The production of calcitriol is stimulated by hypocalcemia and mediated by an increase in PTH and a decrease in plasma [Pi]. Calcitriol increases plasma [Ca^{++}] by actions similar to that of PTH (see preceding list). Calcitonin is also secreted by the parathyroid glands, and its secretion is stimulated by hypercalcemia. Calcitonin decreases plasma [Ca^{++}] primarily by stimulating bone formation (i.e., the deposition of Ca^{++} in bone). Figure 9-2 illustrates the relationship between plasma [Ca^{++}] and plasma levels of PTH and calcitonin.

Conditions that lower PTH levels (i.e., vitamin D deficiency or postsurgical hypoparathyroidism following parathyroidectomy caused by adenoma) reduce plasma [Ca^{++}] and can cause hypocalcemic tetany (intermittent muscular contraction), which is characterized by skeletal muscle spasms. In severe cases hypocalcemic tetany can cause death by asphyxiation. Hypercalcemia can also be lethal, causing cardiac arrhythmia and decreased neuromuscular excitability. Clinically the most common causes of hypercalcemia are primary hyperparathyroidism and malignancy-associated hypercalcemia. Primary hyperparathyroidism results from the overproduction of PTH caused by a tumor of the parathyroid glands. In contrast, malignancy-associated hypercalcemia occurs in 10%-20% of all patients with cancer and is caused by secretion of parathyroid hormone–related peptide (PTHRP), a PTH-like hormone secreted by carcinomas in a variety of organs. Increased levels of PTH and PTHRP cause hypercalcemia and hypercalciuria.

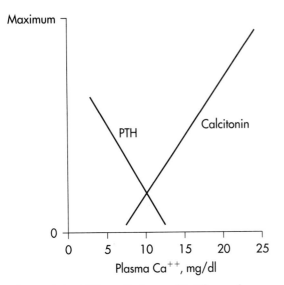

Figure 9-2 ■ **Effect of plasma [Ca^{++}] on plasma levels of PTH and calcitonin.** (Modified from Azria M: *The calcitonins: physiology and pharmacology,* Basel, Switzerland, 1989, Karger.)

During an acidosis the [H$^+$] in plasma is increased. This increase in the [H$^+$] causes more H$^+$ to bind to plasma proteins, HCO_3^-, citrate, Pi, and $SO_4^=$, thereby displacing Ca^{++}. This in turn increases the plasma concentration of ionized Ca^{++}. In contrast, during an alkalosis the [H$^+$] of plasma decreases. Some H$^+$ ions dissociate from plasma proteins, HCO_3^-, citrate, Pi, and $SO_4^=$, in exchange for Ca^{++}, thereby decreasing the plasma concentration of ionized Ca^{++}.

Approximately 50% of the Ca^{++} in plasma is ionized, 45% is bound to plasma proteins (mainly albumin), and 5% is complexed to several anions, including HCO_3^-, citrate, Pi, and $SO_4^=$ (Table 9-2). The pH of the plasma influences this distribution. Acidosis increases the percentage of ionized calcium at the expense of Ca^{++} bound to proteins, whereas alkalosis decreases the percentage of ionized calcium, again by altering Ca^{++} bound to proteins. Thus, individuals with alkalosis are more susceptible to tetany than individuals with acidosis, even when total plasma Ca^{++} levels are reduced. Ca^{++} available for filtration consists of the ionized fraction and that complexed with anions. Thus, about 55% of the Ca^{++} in the plasma is available for glomerular filtration.

Ca^{++} Transport along the Nephron

Normally 99% of the filtered Ca^{++} (i.e., ionized and complexed) is reabsorbed by the nephron.

The proximal tubule reabsorbs 70% of the filtered Ca^{++}. Another 20% is reabsorbed in Henle's loop (mainly the thick ascending limb), approximately 9% is reabsorbed by the distal tubule, and less than 1% is reabsorbed by the collecting duct. About 1% (200 mg/day) is excreted in the urine. This fraction is equal to the net amount absorbed daily by the gastrointestinal tract. Figure 9-3 summarizes the handling of Ca^{++} by the different portions of the nephron.

Cellular Mechanisms of Ca^{++} Reabsorption

Ca^{++} reabsorption by the proximal tubule occurs by two pathways: transcellular and paracellular (Figure 9-4). Ca^{++} reabsorption across the cellular pathway (i.e., transcellular) accounts for 20% of proximal reabsorption. Ca^{++} reabsorption through the cell is an active, two-step process. Ca^{++} diffuses across the apical membrane into the cell down its electrochemical gradient. This gradient is exceptionally steep because the Ca^{++} concentration in the cell is only 0.4 µg/dl, about 10,000-fold less than that in the tubular fluid (6 mg/dl). The cell interior is electrically negative with respect to the luminal side of the apical membrane, and this also favors Ca^{++} entry into the cell, most likely via Ca^{++} channels. Ca^{++} is extruded across the basolateral membrane against its electrochemical gradient. The mechanism for the extrusion of Ca^{++} is thought to occur by a

Ca^{++}-ATPase and a 3Na$^+$-Ca^{++} antiporter. Eighty percent of Ca^{++} is reabsorbed between cells across the tight junctions (i.e., paracellular pathway). This passive, paracellular reabsorption of Ca^{++} occurs by solvent drag along the entire length of the proximal tubule and is also driven by the positive luminal voltage in the second half of the proximal tubule (see Chapter 4). Thus, in the proximal tubule approximately 80% of Ca^{++} reabsorption is paracellular and 20% is transcellular.

Ca^{++} reabsorption by Henle's loop is restricted to the thick ascending limb. Ca^{++} is reabsorbed via a cellular and a paracellular route by mechanisms similar to those described for the proximal tubule, except that Ca^{++} is not reabsorbed by solvent drag in this segment (recall that the thick ascending limb is impermeable to water). In the thick ascending limb, Ca^{++} and Na$^+$ reabsorptions are parallel to each other because of the significant component of Ca^{++} reabsorption that occurs by passive, paracellular mechanisms secondary to Na$^+$ reabsorption and by the generation of the lumen-positive transepithelial voltage (see Chapter 4). **Therefore changes in**

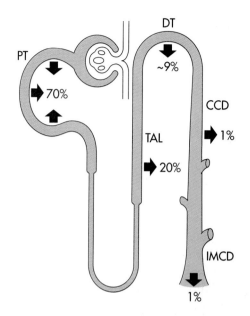

Figure 9-3 ■ Transport pattern of Ca^{++} along the nephron. Percentages refer to the amount of the filtered Ca^{++} reabsorbed by each nephron segment. Approximately 1% of the filtered Ca^{++} is excreted. *PT*, Proximal tubule; *TAL*, thick ascending limb; *DT*, distal tubule; *CCD*, cortical collecting duct; *IMCD*, inner medullary collecting duct.

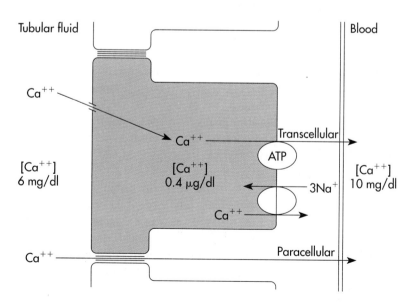

Figure 9-4 ■ Cellular mechanisms of Ca^{++} reabsorption by the proximal tubule. Ca^{++} is reabsorbed by transcellular and paracellular routes. The mechanism of Ca^{++} diffusion into the cell across the apical membrane has not been characterized but is likely to occur via Ca^{++} channels.

T A B L E 9 - 2				
Forms of Ca^{++} and Pi in plasma				
Ion	**mg/dl**	**Ionized**	**Protein-bound**	**Complexed**
Ca^{++}	10 mg/dl	50%	45%	5%
Pi	4 mg/dl	84%	10%	6%

Ca^{++} is bound (i.e., complexed) to various anions in the plasma, including HCO$_3^-$, citrate, Pi, and SO$_4^=$. Pi is complexed to various cations, including Na$^+$ and K$^+$.

Na$^+$ reabsorption also result in parallel changes in Ca^{++} reabsorption by the proximal tubule and the thick ascending limb of Henle's loop.

In the distal tubule, where the voltage in the tubule lumen is electrically negative with respect to the blood, Ca^{++} reabsorption is entirely active because Ca^{++} is reabsorbed against its electrochemical gradient. Ca^{++} reabsorption by the distal tubule is exclusively transcellular, and the mechanism is similar to that in the proximal tubule and thick ascending limb: uptake across the apical membrane by Ca^{++}-permeable ion channels and extrusion across the basolateral membrane by Ca^{++}-ATPase and 3Na$^+$-Ca^{++} antiporter. **Although changes in Na$^+$ and Ca^{++} excretion are usually parallel, because the reabsorption of Ca^{++} and Na$^+$ by the distal tubule is independent and differentially regulated, changes in urinary Ca^{++} and Na$^+$ excretion are not always parallel. For example, thiazide diuretics inhibit Na$^+$ reabsorption by the distal tubule and stimulate Ca^{++} reabsorption by this segment. Accordingly, the net effect of thiazide diuretics is to increase urinary Na$^+$ excretion and reduce urinary Ca^{++} excretion (see Chapter 10 for additional details).**

Regulation of Urinary Ca^{++} Excretion

Urinary Ca^{++} excretion is regulated by PTH, calcitonin, and calcitriol. PTH exerts the most powerful control on renal Ca^{++} excretion and is responsible for maintaining Ca^{++} homeostasis. Overall, this hormone stimulates Ca^{++} reabsorption by the kidneys (i.e., reduces Ca^{++} excretion). Although PTH inhibits the reabsorption of NaCl and fluid (and therefore Ca^{++}) by the proximal tubule, PTH dramatically stimulates Ca^{++} reabsorption by the thick ascending limb of Henle's loop and the distal tubule. As a result, urinary Ca^{++} excretion declines. Calcitonin and calcitriol also stimulate Ca^{++} reabsorption by the kidneys. Calcitonin stimulates Ca^{++} reabsorption by the thick ascending limb of Henle's loop and the distal tubule, but it is quantitatively less important than PTH. Either directly or indirectly, calcitriol enhances Ca^{++} reabsorption by the distal tubule. It is also quantitatively less important than PTH.

In contrast to the hormones that regulate urinary Ca^{++} excretion (i.e., PTH, calcitonin, and calcitriol), several factors disturb Ca^{++} excretion. For example, an increase in plasma [Pi] (e.g., increased dietary intake of Pi) elevates PTH levels and thereby decreases Ca^{++} excretion. In contrast, a decline in the plasma [Pi] (e.g., dietary Pi depletion) has the opposite effect. Changes in the ECF volume alter Ca^{++} excretion mainly by affecting NaCl and fluid reabsorption in the proximal tubule. Contraction of the ECF volume increases NaCl and water reabsorption by the proximal tubule and thereby enhances Ca^{++} reabsorption. Accordingly, urinary Ca^{++} excretion declines. Expansion of the ECF volume has the opposite effect. Acidosis increases Ca^{++} excretion, whereas alkalosis decreases excretion. The regulation of Ca^{++} reabsorption by pH occurs in the distal tubule by an unknown mechanism.

■ PHOSPHATE

Pi is an important component of many organic molecules, including DNA, RNA, ATP, and intermediates of metabolic pathways. It is also a major constituent of bone. Its concentration in plasma is an important determinant in bone formation and resorption. In addition, urinary Pi is an important buffer (titratable acid) for the maintenance of acid-base balance (see Chapter 8). Eighty-six percent of Pi is located in bone, 14% is located in the intracellular fluid, and 0.03% is located in the extracellular fluid (Table 9-1). The

plasma [Pi] is 4 mg/dl (Table 9-2). Approximately 10% of the Pi in the plasma is protein-bound and therefore unavailable for ultrafiltration by the glomerulus. Accordingly, the [Pi] in the ultrafiltrate is 10% less than that in plasma.

Overview of Pi Homeostasis

A general scheme of Pi homeostasis is shown in Figure 9-5. The maintenance of Pi homeostasis depends on two factors:

1. The amount of Pi in the body
2. The distribution of Pi between the intracellular fluid and the ECF compartments

Total body Pi is determined by the relative amount of Pi absorbed by the gastrointestinal tract versus the amount excreted by the kidneys. Pi absorption by the gastrointestinal tract occurs by active and passive mechanisms; it increases as dietary Pi rises, and it is stimulated by calcitriol. Despite changes in Pi intake between 800 and 1500 mg/day, total body Pi balance is maintained by the kidneys, which excrete an amount of Pi

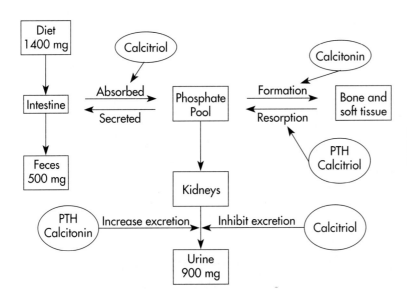

Figure 9-5 ■ Overview of Pi homeostasis. See text for details.

in the urine equal to the amount absorbed by the gastrointestinal tract. **Thus, the kidneys play a vital role in maintaining Pi homeostasis.**

The second factor that maintains Pi homeostasis is the distribution of Pi among bone and the intracellular and extracellular fluid compartments. PTH, calcitriol, and calcitonin regulate the distribution of Pi between bone and the extracellular fluid. The release of Pi from intracellular stores is stimulated by the same hormones (PTH and calcitriol) that release Ca^{++} from this pool. Thus, the release of Pi is always accompanied by a release of Ca^{++}. In contrast, calcitonin increases bone formation and thereby decreases plasma [Pi]. The kidneys also contribute importantly to the regulation of plasma [Pi]. A small increase in plasma [Pi] increases the amount of Pi filtered by the glomerulus. Because the kidneys normally reabsorb Pi at a maximal rate, an increase in the amount filtered leads to a rise in urinary Pi excretion. This in turn elevates urinary Pi excretion to a value above Pi absorption by the gastrointestinal tract, resulting in a net loss of Pi from the body. This loss of Pi causes plasma [Pi] to fall. **Accordingly, the kidneys regulate plasma [Pi].** The maximum reabsorptive rate for Pi is variable and regulated by dietary Pi intake. A high-Pi diet decreases the maximum reabsorptive rate of Pi by the kidneys, and a low-Pi diet increases the maximum reabsorptive rate. This effect of dietary Pi intake on the maximum Pi transport rate of the kidneys is independent of changes in PTH levels.

Pi Transport along the Nephron

Figure 9-6 summarizes Pi transport by the various portions of the nephron. The proximal tubule reabsorbs 80% of the Pi filtered by the glomerulus, and the distal tubule reabsorbs 10%. In contrast, Henle's loop and the collecting duct reabsorb negligible amounts of Pi. Therefore 10% of the filtered load of Pi is excreted.

In patients with chronic renal failure the kidneys cannot excrete Pi, and because of continued Pi absorption by the gastrointestinal tract, Pi accumulates in the body, thereby elevating plasma [Pi]. The increased Pi complexes with Ca^{++}, thereby reducing plasma [Ca^{++}]. Pi accumulation also decreases the production of calcitriol, which reduces Ca^{++} absorption by the intestine, an effect that further decreases plasma [Ca^{++}]. The fall in plasma [Ca^{++}] increases PTH secretion and Ca^{++} release from bone, resulting in osteitis fibrosa cystica (i.e., increased bone resorption with replacement by fibrous tissue, which renders bone more susceptible to fracture). Chronic hyperparathyroidism (i.e., elevated PTH levels) during chronic renal failure can lead to metastatic calcifications in which Ca^{++} and Pi precipitate in arteries (leading to ischemia), soft tissues, and viscera. Deposition of Ca^{++} and Pi in heart and lung tissue may cause myocardial failure and pulmonary insufficiency, respectively. Prevention and treatment of hyperparathyroidism and Pi retention include a low Pi diet or the administration of a "phosphate binder" (i.e., an agent that forms insoluble Pi salts, rendering the Pi unavailable for reabsorption by the gastrointestinal tract). Supplemental Ca^{++} and calcitriol are also used.

Pi reabsorption by the proximal tubule occurs mainly, if not exclusively, by a transcellular route. As shown in Figure 9-7, Pi uptake across the apical membrane occurs by a $2Na^+$-Pi symport mechanism. Pi exits across the basolateral membrane, most likely by a Pi-anion antiporter. The cellular mechanism of Pi reabsorption by the distal tubule has not been characterized.

Regulation of Urinary Pi Excretion

Table 9-3 summarizes the major hormones and factors that regulate urinary Pi excretion. All act on the proximal tubule and either stimulate or inhibit Pi reabsorption. **PTH is the most important hormone that controls Pi excretion.** PTH stimulates cAMP production and inhibits Pi reabsorption by the proximal tubule, thereby increasing Pi excretion. Dietary Pi intake also regulates Pi excretion by mechanisms unrelated to changes in PTH levels. Pi loading increases excretion, whereas Pi depletion decreases excretion. Changes in dietary Pi intake modulate Pi transport by altering the transport

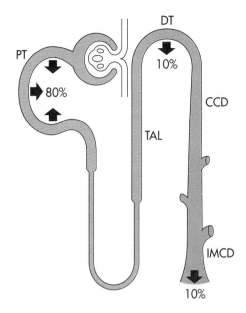

Figure 9-6 ■ **Transport pattern of Pi along the nephron. Pi is reabsorbed primarily by the proximal tubule and distal tubule. Percentages refer to the amount of the filtered Pi reabsorbed by each nephron segment. Approximately 10% of the filtered Pi is excreted.** *PT,* **Proximal tubule;** *TAL,* **thick ascending limb;** *DT,* **distal tubule;** *CCD,* **cortical collecting duct;** *IMCD,* **inner medullary collecting duct.**

T A B L E   9 - 3

Hormones and factors influencing urinary Pi excretion

Increase excretion	Decrease excretion
Increase of PTH	Decrease of PTH
Pi loading	Pi depletion
ECV expansion	ECV contraction
Acidosis	Alkalosis
Glucocorticoids	Growth hormone

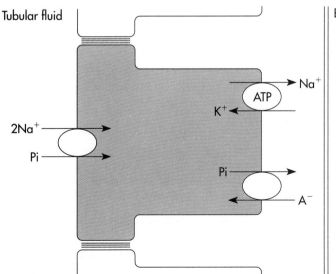

Figure 9-7 ■ **Cellular mechanism of Pi reabsorption by the proximal tubule. The apical transport pathway may operate primarily as a 2Na⁺/Pi symporter. Pi leaves the cell across the basolateral membrane by a Pi-anion antiporter and possibly by a Na⁺/Pi symporter (not shown). A⁻ indicates an anion.**

rate of each 2Na$^+$-Pi symporter and increasing the number of transporters.

ECF volume also affects Pi excretion; volume expansion increases excretion, and volume contraction decreases excretion. The effect of the ECF volume on Pi excretion is indirect and may involve changes in hormone levels other than PTH. Acid-base balance also influences Pi excretion; acidosis increases Pi excretion, and alkalosis decreases Pi excretion. Glucocorticoids increase the excretion of Pi. Glucocorticoids increase the delivery of Pi to the distal tubule and collecting duct by inhibiting proximal tubular Pi reabsorption. This inhibition enables the distal tubule and collecting duct to secrete more H$^+$ and generate more HCO$_3^-$, because Pi is an important urinary buffer (see Chapter 8 for an explanation). Finally, growth hormone decreases Pi excretion.

■ INTEGRATIVE REVIEW OF PTH, CALCITRIOL, AND CALCITONIN ON Ca^{++} AND Pi HOMEOSTASIS

The major stimulus to PTH secretion is hypocalcemia. As summarized in Figure 9-8, PTH has numerous effects on Ca^{++} and Pi homeostasis. PTH stimulates bone resorption (i.e., release of Ca^{++} and Pi from bone), increases urinary Pi excretion, decreases urinary Ca^{++} excretion, and stimulates the production of calcitriol, which stimulates Ca^{++} and Pi absorption by the intestine. **Because changes in Pi handling in bone, intestine, and kidneys tend to balance out, PTH increases plasma [Ca^{++}] while having**

little effect on plasma [Pi]. Overall, a rise in plasma PTH levels increases plasma [Ca^{++}] and decreases plasma [Pi]. A decline in plasma PTH levels has the opposite effect.

Calcitriol also plays an important role in Ca^{++} and Pi homeostasis (Figure 9-9). Calcitriol stimulates Ca^{++} and Pi absorption by the intestine and Ca^{++} and Pi release from bone and decreases Ca^{++} and Pi excretion by the kidneys. The net effect of calcitriol is to increase plasma [Ca^{++}] and [Pi]. Thus, the major stimuli to calcitriol production are hypocalcemia via PTH and hypophosphatemia (i.e., a low plasma [Pi]).

Calcitonin is also an important hormone in Ca^{++} homeostasis because it blocks bone resorption and stimulates Ca^{++} deposition in bone (Figure 9-10). Although calcitonin has a modest direct effect on decreasing urinary Ca^{++} excretion, this is a relatively minor action of the hormone. The major stimulus to calcitonin secretion is an increase in plasma [Ca^{++}]. Because changes in Pi handling in bone, intestine, and kidneys tend to balance out, calcitonin decreases plasma [Ca^{++}] while having little effect on plasma [Pi].

■ SUMMARY

1. Ca^{++} and inorganic phosphate (Pi) are multivalent ions that subserve many important functions. The kidneys, in conjunction with the gastrointestinal tract and bone, play a vital role in regulating plasma Ca^{++} and Pi levels.
2. Plasma Ca^{++} is regulated by parathyroid hormone (PTH), calcitriol, and calcitonin. Ca^{++}

In the absence of glucocorticoids (e.g., Addison's disease), Pi excretion is depressed, as is the ability of the kidneys to excrete titratable acid and generate new HCO$_3^-$. Growth hormone increases the reabsorption of Pi by the proximal tubule. As a result, growing children have a plasma [Pi] elevated above that found in adults, which is important for the formation of bone.

Estrogens defend against PTH-mediated resorption of bone. In estrogen-deficient conditions, most prominently those following menopause, the unabated effect of PTH on bone contributes importantly to the development of osteoporosis. Estrogen-replacement therapy, which should be accompanied by progesterone, is useful for women at high risk for developing osteoporosis.

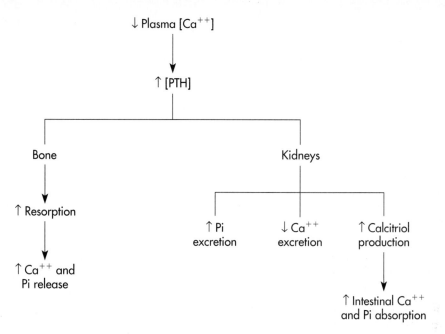

Figure 9-8 ■ Effect of PTH on Ca^{++} and Pi homeostasis. The major stimulus of PTH secretion is hypocalcemia. (Modified from Rose BD, Rennke HG: *Renal pathophysiology: the essentials,* Baltimore, 1994, Williams & Wilkins.)

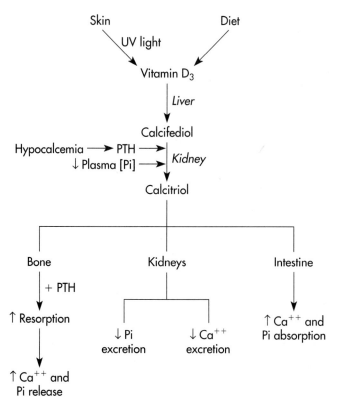

Figure 9-9 ■ Activation of vitamin D$_3$ and its effect on Ca^{++} and Pi metabolism. Hypocalcemia and hypophosphatemia are the major stimuli to the metabolism of calcifediol to calcitriol in the kidneys. The net effect of calcitriol is to increase plasma [Ca^{++}] and [Pi]. (Modified from Rose BD, Rennke HG: *Renal pathophysiology: the essentials,* Baltimore, 1994, Williams & Wilkins.)

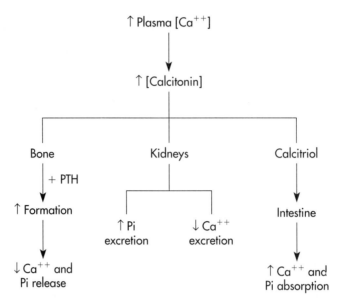

Figure 9-10 ■ **Effect of calcitonin on Ca^{++} and Pi homeostasis. The major stimulus of calcitonin secretion is hypercalcemia. The net effect of calcitonin is to reduce plasma [Ca^{++}]. Thus, to this end, quantitatively the most important effects of calcitonin are to stimulate bone formation and decrease bone resorption. Although calcitonin reduces urinary Ca^{++} excretion and intestinal Ca^{++} absorption, these effects are relatively minor and have little effect on plasma [Ca^{++}].** (Modified from Rose BD, Rennke HG: *Renal pathophysiology: the essentials,* Baltimore, 1994, Williams & Wilkins.)

excretion by the kidneys is determined by the net rate of intestinal Ca^{++} absorption, the balance between bone formation and resorption, and the net rate of Ca^{++} reabsorption by the distal tubule and thick ascending limb (TAL) of Henle's loop. Ca^{++} reabsorption by the TAL is regulated by PTH, calcitriol, and calcitonin, which stimulate Ca^{++} reabsorption.

3. Plasma [Pi] is regulated by the maximum reabsorptive capacity of Pi by the kidneys. A fall in [Pi] stimulates production of calcitriol, which causes the release of Pi from bone into the extracellular fluid. Calcitriol also increases Pi absorption by the intestine and decreases urinary Pi excretion.

KEY WORDS AND CONCEPTS

- Ca^{++} homeostasis
- Pi homeostasis
- PTH
- Calcitriol
- Calcitonin
- Hypocalcemia
- Hypercalcemia
- Regulation of renal Ca^{++} excretion
- Pi homeostasis
- Vitamin D$_3$

■ **SELF-STUDY PROBLEMS**

1. How is Ca^{++} reabsorption in the proximal tubule dependent on Na^+ reabsorption? What would happen to Ca^{++} excretion if a subject was given a diuretic, such as mannitol, that inhibits sodium and water reabsorption by the proximal tubule?

2. What effect would furosemide, an inhibitor of Na^+ reabsorption by the thick ascending limb of Henle's loop, have on urinary Ca^{++} excretion?

3. What would happen to Pi excretion if plasma [Pi] was increased from 4 to 6 mg/dl?

Physiology of Diuretic Action

OBJECTIVES

Upon completion of this chapter the student should be able to answer the following questions:

1. What effects do diuretics have on Na^+ handling by the kidneys?
2. Why do diuretics decrease the volume of the extracellular fluid (ECF) and the effective circulating volume (ECV)?
3. What mechanisms are involved in delivering diuretics into the lumen of the nephron?
4. What is the primary nephron site where each class of diuretics acts, and what is the specific membrane transport protein effected?
5. What are the effects of the various classes of diuretics on the renal handling of K^+, Ca^{++}, HCO_3^-, Pi, and solute-free water?

Diuretics, as the name implies, are drugs that cause an increase in urine output. It is important, however, to distinguish this diuresis from that which occurs following the ingestion of large volumes of water. In the latter case the urine comprises primarily water, and solute excretion is not increased. **In contrast, diuretics result in the enhanced excretion of both solute and water.**

All diuretics have as their common mode of action the inhibition of Na^+ reabsorption by the nephron. Consequently, they cause an increase in the excretion of Na^+, termed *natriuresis.* The effects of diuretics, however, are not limited to Na^+ handling. The renal handling of many other solutes is also influenced, usually as a consequence of alterations in Na^+ transport.

This chapter reviews the various diuretics' cellular mechanisms of action and the nephron sites at which these diuretics act. In addition to their effects on Na^+ handling by the nephron, their effects on the renal handling of other solutes (K^+, Ca^{++}, Pi, and HCO_3^-) and water are also considered.

■ GENERAL PRINCIPLES OF DIURETIC ACTION

The primary action of diuretics is to increase the excretion of Na^+. As described in Chapter 6, alterations in Na^+ excretion by the kidneys result in alterations in the volume of the extracellular fluid (ECF) compartment and the effective circulating volume (ECV). Consequently, diuretics decrease the volume of the ECF and ECV. Indeed, diuretics are commonly given in clinical situations when the ECF compartment is expanded, with the intent of reducing its volume.

Although generally predictable for a particular class of diuretics, the effects of diuretic administration can be quite variable. Several factors are important in determining the overall effect of a particular diuretic:

1. The nephron segment where the diuretic acts
2. The response of nephron segments distal to the site of action of the diuretic
3. The delivery of sufficient quantities of the diuretic to its site of action
4. The volume of the ECF and ECV

Sites of Action of Diuretics

Diuretics act on specific renal tubule–membrane transport proteins. Consequently, the localization of these membrane transport proteins along the nephron determines the diuretic's site of action. Figure 10-1 depicts the nephron sites at which the different classes of diuretics act. The osmotic diuretics act along the proximal tubule and thin descending limb of Henle's loop. The carbonic anhydrase inhibitors act primarily in the proximal tubule. The thick ascending limb of Henle's loop is the site of action of the loop diuretics. The early portion of the distal tubule is the site of action of the thiazide diuretics, and the K+-sparing diuretics act on the late portion of the distal tubule and the cortical collecting duct.

The site of action of a diuretic in turn determines the magnitude of the associated natriuresis. The effect diuretics have on the handling of solutes other than Na+ also depends on the site of action. Examples illustrating this point are given in subsequent sections.

Response of More Distal Nephron Segments

When a diuretic inhibits Na+ reabsorption at one nephron site, it causes an increased delivery of Na+ and water to more distal segments. The

Figure 10-1 ■ **Sites of action of diuretics along the nephron.** *PT,* **Proximal tubule;** *TAL,* **thick ascending limb;** *DT,* **distal tubule;** *CCD,* **cortical collecting duct;** *IMCD,* **inner medullary collecting duct.**

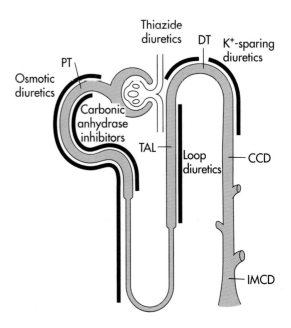

function of these more distal segments and their ability or inability to handle this increased load ultimately determine the overall effect of the diuretic on urinary excretion. Examples of this are considered in detail below with each of the various diuretics.

Adequate Delivery of Diuretics to Their Site of Action

The effect of a diuretic on Na^+ excretion also depends on the delivery of adequate quantities of the drug to its site of action. With the exception of the aldosterone antagonists, which act intracellularly, diuretics act from the lumen of the nephron (carbonic anhydrase inhibitors have both a luminal and intracellular site of action). Diuretics gain access to the lumen by glomerular filtration and through secretion by the **organic anion** and **organic cation secretory systems** located in the proximal tubule (see Chapter 4). Thus, the effect of a diuretic can be blunted if, for example, it is administered with another drug that competes for the same secretory mechanism.

Volume of the ECF and ECV

Finally, the effect of a diuretic depends on the ECF volume and ECV. As described in Chapter 6, when the ECV is decreased, the GFR is reduced, thereby reducing the filtered load of Na^+. In addition, Na^+ reabsorption by the proximal tubule is enhanced. Thus, the effect of a diuretic that acts on the distal tubule would be blunted if administered in the setting of a reduced ECV. Under this condition, the decreased GFR (i.e., decreased filtered load of Na^+), together with enhanced Na^+ reabsorption by the proximal tubule, would result in the delivery of a smaller quantity of Na^+ to the distal tubule. Thus, even if the diuretic completely inhibited Na^+ reabsorption in the distal tubule, the associated natriuresis would be less than would occur if the ECV were normal.

The dependence of diuretic-induced natriuresis on the ECV also explains why the effect of a diuretic is self-limited. As illustrated in Figure 10-2, administration of a diuretic to an individual with fixed Na^+ intake results in a short-lived natriuresis. The transient response reflects the fact

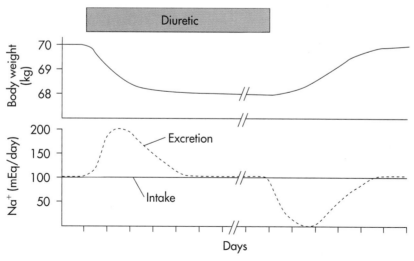

Figure 10-2 ■ Effect of long-term diuretic therapy on renal Na^+ excretion. Because of diuretic-induced natriuresis, ECF and ECV are reduced. This is detected as a decrease in body weight.

that by increasing Na^+ excretion, the diuretic reduces the ECV (detected as a decrease in body weight). Such a fall in the ECV decreases GFR and increases proximal tubular reabsorption. These effects in turn limit the natriuretic response, as described above. After a short period (usually several days), the individual reaches a new steady state, during which Na^+ intake again equals excretion. However, the ECV is decreased. When diuretic therapy is discontinued, renal Na^+ excretion is reduced. After a period of positive Na^+ balance, during which ECV is returned to normal (i.e., return of body weight to its original value), a new steady state is again achieved.

The concept of **steady state** deserves special emphasis. Normally, individuals are in steady state balance with regard to solute (e.g., Na^+) and water, with intake equaling excretion. Administration of a diuretic temporarily disrupts this balance by increasing excretion, and a negative balance exists. However, excretion cannot exceed intake indefinitely, and a new steady state is eventually achieved. In this new steady state, intake and excretion are again balanced, but the ECV is reduced as a result of diuretic-induced excretion of Na^+. Determining whether the individual is in the acute phase (i.e., negative balance) or chronic phase (i.e., steady state) is necessary when attempting to analyze the effects of diuretic therapy. In general, when an individual is on a diuretic for several days or longer, a new steady state is achieved and the ECV is reduced from what it was before diuretic administration.

■ MECHANISMS OF ACTION OF DIURETICS
Osmotic Diuretics

Osmotic diuretics, as the name implies, are agents that inhibit the reabsorption of solute and water by altering osmotic driving forces along the nephron. Unlike the other classes of diuretics, osmotic diuretics do not inhibit a specific membrane transport protein. They simply affect water transport across the cells of the nephron

through the generation of an osmotic pressure gradient. The best example of an exogenous osmotic diuretic is the sugar mannitol. When present in abnormally high concentrations, endogenous substances such as glucose (i.e., in diabetes mellitus) and urea (i.e., in patients with renal disease whose plasma urea levels are elevated) can also act as osmotic diuretics.

Osmotic diuretics (e.g., mannitol) gain access to the tubular fluid by glomerular filtration. Because they are not reabsorbed or only poorly reabsorbed, they remain within the lumen, where they can exert an osmotic pressure inhibiting tubular fluid reabsorption. Osmotic diuretics affect fluid reabsorption in those segments that water easily penetrates (i.e., the proximal tubule and descending thin limb of Henle's loop). Because of the large volumes of filtrate reabsorbed in the proximal tubule (60%-70% of the filtered load), this nephron site is the most important when considering the action of osmotic diuretics.

As described in Chapter 4, reabsorption of tubular fluid by the proximal tubule is essentially an isoosmotic process (i.e., the osmolality of the reabsorbed fluid is slightly hyperosmotic as compared with that of tubular fluid). Solute (primarily NaCl) is actively reabsorbed by the proximal tubule cells. This sets up a small osmotic pressure difference across the tubule, with the lumen being 3 to 5 mOsm/kg H_2O hypoosmotic with respect to the interstitial fluid. Given the fact that water is readily able to cross the proximal tubule, this small osmotic pressure gradient is sufficient to cause water reabsorption. Also, as water flows from the lumen to the interstitium, it brings additional solute with it via solvent drag.

When an osmotic diuretic is present in the tubular fluid, its concentration will increase progressively as a result of NaCl and water reabsorption by the nephron. With this increase in concentration, an osmotic gradient develops opposite to the normal gradient generated by NaCl reabsorption. As a result, both NaCl (solvent drag component) and water reabsorption are reduced. Some of the Na$^+$ that is not reabsorbed by the proximal tubule is reabsorbed downstream by the thick ascending limb. Because Na$^+$ reabsorption by the thick ascending limb increases as NaCl delivery rises, the degree of natriuresis seen with osmotic diuretics is less than expected based on the magnitude of proximal tubule reabsorption. Although Na$^+$ excretion rates as high as 60% of the filtered load have been seen in experimental situations, the usual natriuresis seen in individuals treated with osmotic diuretics is only about 10% of the filtered load.

Carbonic Anhydrase Inhibitors

Carbonic anhydrase inhibitors (e.g., acetazolamide) reduce Na$^+$ reabsorption by their effect on carbonic anhydrase. This enzyme is abundant in the proximal tubule and therefore represents the major site of action of these diuretics. Carbonic anhydrase is also present in other cells along the nephron (e.g., intercalated cells of the collecting duct), and administration of carbonic anhydrase inhibitors affects the activity of the enzyme at these sites as well. However, the effects of these diuretics are almost entirely attributed to their inhibition of the enzyme in the proximal tubule.

As described in Chapter 8, carbonic anhydrase is critical for the reabsorption of HCO$_3^-$ by the proximal tubule. In this segment the enzyme is located within the cell and apical membrane. The intracellular enzyme facilitates the formation of H$^+$ and HCO$_3^-$ from CO$_2$ and H$_2$O. HCO$_3^-$ exits the cell across the basolateral membrane and returns to the blood, whereas H$^+$ is secreted into the tubular fluid. In the tubular fluid, H$^+$ combines with the filtered HCO$_3^-$ to form H$_2$CO$_3$. This is rapidly hydrolyzed to CO$_2$ and H$_2$O by the carbonic anhydrase located in the apical membrane, thus facilitating CO$_2$ and H$_2$O reabsorption. The activity of the apical membrane and intracellular enzymes is decreased by the carbonic

anhydrase inhibitors, which significantly reduces the reabsorption of HCO$_3^-$. Because a significant portion of H$^+$ secretion, and thus HCO$_3^-$ reabsorption, by the proximal tubular cell depends on Na$^+$ (Na$^+$-H$^+$ antiporter in the apical membrane), inhibition of carbonic anhydrase also results in a decrease in Na$^+$ reabsorption.

Approximately one third of all proximal tubular Na$^+$ reabsorption is related to the process of HCO$_3^-$ reabsorption. Inhibition of this process by the carbonic anhydrase inhibitors would therefore be expected to cause a large increase in Na$^+$ excretion (as much as 20% of the filtered load). However, this is not the case; Na$^+$ excretion rates of only 5% to 10% of the filtered load are seen with these diuretics. The reason for this is the same as that described for the osmotic diuretics and relates to the ability of the thick ascending limb to increase its reabsorptive rate when Na$^+$ delivery is increased.

Loop Diuretics

Loop diuretics (e.g., furosemide, bumetanide, and ethacrynic acid) are organic anions that enter the tubular lumen by glomerular filtration and via secretion by the organic anion secretory system of the proximal tubule. They inhibit Na$^+$ reabsorption by the thick ascending limb of Henle's loop by blocking the 1Na$^+$-1K$^+$-2Cl symporter located in the apical membrane of these cells (see Chapter 4). By this action, they not only inhibit Na$^+$ reabsorption but also disrupt the process of countercurrent multiplication. Because of this effect, loop diuretics impair the kidneys' ability both to dilute and to concentrate the urine. Dilution is impaired because solute (NaCl) reabsorption by the water-impermeable thick ascending limb of Henle's loop is inhibited. NaCl reabsorption by the medullary portion of the thick ascending limb is also critical for the generation and maintenance of an elevated medullary interstitial fluid osmolality. Therefore inhibition of transport by the loop diuretics results in a decrease in the osmolality of the medullary interstitial fluid. With a decrease in medullary interstitial fluid osmolality, water reabsorption from the collecting duct is impaired, and the concentrating ability of the kidneys is reduced. Water reabsorption from the descending thin limb of Henle's loop is also impaired by loop diuretics, again because of the decrease in medullary interstitial fluid osmolality. This decrease in descending thin limb reabsorption accounts in part for the increase in water excretion seen with loop diuretics.

Loop diuretics are the most potent diuretics available, increasing the excretion of Na^+ to 25% of the filtered load. This large natriuresis reflects the fact that the thick ascending limb normally reabsorbs approximately 20% to 25% of the filtered load of Na^+, and the downstream segments have a limited capacity, at least acutely, to compensate for the increased delivered load of Na^+ received as a result of the diuretics' actions.

Thiazide Diuretics

Like the loop diuretics, **thiazide diuretics** (e.g., chlorothiazide, metolazone)[38] are organic anions that gain access to the tubular lumen by filtration and secretion in the proximal tubule. They act to inhibit Na^+ reabsorption in the early portion of the distal tubule by blocking the Na^+-Cl^- symporter in the apical membrane of these cells (see Chapter 4). Because water cannot cross this portion of the nephron, it is a site where the urine is diluted. Therefore thiazides reduce the ability to dilute the urine maximally by inhibiting NaCl reabsorption. Natriuresis with thiazide diuretics is 5% to 10% of the filtered load.

---

38 Metolazone is not in the same chemical class of drugs as the thiazides. However, because its site of action is the same, it is grouped with this class of diuretics.

K+-Sparing Diuretics

The **K+-sparing diuretics** act on the region of the nephron where K^+ secretion occurs (late portion of the distal tubule and cortical collecting duct). They produce a small natriuresis (3% of the filtered load), reflecting the amount of Na^+ reabsorbed by this region of the nephron. As the name implies, their utility lies in their ability to inhibit K^+ secretion by this region of the nephron.

There are two classes of K+-sparing diuretics: one acts by antagonizing aldosterone's action on the principal cell of the collecting duct (e.g., spironolactone), whereas the other class blocks the entry of Na^+ into these same cells through the Na^+-selective channels in the apical membrane (e.g., amiloride, triamterene). Amiloride and triamterene are organic cations that enter the tubular lumen by glomerular filtration and secretion by the organic cation secretory system of the proximal tubule.

The reabsorption of Na^+ and the secretion of K^+ by the principal cell of the collecting duct are stimulated by aldosterone. Aldosterone acts by increasing the number of functional Na^+ and K^+ channels in the apical membrane and the levels of Na^+-K^+-ATPase in the basolateral membrane (see Chapters 6 and 7). By this action, Na^+ entry into the cell from the lumen is enhanced, as is its extrusion from the cell across the basolateral membrane. Similarly the blood-to-lumen movement of K^+ is enhanced. In the presence of an aldosterone antagonist, these effects are reversed and both Na^+ reabsorption and K^+ secretion are reduced.

The ability of the Na^+ channel blockers amiloride and triamterene to inhibit Na^+ reabsorption and K^+ secretion is similar to that of spironolactone, but the cellular mechanism is different. Amiloride and triamterene interact directly with the Na^+-selective channel in the apical membrane of the principal cell and block the entry of Na^+. With decreased Na^+ entry, there is decreased Na^+ extrusion across the basolateral membrane via Na^+-K^+-ATPase. This in turn reduces cellular K^+ uptake and ultimately its secretion into the tubular fluid. The blockade of the apical membrane Na^+ channels also alters the electrical profile across the luminal membrane, with the voltage across this membrane increasing in magnitude. Because of this voltage change, the electrochemical gradient for K^+ movement out of the cell is reduced. This membrane voltage effect also contributes to the inhibition of K^+ secretion.

■ EFFECT OF DIURETICS ON THE EXCRETION OF WATER AND OTHER SOLUTES

Through their effects on Na^+ handling along the nephron, diuretics also influence the handling of water and other solutes. Table 10-1 summarizes the effects of the various diuretics on the handling of some of these solutes and the ability of

the kidneys to excrete (C_{H_2O}) and reabsorb ($T^C_{H_2O}$) solute-free water.

Solute-Free Water

As discussed in Chapter 5, the ability of the kidneys either to excrete or to reabsorb solute-free water depends on several factors. With regard to the action of diuretic agents the factors of concern are as follows:

1. The normal function of the nephron segments (particularly the thick ascending limb)
2. The delivery of adequate solute to Henle's loop
3. The maintenance of a hyperosmotic medullary interstitium (reabsorption of solute-free water only)

The thick ascending limb of Henle's loop is the most important site for the separation of solute and water. As noted above, this separation not only dilutes the tubular fluid but, by estab-

TABLE 10-1

Urinary excretion of water and some solutes with diuretics

Diuretic	Na^+ excretion (%)*	K^+ excretion	HCO_3^- excretion	Ca^{++} excretion	C_{H_2O}	$T^C_{H_2O}$
Osmotic diuretic	10	↑	↑	↑	↑	↑
Acetazolamide	5-10	↑	↑	↑	↑	↑
Bumetanide	25	↑	↓	↑	↓	↓
Ethacrynic acid	25	↑	↓	↑	↓	↓
Furosemide	25	↑	↓	↑	↓	↓
Chlorothiazide	5-10	↑	↓	↓	↓	Unchanged
Metolazone	5-10	↑	↓	↓	↓	Unchanged
Amiloride	3	↓	↑	Unchanged†	Unchanged	Unchanged
Spironolactone	3	↓	↑	Unchanged†	Unchanged	Unchanged
Triamterene	3	↓	↑	Unchanged†	Unchanged	Unchanged

*Percent of filtered load excreted into the urine.
†Ca^{++} excretion does decrease slightly with K^+-sparing diuretics, but the effect is insignificant.
All the effects (except HCO_3^- excretion) reflect the initial effect of the diuretic. The effects of the loop and thiazide diuretics on HCO_3^- excretion occur with prolonged use of these drugs and are secondary to the diuretic-induced decrease in effective circulating volume.

lishing a hyperosmotic medullary interstitium, allows for water reabsorption from the collecting duct and thus concentration of the urine. Inhibition of thick ascending limb reabsorption by loop diuretics therefore results in inhibition of both C_{H_2O} and $T^C_{H_2O}$.

The early portion of the distal tubule is also a site of solute and water separation and thus tubular fluid dilution. Accordingly, inhibition of transport by the thiazide diuretics impairs dilution of the urine and thus reduces C_{H_2O}. Thiazide diuretics impair urine dilution to a lesser degree than do loop diuretics, reflecting the difference in NaCl reabsorptive capacity between the distal tubule (5%-10% of the filtered load) and the thick ascending limb (25% of the filtered load). In contrast to the loop diuretics, thiazide diuretics do not significantly impair the ability of the kidneys to concentrate the urine. As already noted, concentration of the urine requires a hyperosmotic medullary interstitium so that water can be reabsorbed from the collecting duct in the presence of ADH. Because thiazide diuretics act on distal tubules that are located in the cortex, their action at this site does not appreciably alter the medullary interstitial osmotic gradient. Consequently, urine-concentrating ability, and thus the generation of $T^C_{H_2O}$, is unaffected by thiazide diuretics.

The action of diuretics in the proximal tubule (osmotic diuretics and carbonic anhydrase inhibitors) results in an increase in the delivery of NaCl and water to Henle's loop. In view of the thick ascending limb's ability to increase its transport rate in response to an increased delivered load of NaCl, the separation of solute and water increases. As a result, these diuretic agents increase the ability of the kidneys to produce either C_{H_2O} or $T^C_{H_2O}$.

Although the late portion of the distal tubule and the collecting duct are able to dilute the luminal fluid in the absence of ADH, Na$^+$ transport in these segments is not of sufficient magnitude to contribute significantly to the generation of C_{H_2O}. Consequently, the K$^+$-sparing diuretics do not appreciably alter this parameter or the kidneys' ability to generate $T^C_{H_2O}$.

K$^+$ Handling

One of the major consequences of diuretic use (excluding the K$^+$-sparing diuretics) is increased excretion of K$^+$. This can be of sufficient magnitude to result in hypokalemia. The basis for this diuretic-induced increase in renal K$^+$ excretion lies in the fact that when a diuretic inhibits Na$^+$ and water reabsorption in segments upstream from the late portion of the distal tubule and cortical collecting duct (K$^+$ secretory site of the nephron), tubular fluid flow rate increases. The increased tubular fluid flow rate stimulates K$^+$ secretion at this site (see Chapter 7). In addition, by their action on Na$^+$ balance, diuretics decrease the ECV. This in turn leads to increased secretion of aldosterone by the adrenal cortex (see Chapter 6), which acts at this site to stimulate K$^+$ secretion. The K$^+$-sparing diuretics prevent the increase in K$^+$ excretion caused by the other diuretics; therefore they are usually given in combination with these other diuretics to prevent or at least minimize the development of hypokalemia.

Trimethoprim is an antibiotic used to treat *Pneumocystis carinii* infections. *P. carinii* infections are frequently seen in individuals whose immune systems are compromised (e.g., individuals with acquired immunodeficiency syndrome [AIDS]). Hyperkalemia may occur in individuals treated with trimethoprim and is a result of reduced renal K$^+$ excretion. K$^+$ excretion is reduced because trimethoprim inhibits K$^+$ secretion by the principal cells of the late distal tubule and cortical collecting duct. The mechanism for this inhibition of K$^+$ secretion is similar to that of amiloride and triamterene (i.e., inhibition of the Na$^+$ channel in the apical membrane of the cell).

HCO_3^- Handling

By inhibiting HCO_3^- reabsorption in the proximal tubule and thereby increasing HCO_3^- excretion, carbonic anhydrase inhibitors can result in the development of a metabolic acidosis. With this acidosis the filtered load of HCO_3^- is reduced (i.e., the plasma $[HCO_3^-]$ is reduced). This results in less HCO_3^- available for reabsorption, which diminishes the effectiveness of carbonic anhydrase inhibitors.

Although only carbonic anhydrase inhibitors directly alter HCO_3^- handling by the nephron, all diuretics can secondarily affect systemic acid-base balance. Both loop and thiazide diuretics can induce a metabolic alkalosis, which is a consequence of the decrease in ECV that accompanies their use. With a decrease in the ECV, Na^+ is more avidly reabsorbed in the proximal tubule (see Chapter 6). Because HCO_3^- is reabsorbed together with Na^+ in this segment, proximal tubule HCO_3^- reabsorption increases. Additionally the reduction in ECV stimulates aldosterone secretion by the adrenal cortex. As discussed in Chapter 8, aldosterone stimulates H^+ secretion by intercalated cells of the collecting duct. Because proximal tubule HCO_3^- reabsorption is increased, virtually none of the filtered load of HCO_3^- reaches the collecting duct. Therefore the increased H^+ secretion that occurs in the collecting duct results in the production of new HCO_3^- as the H^+ is excreted with non-HCO_3^- urinary buffers (e.g., ammonia and titratable acid). This new HCO_3^- is added to the plasma and produces a metabolic alkalosis.

By inhibiting Na^+ reabsorption in the late portion of the distal tubule and cortical collecting duct, K^+-sparing diuretics secondarily inhibit H^+ secretion and can lead to the development of a metabolic acidosis. H^+ secretion is facilitated by a lumen-negative transepithelial voltage. Normally, Na^+ reabsorption in these nephron segments results in the generation of such a voltage. By inhibiting Na^+ reabsorption and thus the negative luminal voltage, K^+-sparing diuretics reduce H^+ secretion. With reduced H^+ secretion, insufficient quantities of net acid are excreted and a metabolic acidosis ensues.

Ca^{++} and Pi Handling

With the exception of K^+-sparing diuretics, all the diuretics can significantly alter Ca^{++} handling by the kidney. With inhibition of proximal tubule solute and water reabsorption (osmotic diuretics and carbonic anhydrase inhibitors), there is reduced reabsorption of Ca^{++} and thus increased excretion. The amount of Ca^{++} excreted is less than expected from inhibition of proximal tubule transport. This again reflects the ability of the downstream segments (particularly the thick ascending limb of Henle's loop) to increase reabsorption following an increased delivered load. The mechanism by which these diuretics inhibit proximal tubule Ca^{++} reabsorption is related to their ability to reduce solvent drag (see Chapter 9). With the use of carbonic anhydrase inhibitors, increased Ca^{++} excretion occurs in the setting of an alkaline urine (increased urinary $[HCO_3^-]$). Because Ca^{++} is less soluble in alkaline urine, the potential exists for the formation of Ca^{++}-containing renal stones.

Loop diuretics also increase Ca^{++} excretion, an action explained by the effect of these diuretics on the transepithelial voltage of the thick ascending limb of Henle's loop. Normally the transepithelial voltage of this segment is oriented lumen-positive (see Chapter 4), providing a driving force for the movement of Ca^{++} from the lumen to blood through the paracellular pathway (see Chapter 9). When transport of NaCl by Henle's loop is blocked by loop diuretics, this lumen-positive voltage is abolished and the driving force for Ca^{++} reabsorption is reduced. Normally Henle's loop reabsorbs about 20% of the filtered load of Ca^{++} (see Chapter 9). Inhibition of Ca^{++} reabsorption by loop diuretics can therefore have a significant effect on overall Ca^{++} balance. For this reason, loop diuretics are frequently used to treat hypercalcemia. Despite this action of loop diuretics, hypercalcemia can occur with their long-term use. The mechanism responsible for this effect is related to the diuretic-induced decrease in the ECV. When the ECV is decreased, proximal tubule reabsorption is enhanced, which in turn increases Ca^{++} reabsorption at this site and therefore decreases urinary Ca^{++} excretion.

Thiazide diuretics stimulate Ca^{++} reabsorption by the cells of the distal tubule and thus reduce Ca^{++} excretion. The distal tubule normally reabsorbs approximately 9% of the filtered load of Ca^{++} (see Chapter 9). The reabsorption of Ca^{++} at this site is an active, transcellular process involving entry of Ca^{++} into the cell via channels in the apical membrane and extrusion from the cell across the basolateral membrane by Ca^{++}-ATPase and 3Na$^+$-Ca^{++} antiporter. The thiazide diuretics, by inhibiting the entry of NaCl into the cell, cause the membrane potential to hyperpolarize (i.e., the cell interior becomes more electrically negative).[39] This hyperpolarization in turn increases the amount of time the apical membrane Ca^{++} channels are open, as well as increasing the electrochemical gradient for Ca^{++} entry into the cell. The net effect is an increase in Ca^{++} reabsorption. (The increased entry of Ca^{++} into the cell is matched by an increased extrusion across the basolateral membrane by the Ca^{++}-ATPase and 3Na$^+$-Ca^{++} antiporter.) Because thiazides reduce urinary Ca^{++} excretion, they are sometimes used to lower the incidence of Ca^{++}-containing stone formation in individuals who normally excrete high levels of Ca^{++} in their urine.

---

[39] Hyperpolarization of the membrane potential occurs as a result of a decrease in the intracellular [Cl$^-$]. The basolateral membrane of the distal tubule cell contains Cl$^-$ channels; thus, the membrane potential is determined in part by the Cl$^-$ equilibrium potential. A decrease in the intracellular [Cl$^-$] increases the magnitude of this equilibrium potential (i.e., it becomes more negative).

The K$^+$-sparing diuretics increase Ca^{++} reabsorption by the cortical collecting duct. However, the magnitude of this effect is small, and its mechanism is not completely understood.

With the exception of the K$^+$-sparing diuretics, all diuretics acutely increase Pi excretion. However, the cellular mechanisms for this effect are not completely understood. The effect is modified, however, with long-term diuretic therapy. With the decrease in ECV that accompanies long-term diuretic use, proximal tubule Na$^+$ reabsorption is stimulated. Because the proximal tubule reabsorbs the largest portion of the filtered load of Pi and because this reabsorptive process is coupled with Na$^+$ (see Chapters 4 and 9), Pi excretion is reduced in this setting.

■ SUMMARY

1. Diuretics inhibit solute (primarily NaCl) transport at various sites along the nephron. As a result of their action, the excretion of solute and water by the kidneys increases.
2. By increasing the excretion of NaCl by the kidneys, diuretics cause a decrease in ECV and the volume of the ECF. This decreased ECF volume results in a loss of body weight.
3. The ability of a particular diuretic to increase solute and water excretion depends upon several factors, including the nephron segment where the diuretic acts, the ability of nephron segments distal to the diuretic's site of action to increase their reabsorption of solute and water, the delivery of sufficient quantities of the diuretic to its site of action, and the ECV.
4. Osmotic diuretics inhibit solute and water reabsorption in the proximal tubule and descending thin limb of Henle's loop. Quantitatively the proximal tubule is the more important site of action.
5. Carbonic anhydrase inhibitors act primarily in the proximal tubule to inhibit Na$^+$, HCO$_3^-$, and water reabsorption.

6. Loop diuretics inhibit NaCl reabsorption by the thick ascending limb of Henle's loop. They are the most potent diuretics and can increase Na^+ excretion to as much as 25% of the filtered load.

7. Thiazide diuretics inhibit NaCl reabsorption in the distal tubule. They also stimulate Ca^{++} reabsorption at this site.

8. K^+-sparing diuretics act at the late portion of the distal tubule and the cortical collecting duct. They inhibit Na^+ reabsorption and in doing so inhibit K^+ secretion. Their most important use is related to their ability to reduce renal K^+ excretion.

9. Osmotic diuretics and carbonic anhydrase inhibitors increase the ability of the kidneys to excrete and reabsorb solute-free water. The loop diuretics impair both solute-free water reabsorption and excretion, while the thiazide diuretics impair only solute-free water excretion. The K^+-sparing diuretics do not have a significant effect on solute-free water excretion.

10. All diuretics, with the exception of the K^+-sparing diuretics, increase the renal excretion of K^+. This effect is in response to increased delivery of tubular fluid to the K^+ secretory portion of the nephron (distal tubule and cortical collecting duct) and increased aldosterone levels secondary to the diuretic-induced decrease in the ECV.

11. The carbonic anhydrase inhibitors and K^+-sparing diuretics can induce a metabolic acidosis. The loop diuretics and thiazide diuretics can cause a metabolic alkalosis.

■ **KEY WORDS AND CONCEPTS**

- Natriuresis
- Steady state
- Organic anion and organic cation secretory systems

- Osmotic diuretics
- Carbonic anhydrase inhibitors
- Loop diuretics
- Thiazide diuretics
- K^+-sparing diuretics

■ **SELF-STUDY PROBLEMS**

1. Diuretics are administered to two groups of individuals: Group 1 subjects are water loaded and produce dilute urine, whereas Group 2 subjects are water deprived and produce concentrated urine. After control urine and plasma samples are obtained, each individual receives one of three diuretics, and urine and plasma samples are again obtained. Calculate C_{H_2O} and $T^C_{H_2O}$. Based on the effect of the diuretics on these parameters, identify the class of diuretic administered. (See table on p. 182.)

2. Patients with nephrogenic diabetes insipidus can obtain symptomatic relief from their polyuria with long-term use of a thiazide diuretic. What is the mechanism by which long-term thiazide therapy produces a decrease in urine volume in these patients?

3. An individual takes a thiazide diuretic as partial therapy for hypertension. Before therapy, plasma $[K^+]$ is 4 mEq/L. After several months of therapy, the individual's blood pressure is reduced and plasma $[K^+]$ is 3 mEq/L.
   a. By what mechanism could the diuretic lead to a decrease in blood pressure?
   b. By what mechanism did the plasma $[K^+]$ fall? What other classes of diuretics would produce this effect?
   c. What can be done to increase the plasma $[K^+]$ to the level it was before diuretic therapy was initiated?

4. The antibiotic penicillin is secreted into the urine by the organic anion secretory system of the proximal tubule. If an individual taking a thiazide diuretic for hypertension develops an infection requiring penicillin, what effect, if any, could this have on the action of the diuretic?

Condition	P_{osm} (mOsm/kg H_2O)	U_{osm} (mOsm/kg H_2O)	$\dot{V}$ (ml/min)	C_{H_2O} (ml/min)	$T^c_{H_2O}$ (ml/min)
Water Diuresis					
Before diuretic A	285	70	10	_____	_____
After diuretic A	284	125	16	_____	_____
Before diuretic B	286	65	12	_____	_____
After diuretic B	286	200	19	_____	_____
Before diuretic C	284	70	11	_____	_____
After diuretic C	285	195	15	_____	_____
Antidiuresis					
Before diuretic A	288	1,200	0.6	_____	_____
After diuretic A	289	450	12	_____	_____
Before diuretic B	290	1,100	0.7	_____	_____
After diuretic B	288	300	13	_____	_____
Before diuretic C	287	1,200	0.7	_____	_____
After diuretic C	290	355	10	_____	_____

Diuretic A: _____

Diuretic B: _____

Diuretic C: _____

11

Physiologic Adaptation to Nephron Loss

OBJECTIVES

Upon completion of this chapter the student should be able to answer the following questions:

1. What changes in structure and function do nephrons undergo to compensate for the loss of other nephrons to disease processes?
2. What is the "intact nephron hypothesis," and how does it help explain the adaptation of nephrons to the loss of other nephrons to disease processes?

3. How is steady state balance maintained as the number of functioning nephrons is reduced by disease?
4. What are the adaptive responses of the nephrons for the maintenance of steady state balance of water, Na^+, K^+, pH, HCO_3^-, Ca^{++}, and Pi?
5. What happens to steady state balance when the limits of the adaptive response to nephron loss are exceeded?

The nephrons of the kidneys have a remarkable ability to adapt their function and are able to do so under a wide range of conditions. The preceding chapters have focused on how nephrons regulate their function and respond to the homeostatic needs of the healthy individual. However, further insight into the function of the nephrons and, in particular, the range over which physiologic adaptation can occur may be gained by considering how nephrons respond to disease processes. A number of disease processes can have an impact on the kidneys and impair their function. Some of these processes are reversible

and may impair renal function only temporarily (e.g., decreased renal perfusion secondary to hemorrhage, obstruction of the ureter by a renal stone), whereas others permanently impair renal function by reducing the number of nephrons (e.g., diabetes mellitus, hypertension). This chapter examines the physiologic response of nephrons as their number is reduced by disease processes.[40] It is intended to emphasize physiologic

_____

40 In this context, any process that results in a permanent loss of nephrons is termed *renal disease*.

183

principles already discussed and introduce students to some new pathophysiologic principles.

■ MAINTENANCE OF STEADY STATE BALANCE

As noted in the preceding chapters, the kidneys have the capacity to vary the excretion of many solutes and water over a wide range. This capacity to regulate excretion is essential for the maintenance of steady state fluid and electrolyte balance in the face of wide fluctuations in dietary intake.

With appropriate diets, individuals with renal disease are able to maintain **steady state balance** (i.e., intake = excretion) for most electrolytes and water even if their kidneys have only 10% to 15% of the full complement of nephrons. Beyond this point, steady state balance is increasingly difficult to achieve, and therapies to replace renal function (e.g., hemodialysis, kidney transplantation) must be initiated.

Steady state balance can be achieved as long as the excretory capacity of the kidneys is sufficient to accommodate dietary intake. If renal excretory capacity is reduced by disease, dietary intake must also be reduced accordingly. Figure 11-1 illustrates ranges for excretion of water and Na^+. In a healthy individual with normal functioning kidneys, water excretion, and thus water intake, can be varied from as little as 0.5 L/day to as much as 18 L/day. However, as nephrons are lost to disease, this range narrows. When the total number of nephrons is only 10% to 15% of normal the excretory range is 1 to 4 L/day (see Figure 11-1). Thus, ingestion of less than 1 L/day of water leads to negative water balance, and body fluid osmolality increases. Conversely, positive water balance occurs if water intake exceeds 4 L/day, and body fluid osmolality decreases. A similar narrowing of the regulatory range is seen for Na^+. Normal kidneys can virtually eliminate all Na^+ from the urine or increase excretion to

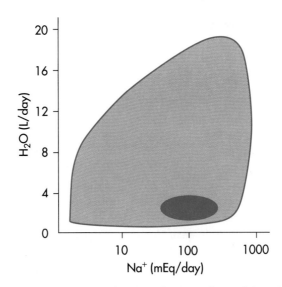

Figure 11-1 ■ Ranges for excretion of water and Na^+ with normal renal function (shaded area) and with renal disease in which the kidneys have only 10% to 15% of the normal number of nephrons (filled area). Steady state balance for both water and Na^+ can be achieved if dietary ingestion is matched to the excretory ability of the kidneys. See text for details. (Modified from Meyer TW, Baboolal K, Brenner BM: *Nephron adaptation to injury.* In Brenner BM, editor: *The kidney,* ed 5, Philadelphia, 1996, WB Saunders.)

nearly 1000 mEq/day. However, as nephrons are lost, this range is reduced. With only 10% to 15% of the normal number of nephrons, Na⁺ excretion can vary only between 75 and 200 mEq/day. Consequently, a diet containing less than 75 mEq/day of Na⁺ leads to a decrease in the effective circulating volume (ECV), whereas ingestion of more than 200 mEq/day of Na⁺ expands the ECV.

Steady state balance may be achieved with or without a change in the plasma concentration of the solute. Table 11-1 summarizes how the plasma concentrations of various solutes change with **progressive nephron loss.**

The maintenance of steady state balance for a substance that is excreted largely by glomerular filtration (e.g., creatinine, urea) is achieved at progressively higher plasma concentrations. The reason for this can be understood by considering the following equation:

$$U_x \times \dot{V} = GFR \times P_x \qquad (11\text{-}1)$$

where $U_x \times \dot{V}$ is the excretion rate of the substance, and P_x is its concentration in the plasma (see also Chapter 3). If production or intake of x is constant, its plasma concentration must increase as the GFR decreases in order to maintain a constant rate of excretion. Because of this relationship, the plasma concentration of a substance excreted primarily by filtration alone (e.g., creatinine) increases progressively with decreasing GFR (Figure 11-2).

In contrast to creatinine, the plasma concentration of a number of solutes (e.g., Na⁺, K⁺) can be maintained at a relatively constant level even as GFR declines. For these solutes, excretion does not solely depend on the glomerular filtration rate but also reflects tubular transport. It is the ability of the nephrons to alter transport rates for these solutes that allows for greater control of the plasma concentration.

T A B L E 1 1 - 1

Regulation of some solutes with progressive nephron loss

Little or no regulation: Plasma concentrations increase as nephrons are lost.
- Creatinine
- Urea

Partial regulation: Plasma concentrations can be maintained until 50% to 70% of nephrons are lost.
- HCO_3^-
- Ca^{++}
- Pi

Near-complete regulation: Plasma concentrations can be maintained until 75% to 90% of nephrons are lost.
- Water (P_{osm})
- Na⁺
- K⁺

The ability to regulate the plasma concentration of a solute may also require adjustments in dietary intake.

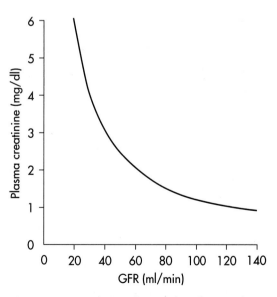

Figure 11-2 ■ **Relationship of the plasma creatinine concentration to the glomerular filtration rate (GFR). The plasma creatinine concentration doubles each time the GFR is reduced by half.**

■ STRUCTURAL AND FUNCTIONAL ADAPTATION TO NEPHRON LOSS

The ways in which diseased kidneys function to maintain fluid and electrolyte balance in the face of a reduced number of nephrons are described by the **intact nephron hypothesis.** This hypothesis recognizes that the structure and function of the remaining nephrons may be altered as compared with those of undiseased kidneys. However, the hypothesis assumes that glomeruli do not filter fluid into nonfunctioning tubules, and normal tubules do not function with nonfiltering glomeruli. Thus, according to the intact nephron hypothesis, the physiologic response of diseased kidneys results from the ability of the remaining nephrons to function essentially as intact nephron units, albeit in an abnormal environment.

Structural Changes

The adult kidney does not have the capacity to regenerate nephrons. However, as nephrons are lost, the remaining nephrons compensate by undergoing hypertrophy.[41] This hypertrophy is seen along the entire nephron. The glomeruli can increase in diameter by approximately 50%. The cells of the proximal tubule can also increase in size, resulting in an increase in both tubule diameter and tubule length. Similar changes may also be seen in the distal portions of the nephron, although the hypertrophy is not as marked as that seen in the proximal tubule.

The signals and factors responsible for this hypertrophic response are incompletely understood. Initial efforts to understand this phenomenon focused on the increased "work" imposed on the **remaining functioning nephrons** as they try to maintain steady state balance for various solutes. Unfortunately, this

concept of work hypertrophy provides little insight into the underlying mechanisms that couple the increased work load to the process of hypertrophy. Increasing evidence suggests that several autocrine, paracrine, and endocrine factors play roles in this adaptive response (e.g., angiotensin II, transforming growth factor [TGF-β], insulin-like growth factor).

Membrane transporter (e.g., Na^+-K^+-ATPase) activity in remaining functional nephrons increases in accordance with the structural hypertrophy. Many enzymes also increase their activity in the hypertrophied remaining functional nephrons. For example, the enzymes responsible for the metabolism of glutamine to ammonium in the proximal tubule increase, which allows the remaining functioning nephrons to excrete more net acid as ammonium in an effort to maintain acid-base balance (see below).

Functional Changes

The hypertrophic response of the kidneys to the loss of nephrons has several functional consequences. These functional adaptations, occurring at both the glomerulus and tubule, are important for the kidneys' ability to maintain fluid and electrolyte balance.

Glomerulus Hypertrophy of the remaining functional glomeruli results in an increase in their filtration rate. Thus, whereas whole kidney glomerular filtration rate (GFR) declines because of the loss of nephrons, the **single nephron glomerular filtration rate (SNGFR)** increases.

SNGFR increases secondary to an increase in the glomerular capillary hydrostatic pressure (P_{GC}). This increase in P_{GC} is thought to be mediated by dilation of the afferent arterioles, which appears to be mediated by the local release of vasoactive substances. One likely group of vasoactive mediators is the prostaglandins, because administration of nonsteroidal antiinflammatory agents, which act by inhibiting prostaglandin synthesis, can reduce renal plasma flow and GFR in

---

41 *Hypertrophy* refers to an increase in size of existing cells. Hyperplasia (increased numbers of cells) also occurs but to a lesser degree than hypertrophy.

individuals with renal disease, especially those individuals whose ECV is also reduced (see Chapter 3). Additional mediators are probably involved as well, although these have not yet been identified.

Because glomerular volume is increased, an increase in the surface area available for filtration might be expected to contribute to the increase in SNGFR. However, measurements in animal model systems have not revealed significant changes in the glomerular filtration coefficient (K_f). Because K_f depends on both surface area and intrinsic permeability, it would appear that although the area available for filtration is increased, the permeability of the filtration barrier is decreased. The net effect is no change in the K_f.

The increase in SNGFR in the remaining functioning nephrons can be viewed as a beneficial adaptation because an increase in SNGFR would enhance the ability of the kidneys to excrete various substances (e.g., creatinine and urea). However, hyperfiltration, and in particular the elevated P_{GC}, appears to damage the glomerulus. The increase in P_{GC} causes the capillary walls to thicken, eventually resulting in scarring and obliteration of the glomerulus. This hyperfiltration-induced obliteration of glomeruli contributes to the progressive loss of renal function.

Therapy is now directed at reducing P_{GC} in the glomeruli of remaining functioning nephrons in an attempt to minimize capillary wall thickening and scarring. Angiotensin-converting enzyme (ACE) inhibitors have shown some promise in this regard. When patients with diseases that cause progressive nephron loss are treated with ACE inhibitors, the rate of nephron loss is slowed. This beneficial effect would seem to indicate that angiotensin II is somehow involved in the elevation of P_{GC} normally seen in the remaining functioning nephrons.

Proximal Tubule Several important functional adaptations of the proximal tubule have been identified. The first is an increased capacity to reabsorb the glomerular filtrate. This increased reabsorptive capacity parallels proximal tubule hypertrophy and, more importantly, is matched to the increase in SNGFR. Thus, glomerulotubular balance (GT balance) remains intact. The maintenance of GT balance allows the proximal tubule to reabsorb the increased filtered load of several important constituents of the glomerular filtrate (e.g., glucose, amino acids) that might otherwise be lost in the urine. Second, glutamine metabolism by the proximal tubule is increased. As noted previously and discussed in more detail later, this allows for increased excretion of net acid as ammonium by each remaining functional nephron. Finally, Pi reabsorption by the proximal tubule is reduced. The reduction in Pi reabsorption is mediated in part by elevated levels of parathyroid hormone (PTH). The adaptive advantage of this change in proximal tubule Pi reabsorption is considered in more detail later.

Loop of Henle The capacity of the loop of Henle to reabsorb NaCl is enhanced in the remaining functioning nephrons. Because reabsorption of NaCl at this site results in the separation of solute and water, the capacity to either excrete or reabsorb solute-free water at the single nephron level is enhanced. However, structural changes can occur in the medulla as a result of disease processes (e.g., scarring and obliteration of vasa recta), impairing the ability of the loop of Henle and vasa recta to maintain the hyperosmotic medullary interstitial gradient. In this situation the overall ability of the kidneys to concentrate the urine is impaired.

Distal Tubule and Collecting Duct With progressive nephron loss the capacity of both the distal tubule and the cortical collecting duct to secrete K^+ increases. This increase in secretory capacity plays an important role in allowing the remaining functioning nephrons to maintain

K+ balance even when 85% to 90% of nephrons have been lost.

■ SOLUTE AND WATER TRANSPORT BY THE REMAINING FUNCTIONING NEPHRONS

As nephrons are lost to disease, the remaining functional nephrons must excrete increasingly more solute and water in order to maintain steady state balance. For example, a tenfold reduction in the number of nephrons would require a tenfold increase in the excretion of a substance by the remaining functioning nephrons.

As already noted, the adaptive response of diseased kidneys is quite effective, and steady state balance can be maintained for many solutes and water even with only 10% to 15% of the normal number of nephrons, provided appropriate modifications of the diet occur. However, there are limits to the adaptive response in terms of both

the range of excretion rate and the time course of the excretory response to dietary challenge. Thus, rapid excretion of a large solute or water load does not occur, and patients with renal disease are more prone to fluid and volume overload (increased effective circulating volume), hyperkalemia, and acidosis. Similarly the kidneys cannot adapt quickly and completely to marked reductions in intake of solutes and water. Therefore patients with renal disease are also more prone to dehydration and depletion of their effective circulating volume. Table 11-2 summarizes changes in the plasma levels of some solutes as nephrons are lost to disease. Also summarized are some functional parameters of the kidneys.

Sodium

In a normal individual the renal excretion of the daily intake of Na^+ (150 mEq/day) occurs with a

TABLE 11-2

Effects of progressive nephron loss on the plasma concentration of some solutes and urine concentrating ability

	GFR (% of normal)				
	100	65	33	20	10
Plasma [Na^+]-mEq/L	140	140	140	138	136
Plasma [K^+]-mEq/L	4	4	4	4.5	5.5
Plasma [Ca^{++}]-mg/dl	10	10	10	8.7	8.2
Plasma [Pi]-mg/dl	4	4.2	4.3	5.2	5.8
Plasma [HCO_3^-]-mEq/L	24	24	22	16	13
Plasma [creatinine]-mg/dl	1	1.6	3.1	5.0	10.4
Plasma BUN-mg/dl	14	18	29	46	82
Plasma pH	7.4	7.4	7.37	7.3	7.26
P_{osm}-mOsm/kg H_2O	290	292	295	300	310
Max. U_{osm}-mOsm/kg H_2O	1200	1000	500	350	310
Min. U_{osm}-mOsm/kg H_2O	50	50	70	200	310

The values used here illustrate the direction and typical changes that occur with progressive nephron loss. The values for a given individual may vary from those listed. *BUN*, Blood urea nitrogen.

fractional excretion (amount excreted/amount filtered $\times$ 100) of less than 1%. To maintain Na^+ balance with this same diet, fractional excretion rates must increase as the total number of nephrons decreases. For example, if the GFR is reduced to 10% of normal, fractional excretion would have to increase to 6% (Table 11-3).

With moderate degrees of renal impairment the adaptation to increase the fractional excretion of Na^+ appears to occur in the distal tubule and collecting duct. As noted previously, GT balance operates under these conditions. Thus, despite the increased filtered load of Na^+, proximal tubule reabsorption is increased proportionately. Because fractional Na^+ excretion is increased, distal tubule and collecting duct reabsorption must be reduced. The mechanisms for this reduction in Na^+ reabsorption by the distal tubule and collecting duct are not understood. Current theories have focused on the role of circulating natriuretic substances such as ANP and urodilatin, although other natriuretic substances may also be involved.

With more advanced degrees of nephron loss, fractional Na^+ reabsorption by the proximal tubule is reduced. Under this setting the entire nephron contributes to the increase in fractional Na^+ excretion. The mechanism underlying the decrease in proximal tubule fractional Na^+ reabsorption has been attributed to the presence of an osmotic diuresis in the remaining functioning nephrons. This osmotic diuresis results from the increased concentration of poorly reabsorbed solutes in the glomerular filtrate (e.g., creatinine, urea).

With increasing nephron loss the ability of the kidneys to respond to increases in Na^+ intake becomes progressively more impaired. This is not surprising, given the fact that each remaining nephron functions closer and closer to its maximum capacity as nephrons are progressively lost to disease. When these nephrons are challenged beyond their capacity, the patient experiences positive Na^+ balance with expansion of effective circulating volume. Depending on the magnitude of this expansion, the patient may exhibit signs of generalized and pulmonary edema (see Chapter 6).

As the number of functioning nephrons is reduced, the capacity to conserve Na^+ decreases. Normally the renal excretion of Na^+ can be reduced to 1 or 2 mEq/day. However, the osmotic diuresis that develops in the remaining functioning nephrons necessitates the loss of increasingly larger quantities of Na^+. As a result, patients with renal failure can develop negative Na^+ balance, with a decrease in effective circulating volume if Na^+ intake is restricted.

TABLE 11-3

Na^+ balance with progressive nephron loss

	GFR (% of normal)				
	100	**65**	**33**	**20**	**10**
Plasma [Na^+]-mEq/L	140	140	140	138	134
Na^+ excretion rate*-mEq/day	150	150	150	150	150
Filtered load of Na^+-mEq/day	25,200	16,380	8316	4968	2412
Fractional excretion of Na^+-%	0.6	0.9	1.8	3	6

*Daily ingestion of Na^+ = 150 mEq.

Water

As nephrons are lost, the ability to regulate water balance and therefore the osmolality of the body fluids is impaired (see Figure 11-1). Concomitantly, the range of urine osmolality becomes narrower, leading ultimately to the production of urine with an osmolality near that of plasma (see Table 11-2).

The production of smaller volumes of urine with an osmolality similar to plasma results from the osmotic diuresis that develops in the remaining functioning nephrons. With the increased tubular flow induced by the osmotic diuresis, there is almost no change in the composition of the tubular fluid as it flows through the remaining functioning nephrons. In addition, disease-induced structural changes in the kidney, especially the renal medulla, can impair the countercurrent multiplication process. Without countercurrent multiplication the medullary interstitial osmotic gradient cannot be established, and water reabsorption from the collecting duct in the presence of ADH is therefore impaired.

Whole kidney C_{H_2O} and $T^c_{H_2O}$ are decreased as nephrons are lost. However, at the level of the remaining functioning nephrons the separation of solute and water (and thus C_{H_2O} and $T^c_{H_2O}$) is actually increased. The increase in these parameters reflects an increased capacity for NaCl reabsorption by the thick ascending limb of Henle's loop and increased delivery of solute and water to this segment, secondary to the osmotic diuresis. Thus, with advancing renal failure, C_{H_2O} and $T^c_{H_2O}$ per nephron are increased. However, because of the reduced number of nephrons and the reduced medullary interstitial osmotic gradient, whole kidney C_{H_2O} and $T^c_{H_2O}$ are decreased.

For the individual with reduced renal function, these changes in water handling by the kidneys mean that water intake must be carefully monitored. Ingestion of too much solute-free water results in the development of positive water balance (intake > excretion) and a decrease in

P_{osm}. Conversely, ingestion of inadequate amounts of water leads to negative water balance and an increase in P_{osm}.

Acid-Base

As indicated in Table 11-1, regulation of acid-base balance becomes impaired when 50% to 70% of nephrons are lost. This reflects the fact that excretion of net acid by the remaining functioning nephrons is reduced below levels necessary to balance the amount of nonvolatile acid generated through metabolism.

Net acid excretion by the kidney equals the amount of new HCO_3^- generated and reflects the amount of H^+ excreted as titratable acid and NH_4^+, minus the amount of HCO_3^- excreted:

$$NAE = (U_{NH_4^+} \times \dot{V}) + (U_{TA} \times \dot{V}) - (U_{HCO_3^-} \times \dot{V}) \quad \text{(11-2)}$$

A reduction in net acid excretion can occur by a defect in HCO_3^- reabsorption, an inability maximally to acidify the urine, and a decrease in the production of urinary buffers. With progressive nephron loss, net acid excretion is reduced primarily because ammonium is generated in insufficient quantities by the remaining functioning nephrons. At the level of each nephron, ammonium generation is actually increased because the developing systemic acidosis stimulates the enzymes responsible for glutamine metabolism. However, despite this adaptive response the reduced number of remaining functioning nephrons results in an overall decrease in the production and excretion of this important urinary buffer. In general, HCO_3^- reabsorption by the proximal tubule and H^+ secretion by the collecting duct are relatively normal in the remaining functioning nephrons.

As nephron loss progresses and hyperkalemia develops (see p. 191), the amount of ammonium generated by the remaining functioning nephrons is reduced. This reduction in ammonium production is caused by hyperkalemia (see Chapter 8).

The metabolic acidosis seen with chronic renal disease is associated with an increase in the anion gap (see Chapter 8). The anion gap increases because the salts of the nonvolatile acids are not adequately excreted by the kidneys and accumulate in the body fluids (e.g., $SO_4^=$, organic anions). As HCO_3^- is consumed in the titration of these metabolically produced nonvolatile acids, the associated anions, which are unmeasured when determining the anion gap, increase in concentration and thereby increase the anion gap.

Potassium

Potassium balance is relatively well maintained with progressive nephron loss. As indicated in Table 11-1, plasma [K^+] can be maintained with as few as 10% to 15% of the normal number of nephrons.[42]

In both normal and diseased kidneys, renal K^+ handling reflects reabsorption of K^+ in the proximal tubule and loop of Henle and secretion in the distal tubule and collecting duct. With progressive nephron loss, K^+ secretion by the distal tubule and collecting duct increases in the remaining functioning nephrons. This adaptive response results from increased tubular fluid flow rate secondary to the osmotic diuresis. In addition, the capacity of the principal cells of the distal tubule and collecting duct to secrete K^+ is enhanced. In response to transient elevations in the plasma [K^+] following a K^+ load, the principal cells increase the activity of the Na^+-K^+-ATPase in the basolateral membrane. In addition, the ability of K^+ to cross the apical membrane increases. Together these changes result in increased cellular uptake of K^+ and increased secretion from cell to tubule lumen. These adaptive changes in

the principal cell do not require elevations in aldosterone levels.

Calcium and Phosphate

Abnormalities in Ca^{++} and Pi homeostasis with progressive nephron loss are complex and involve not only the kidneys but also the gastrointestinal tract, PTH, and calcitriol. In general, patients with progressive nephron loss develop positive Pi balance because of decreased excretion of Pi. In contrast, patients develop negative Ca^{++} balance with progressive nephron loss primarily because of decreased gastrointestinal absorption (see p. 192).

In normal kidneys, Pi handling involves filtration at the glomerulus and reabsorption primarily by the proximal tubule and Henle's loop (see Chapter 9). As renal failure progresses, the filtered load of Pi in functioning nephrons increases as SNGFR increases. Reabsorption of Pi by the remaining functioning nephrons is also reduced. Thus, each remaining functioning nephron excretes a larger fraction of the filtered Pi load. Despite these adaptive responses, Pi retention ultimately develops and the plasma [Pi] increases. This increase in plasma [Pi] is associated with a reciprocal decrease in plasma [Ca^{++}] (see Chapter 9).

The adaptation of the kidneys to maintain Pi homeostasis illustrates the **trade-off hypothesis.** The trade-off hypothesis simply states that a beneficial adaptive response by the kidneys may result in or be associated with an undesirable effect on other tissues or organ systems. In the case of Pi homeostasis the "trade-off" is the development of hyperparathyroidism and decreased bone mineralization (see Chapter 9). According to this hypothesis, reductions in GFR secondary to nephron loss result in small increases in the plasma [Pi]. The elevation in plasma [Pi] and the associated decrease in ionized [Ca^{++}] (because Pi complexes with Ca^{++}) consequently increase PTH secretion by the parathyroid glands. PTH

---

42 With progressive renal insufficiency, the descending colon increases K^+ secretion into the feces. This helps maintain K^+ homeostasis in patients with advanced renal disease.

acts on the proximal tubule to inhibit the reabsorption of Pi, thereby increasing Pi excretion by each remaining functioning nephron. Thus, renal Pi excretion is maintained, but PTH levels are elevated (secondary hyperparathyroidism). Because PTH also acts on bone to increase Ca^{++} release and thereby maintain the plasma $[Ca^{++}]$, the elevated PTH levels have the undesirable effect of demineralizing bone (see Chapter 9). Demineralization of the bone is further exacerbated by the systemic acidosis that develops with decreased renal excretion of net acid. As acidosis develops, H^+ is buffered by the bone, resulting in demineralization (see Chapter 8).

As discussed in Chapter 9, the kidneys are the primary site for the production of calcitriol. The primary action of this hormone is to stimulate absorption of Ca^{++} by the gastrointestinal tract. With progressive nephron loss the production of calcitriol is reduced. Consequently, intestinal Ca^{++} absorption is reduced, and negative Ca^{++} balance results.

■ SUMMARY

1. According to the intact nephron hypothesis, as nephrons are lost to disease, the remaining glomeruli and nephrons function as an intact unit (i.e., filtering glomeruli are not attached to nonfunctioning nephrons, and functioning nephrons are not attached to nonfiltering glomeruli).
2. As the number of nephrons is reduced, the range over which the kidneys can regulate the excretion of solutes and water is also reduced. In addition, the kidneys are unable to respond rapidly to changes in dietary intake. Consequently, individuals with renal disease are more prone to develop fluid, electrolyte, and acid-base disorders.
3. Steady state balance for many solutes and water can be maintained with renal disease pro-

vided that intake and excretion can be matched. Because the excretory capacity of diseased kidneys is limited, dietary intake of many substances must also be limited.
4. According to the trade-off hypothesis, adaptations required to maintain the excretory capacity of diseased kidneys may lead to undesirable effects on other organs (e.g., the development of secondary hyperparathyroidism).

■ KEY WORDS AND CONCEPTS

- Steady state balance
- Intact nephron hypothesis
- Nephron hypertrophy
- Single nephron glomerular filtration rate (SNGFR)
- Glomerular hyperfiltration
- Trade-off hypothesis
- Progressive nephron loss
- Remaining functioning nephrons

■ SELF-STUDY PROBLEMS

1. Indicate how each parameter listed changes with progressive nephron loss at the level of both the single functioning nephron and the kidneys overall (i.e., increase, decrease, or no change).

	Single nephron	Whole kidney
GFR	_____	_____
Fractional Na^+ excretion	_____	_____
C_{H_2O}	_____	_____
$T^c_{H_2O}$	_____	_____
Pi excretion	_____	_____
Ammonium excretion	_____	_____

2. Two individuals ingest a diet containing 150 mEq/day of Na^+. Individual A has normal renal function (GFR = 180 L/day). Individual B has renal disease (GFR = 50 L/day).

   a. Assuming both individuals are in steady state Na^+ balance, what are their respective Na^+ excretion rates?

      Individual A = _____ mEq of Na^+/day
      Individual B = _____ mEq of Na^+/day

   b. Assuming both individuals have a plasma $[Na^+]$ of 140 mEq/L, what fraction of the filtered load of Na^+ (FE_{Na}) do they excrete?

      Individual A = _____ %
      Individual B = _____ %

3. Total solute excretion by an individual with renal disease is 500 mOsm/day. If the kidneys of this individual can excrete only urine having an osmolality between 200 and 400 mOsm/kg H_2O, what does the daily water intake have to be in order to prevent the osmolality of the body fluids from changing? Assume water is not lost by other routes.

   Minimum water intake = _____ L/day
   Maximum water intake = _____ L/day

Additional Reading

■ GENERAL

Brenner BM, editor: *The kidney,* ed 5, Philadelphia, 1996, WB Saunders. (A two-volume, comprehensive text on the kidney. Includes sections on normal physiology, pathophysiology, and clinical nephrology. Each chapter is written by experts in the field and includes an extensive list of references.)

Narins RG, editor: *Clinical disorders of fluid and electrolyte metabolism,* ed 5, New York, 1994, McGraw-Hill. (A multiauthored text on fluid electrolyte and acid-base disorders. Each section also includes a review of the underlying physiologic concepts and principles.)

Rose BD: *Clinical physiology of acid-base and electrolyte disorders,* ed 4, New York, 1994, McGraw-Hill. (A clearly written book that discusses fluid and electrolyte disorders from basic physiologic principles.)

Schlondorff D, Bonventre JV, editors: *Molecular nephrology,* New York, 1995, Marcel Dekker. (A multiauthored review of the latest advances in the study of renal function. Emphasis is on information obtained from molecular biologic approaches applied to the study of normal renal function as well as some disease states.)

Schrier RW, Gottschalk CW, editors: *Diseases of the kidney,* ed 5, Boston, 1993, Little, Brown & Co. (A three-volume, comprehensive text on pathophysiology and clinical nephrology. Each chapter is written by experts in the field and includes an extensive list of references.)

Seldin DW, Giebisch G, editors: *The kidney: physiology and pathophysiology,* ed 2, New York, 1992, Raven Press. (A three-volume, comprehensive text on the kidney, similar in many ways to the Brenner text. Includes sections on normal physiology, pathophysiology, and clinical nephrology. Each chapter is written by experts in the field and includes an extensive list of references.)

Windhager EE, editor: *Handbook of physiology. Section 8, Renal physiology,* New York, 1992, Oxford University Press. (A two-volume, critical, comprehensive presentation of physiologic observations and concepts.)

■ CHAPTER 1

Fanestil DD: *Compartmentation of body water.* In Narins RG, editor: *Clinical disorders of fluid and electrolyte metabolism,* ed 5, New York, 1994, McGraw-Hill. (Reviews the techniques for measuring the volumes of the body fluid compartments. Regulation of cell volume under normal and pathophysiologic conditions is also considered.)

Rose BD: *Clinical physiology of acid-base and electrolyte disorders,* ed 4, New York, 1994, McGraw-Hill. (Chapter 1 discusses the basic principles of ions in solution. The volume and composition of the various body fluid compartments are also described. Chapter 7 deals with the exchange of water across cell membranes and capillaries.)

■ CHAPTER 2

Bradley WE: *Physiology of the urinary bladder.* In Walsh PC, Gittes RF, Perlmutter AD, Stamey TA, editors: *Cambell's Urology,* ed 5, Philadelphia, 1986, WB Saunders. (A very thorough treatise on the physiology of the lower urinary tract.)

Kriz W, Bankir L: A standard nomenclature for structures of the kidney, *Am J Physiol* 254: F1, 1988. (A complete review of renal nomenclature, providing most synonyms for each structure. Does not, however, contain any references.)

Kriz W, Kaissling B: *Structural organization of the mammalian kidney.* In Seldin DW, Giebisch G, editors: *The kidney: physiology and pathophysiology,* New York, 1992, Raven Press. (A complete and detailed review of renal structure with numerous references.)

195

Tanagho EA: *Anatomy of the lower urinary tract.* In Walsh PC, Gittes RF, Perlmutter AD, Stamey TA, editors: *Cambell's Urology,* ed 5, Philadelphia, 1986, WB Saunders. (A very thorough treatise on the anatomy of the lower urinary tract.)

Tanagho EA: *Anatomy of the genitourinary tract.* In Tanagho EA, McAnich JW, editors: *Smith's General Urology,* ed 14, Norwalk, 1995, Appleton & Lange. (One of the standard texts on urology for medical students and urology residents. Very concise, with numerous illustrations.)

Tisher CC, Madsen KM: *Anatomy of the kidney.* In Brenner BM, editor: *The kidney,* ed 4, Philadelphia, 1996, WB Saunders. (A complete and detailed review of renal structure and ultrastructure. Superb electron micrographs.)

Tucker MS, Stafford SJ: *Disorders of micturition.* In Schrier RW, Gottschalk CW: *Diseases of the kidney,* ed 5, Boston, 1993, Little, Brown & Co. (A review of the anatomy of the bladder and the physiology and pathophysiology of micturition.)

■ CHAPTER 3

Arendshorst WJ, Navar LG: *Renal circulation and glomerular hemodynamics.* In Schrier RW, Gottschalk CW: *Diseases of the kidney,* ed 5, Boston, 1993, Little, Brown & Co. (A comprehensive review of renal hemodynamics and its regulation.)

Carlson JA, Harrington JT: *Laboratory evaluation of renal function.* In Schrier RW, Gottschalk CW, editors: *Diseases of the kidney,* ed 5, Boston, 1992, Little, Brown & Co. (Describes the general approach for the clinical evaluation of renal function. The use of creatinine clearance for the measurement of glomerular filtration rate is discussed.)

Dworkin LD, Brenner BM: *Biophysical basis of glomerular filtration.* In Seldin DW, Giebisch G, editors: *The kidney: physiology and pathophysiology,* ed 2, New York, 1992, Raven Press. (A complete review of the biophysics of glomerular filtration.)

Dworkin LD, Brenner BM: *The renal circulations.* In Brenner BM editor: *The kidney,* ed 5, Philadelphia, 1996, WB Saunders. (Superb illustrations of the renal circulatory system. A very detailed review of the anatomy of the vasculature.)

Koushanpour E, Kriz W: *Renal physiology,* ed 2, Berlin, 1986, Springer-Verlag. (Chapter 7 describes the use of inulin and creatinine to measure the glomerular filtration rate and PAH to measure renal plasma flow.)

Maddox DA, Brenner BM: *Glomerular ultrafiltration.* In Brenner BM, editor: *The kidney,* ed 5, Philadelphia, 1996, WB Saunders. (An advanced review of glomerular ultrafiltration with complete presentations of hormonal regulation of GFR and RBF, autoregulation of GFR, and tubuloglomerular feedback.)

Schuster VL, Seldin DW: *Renal clearance.* In Seldin DW, Giebisch G, editors: *The kidney: physiology and pathophysiology,* ed 2, New York, 1992, Raven Press. (An in-depth review of the concept of renal clearance as applied to the normal and diseased kidney.)

Ulfendahl HR, Wolgast M: *Renal circulation and lymphatics.* In Seldin DW, Giebisch G, editors: *The kidney: physiology and pathophysiology,* ed 2, New York, 1992, Raven Press. (A review of the functional aspects of the renal circulation, including autoregulation of RBF and the pathophysiology of the renal circulation.)

■ CHAPTER 4

Berry CA, Ives HE, Rector FC Jr: *Renal transport of glucose, amino acids, sodium, chloride, and water.* In Brenner BM, editor: *The kidney,* ed 5, Philadelphia, 1996, WB Saunders. (A complete and up-to-date review of solute transport along the nephron.)

Byrne JH, Schultz SG: *An introduction to membrane transport and bioelectricity.* New York, 1988, Raven Press. (A clearly written book reviewing the principles of membrane transport and bioelectricity, without the use of complex and complicated mathematics. Intended for medical students and beginning graduate students.)

Prichard JB, Miller DS: *Proximal tubular transport of organic anions and cations.* In Seldin DW, Giebisch G, editors: *The kidney: physiology and pathophysiology,* ed 2, New York, 1992, Raven Press. (An in-depth review of organic anion and cation transport by the proximal tubule.)

■ CHAPTER 5

Fitzsimmons JT: *Physiology and pathophysiology of thirst and sodium appetite.* In Seldin DW, Giebisch G, editors: *The kidney: physiology and pathophysiology,* ed 2, New York, 1992, Raven Press. (A detailed review of the physiology and pathophysiology of thirst.)

Harris HW Jr, Zeidel ML: *Cell biology of vasopressin.* In Brenner BM, editor: *The kidney,* ed 5, Philadelphia, 1996, WB Saunders. (A detailed and up-to-date review of the actions of ADH on its target cells. Emphasis is on the membrane and biochemical events associated with ADH action.)

Lassiter WE, Gottschalk CW: *Regulation of water balance: urine concentration and dilution.* In Schrier RW, Gottschalk CW, editors: *Diseases of the kidney,* ed 5, Boston, 1992, Little, Brown & Co. (A comprehensive review of the physiology of water balance and the mechanisms of water transport by the kidneys.)

Knepper MA, Rector FC Jr: *Urine concentration and dilu-tion.* In Brenner BM, editor: *The kidney,* ed 5, Philadelphia, 1996, WB Saunders. (A detailed and up-to-date review of the urine concentration and dilution process. Summarizes current research findings and identifies unresolved questions.)

Robertson GL: *Regulation of vasopressin secretion.* In Seldin DW, Giebisch G, editors: *The kidney: physiology and pathophysiology,* ed 2, New York, 1992, Raven Press. (A comprehensive review of the control of ADH secretion. A discussion of the physiology of thirst is also presented.)

Robertson GL, Berl T: *Pathophysiology of water metabolism.* In Brenner BM, editor: *The kidney,* ed 5, Philadelphia, 1996, WB Saunders. (Reviews the control of ADH secretion and the thirst system. Also includes a discussion of disorders of water balance.)

Roy DR, Layton HE, Jamison RL: *Countercurrent mechanism and its regulation.* In Seldin DW, Giebisch G, editors: *The kidney: physiology and pathophysiology,* ed 2, New York, 1992, Raven Press. (A detailed review of the function of Henle's loop and how it functions as a countercurrent multiplier for the production of dilute and concentrated urine.)

Teitelbaum I, Kelleher SP, Berl T: *Diabetes insipidus and the syndrome of inappropriate antidiuretic hormone secretion.* In Brenner BM, editor: *The kidney,* ed 5, Philadelphia, 1996, WB Saunders. (A comprehensive discussion of disorders of ADH secretion and action.)

■ CHAPTER 6

Brenner BM and others: Diverse biological actions of atrial natriuretic peptide, *Physiol Rev* 70: 665, 1990. (A comprehensive review of the actions of ANP. Considerable detail about the cellular mechanisms of action on the kidneys and other organs.)

Gonzalez-Campoy JM, Knox FG: *Integrated responses of the kidney to alterations in extracellular fluid volume.* In Seldin DW, Giebisch G, editors: *The kidney: physiology and pathophysiology,* ed 2, New York, 1992, Raven Press. (A review of the responses of the kidneys to alterations in the ECV.)

Gunning ME, Ingelfinger JR, King AJ, Brenner BM: *Vasoactive peptides and the kidney.* In Brenner BM, editor: *The kidney,* ed 5, Philadelphia, 1996, WB Saunders. (A complete review of ANP and urodilatin and their roles in controlling renal Na^+ excretion.)

Hall JE, Brands MW: *The renin-angiotensin-aldosterone systems: renal mechanisms and circulatory homeostasis.* In Seldin DW, Giebisch G, editors: *The kidney: physiology and pathophysiology,* ed 2, New York, 1992, Raven Press. (A review of renin secretion and the actions of angiotensin II and aldosterone on the kidneys.)

Miller JA, Tobe SW, Skorecki KL: *Control of extracellular fluid volume and the pathophysiology of edema.* In Brenner BM, editor: *The kidney,* ed 5, Philadelphia, 1996, WB Saunders. (A complete and up-to-date review of the control of renal Na^+ handling and the relationship to the volume of the extracellular fluid compartment.)

Palmer BF, Alpern RJ, Seldin DW: *Pathophysiology of edema formation.* In Seldin DW, Giebisch G, editors: *The kidney: physiology and pathophysiology,* ed 2, New York, 1992, Raven Press. (An excellent review of edema formation. Discusses events at the level of the capillary and the role of the kidneys.)

Rose BD, Rennke HG: *Regulation of salt and water balance.* In Rose BD, Rennke HG: *Renal pathophysiology: the essentials,* Baltimore, 1994, Williams & Wilkins. (An excellent introduction to the pathophysiology of Na^+ balance.)

■ CHAPTER 7

Giebisch G, Malnic G, Berliner RW: *Control of renal potassium excretion.* In Brenner BM, editor: *The kidney,* ed 5, Philadelphia, 1996, WB Saunders. (A detailed review of the cellular mechanisms of K^+ transport and the factors and hormones regulating urinary potassium excretion.)

Rose BD, Rennke HG: *Disorders of potassium balance.* In Rose BD, *Rennke HG: Renal pathophysiology: the essentials,* Baltimore, 1994, Williams & Wilkins. (An excellent introduction to the pathophysiology of K^+ balance and the role of the kidneys.)

Seldin DW, Giebisch G, editors: *The regulation of potassium balance,* New York, 1989, Raven Press. (Fourteen chapters on all aspects of K^+ homeostasis. Seven chapters on normal K^+ metabolism and seven on abnormal K^+ metabolism. A first-rate reference for the advanced student or clinician.)

Stanton BA, Giebisch G: *Renal potassium transport.* In Windhager EE, editor: *Handbook of physiology, section 8, Renal physiology,* ed 2, New York, 1992, Oxford University Press. (A detailed review of K^+ homeostasis.)

Wright FS, Giebisch G: *Regulation of potassium excretion.* In Seldin DW, Giebisch G, editors: *The kidney: physiology and pathophysiology,* ed 2, New York, 1992, Raven Press. (A review of renal K^+ handling and its regulation.)

■ CHAPTER 8

Alpern RJ, Emmett M, Seldin DW: *Metabolic alkalosis.* In Seldin DW, Giebisch G, editors: *The kidney: physiology and pathophysiology,* ed 2, New York, 1992, Raven Press. (A review of the physiology and pathophysiology of metabolic alkalosis.)

Alpern RJ, Rector FC Jr: *Renal acidification mechanisms.* In Brenner BM, editor: *The kidney,* ed 5, Philadelphia, 1996, WB Saunders. (A comprehensive review of renal H^+, HCO_3^-, and NH_4^+ handling.)

DuBose TD Jr, Cogan MG, Rector FC Jr: *Acid-base disorders.* In Brenner BM, editor: *The kidney,* ed 5, Philadelphia, 1996, WB Saunders. (Reviews the etiology and pathophysiology of metabolic acidosis and alkalosis. The approach to diagnosis of acid-base disorders in general is also provided.)

Emmett M, Alpern RJ, Seldin DW: *Metabolic acidosis.* In Seldin DW, Giebisch G, editors: *The kidney: physiology and pathophysiology,* ed 2, New York, 1992, Raven Press. (A review of the physiology and pathophysiology of metabolic acidosis.)

Flessner MF, Knepper MA: *Renal acid-base transport.* In Seldin DW, Giebisch G, editors: *The kidney: physiology and pathophysiology,* ed 2, New York, 1992, Raven Press. (A complete review of H^+ transport by the various segments of the nephron.)

Halperin ML and others: *Biochemistry and physiology of ammonium excretion.* In Seldin DW, Giebisch G, editors: *The kidney: physiology and pathophysiology,* ed 2, New York, 1992, Raven Press. (A complete discussion of ammonium production by the kidneys and the important role it plays in the excretion of nonvolatile acid.)

Hamm LL, Alpern RJ: *Cellular mechanisms of renal tubular acidification.* In Seldin DW, Giebisch G, editors: *The kidney: physiology and pathophysiology,* ed 2, New York, 1992, Raven Press. (A comprehensive review of H^+ secretory mechanisms in the various segments of the nephron.)

Madias NE, Cohen JJ: *Respiratory alkalosis and acidosis.* In Seldin DW, Giebisch G, editors: *The kidney: physiology and pathophysiology,* ed 2, New York, 1992, Raven Press. (A review of the physiology and pathophysiology of respiratory acid-base disorders.)

Rose BD, Rennke HG: *Acid-base physiology and metabolic alkalosis.* In Rose BD, Rennke HG: *Renal pathophysiology: the essentials,* Baltimore, 1994, Williams & Wilkins. (An excellent introduction to the pathophysiology of acid-base balance.)

Rose BD, Rennke HG: *Metabolic acidosis.* In Rose BD, Rennke HG: *Renal pathophysiology: the essentials,* Baltimore, 1994, Williams & Wilkins. (An excellent introduction to the pathophysiology of acid-base balance and the use of the anion gap.)

Seldin DW, Giebisch G, editors: *The regulation of acid-base balance,* New York, 1990, Raven Press. (This book covers all aspects of whole body acid-base balance, including the processes of buffering and respiratory compensation. The major emphasis is on the role of the kidney.)

■ CHAPTER 9

Berndt TJ, Knox FG: *Renal regulation of phosphate excretion.* In Seldin DW, Giebisch G, editors: *The kidney: physiology and pathophysiology,* ed 2, New York, 1992, Raven Press. (A thorough review of Pi excretion by the kidneys.)

Friedman PA, Gesek FA: Cellular calcium transport in renal epithelia: measurement, mechanisms, and regulation. *Physiol Rev* 75 (3): 429-471, 1995. (A comprehensive review of calcium transport along the nephron and its regulation by PTH, PTHRP, calcitonin, and calcitriol.)

Knochel JP, Agarwal R: *Hypophosphatemia and hyperphosphatemia.* In Brenner BM, editor: *The kidney,* ed 5, Philadelphia, 1996, WB Saunders. (A detailed review of the pathophysiology of Pi homeostasis.)

Suki WN, Rouse D: *Renal transport of calcium, magnesium, and phosphate.* In Brenner BM, editor: *The kidney,* ed 5, Philadelphia, 1996, WB Saunders. (A detailed review of renal and extrarenal mechanisms of Ca^{++} and Pi homeostatic mechanisms.)

Sutton RAL, Dirks JH: *Disturbances of calcium and magnesium metabolism.* In Brenner BM, editor: *The kidney,* ed 5, Philadelphia, 1996, WB Saunders. (A detailed review of the pathophysiology of Ca^{++} homeostasis.)

■ CHAPTER 10

Dillingham MA, Schrier RW, Greger R: *Mechanisms of diuretic action.* In Schrier RW, Gottschalk CW, editors: *Diseases of the kidney,* ed 5, Boston, 1993, Little, Brown & Co. (A comprehensive review of the mechanisms and sites of action of the various classes of diuretics.)

Fliser D, Ritz E: Clinical problems of diuretics, *Clin Invest* 72: 708-710, 1994. (A short review of the side effects and problems associated with diuretic use.)

Rose BD: Resistance to diuretics, *Clin Invest* 72: 722-724, 1994. (A short review of the factors that contribute to the development of diuretic resistance.)

Rose BD, Rennke HG: *Edematous states and the use of diuretics.* In Rose BD, Rennke HG: *Renal pathophysiology: the essentials,* Baltimore, 1994, Williams & Wilkins. (An excellent introduction to the use of diuretics, especially in the presence of edema.)

Suki WN, Eknoyan G: *Physiology of diuretic action.* In Seldin DW, Giebisch G, editors: *The kidney: physiology and pathophysiology,* ed 2, New York, 1992, Raven Press. (A review of the physiology of diuretic action.)

Wilcox CS: *Diuretics.* In Brenner BM, editor: *The kidney,* ed 5, Philadelphia, 1996, WB Saunders. (A comprehensive review of the physiology and clinical use of diuretics.)

■ CHAPTER 11

Fine LG and others: *Pathophysiology and nephron adaptation in chronic renal failure.* In Seldin DW, Giebisch G, editors: *The kidney: physiology and pathophysiology,* ed 2, New York, 1992, Raven Press. (A review of the physiology and pathophysiology of renal failure, with a focus on how remaining functioning nephrons adapt to preserve fluid and electrolyte balance.)

Meyer TG, Boboolal K, Brenner BM: *Nephron adaptation to renal injury.* In Brenner BM, editor: *The kidney,* ed 5, Philadelphia, 1996, WB Saunders. (A comprehensive review of the response of nephrons to injury and the compensatory adaptation to nephron loss.)

Mitch WE, Stein JH, editors: *The progressive nature of renal disease,* ed 2. *Contemporary issues in nephrology,* vol 26, New York, 1992, Churchill Livingstone. (A single volume devoted to the most recent advances in understanding the progressive loss of renal function in disease.)

Integrative Case Studies

■ CASE 1

A 65-year-old man had a myocardial infarction 4 months ago and is now seen by his physician for fatigability, shortness of breath, and swelling of the ankles. On physical examination he is found to have distended neck veins and pitting edema of the ankles. His breathing is rapid (20 breaths/min), and rales (i.e., fluid in the lungs) are heard bilaterally at the bases of the lungs. He is afebrile, with a pulse rate of 110 beats/min and a blood pressure of 110/70. Since his myocardial infarction he has been taking a cardiac glycoside and a thiazide diuretic. A blood sample is obtained, and the following abnormalities are noted:

Serum $[Na^+]$	$= 130$ mEq/L
Serum $[K^+]$	$= 3.0$ mEq/L
Serum $[HCO_3^-]$	$= 30$ mEq/L
Serum [creatinine]	$= 1.7$ mg/dl

Questions

1a. Is the extracellular fluid (ECF) volume in this man increased or decreased relative to normal? What evidence in the physical examination supports your conclusion?

1b. Is the effective circulating volume (ECV) in this man increased or decreased from normal? What laboratory test could you perform to support your conclusion?

1c. How would you characterize renal Na^+ handling in this man? What evidence in the physical examination supports this conclusion?

1d. What is the mechanism for the development of hyponatremia in this man?

1e. What is the mechanism for the development of hypokalemia in this man?

1f. What type of acid-base disturbance does this man have? What is the mechanism for the development of this disorder?

1g. What is the significance of the elevated serum [creatinine]?

1h. The physician treating this man prescribes a loop diuretic in addition to the thiazide diuretic in order to further reduce Na^+ retention and reduce his edema. What effect will this treatment have on the man's ECV? What is the potential effect of this treatment on the man's serum Na^+, K^+, HCO_3^-, and creatinine concentrations?

■ CASE 2

A 49-year-old woman sees her physician with weakness, fatigability, and loss of appetite. During the past month she has lost 7 kg (15 lb). On physical examination she is found to have hyperpigmentation, especially of the oral mucosa and gums. She is hypotensive, and her blood pressure falls when she assumes an upright posture (BP = 100/60 mm Hg supine and 80/50 mm Hg erect). The following laboratory data are obtained:

$$\begin{aligned}
\text{Serum } [Na^+] &= 130 \text{ mEq/L} \\
\text{Serum } [K^+] &= 6.5 \text{ mEq/L} \\
\text{Serum } [HCO_3^-] &= 20 \text{ mEq/L}
\end{aligned}$$

Questions

2a. The plasma level of what hormone(s) would be expected to be below normal in this woman?

2b. What is the cause of this woman's hypotension?

2c. What is the mechanism for development of hyponatremia in this woman?

2d. Why does this woman have hyperkalemia?

2e. What is the expected acid-base disturbance in this woman, and what is the cause?

■ CASE 3

An 18-year-old man with insulin-dependent diabetes mellitus (Type I) is seen in the emergency department. He reports not taking his insulin during the previous 24 hours because he did not feel well and was not eating. He now has weakness, nausea, thirst, and frequent urination. On physical examination he is found to have deep and rapid respirations (Kussmaul's respirations). At 2:00 AM the following laboratory data are obtained:

$$\begin{aligned}
\text{Plasma } [Na^+] &= 135 \text{ mEq/L} \\
\text{Serum } [Cl^-] &= 99 \text{ mEq/L} \\
\text{Serum } [K^+] &= 8.0 \text{ mEq/L} \\
\text{Serum } [HCO_3^-] &= 7 \text{ mEq/L} \\
\text{Blood pH} &= 6.99 \\
\text{Arterial } P_{CO_2} &= 30 \text{ mm Hg} \\
\text{Serum [glucose]} &= 1200 \text{ mg/dl}
\end{aligned}$$
Urine contains glucose and ketones

After being diagnosed with diabetic ketoacidosis, the man is admitted to the hospital. Saline is administered intravenously, and insulin therapy begun. At 3:00 AM, HCO_3^- is administered with more insulin. The results of therapy are illustrated in Table 1.

Questions

3a. What type of acid-base disorder does this man have? Would you expect the anion gap to be normal?

3b. Why did this man develop hyperkalemia?

3c. Explain why serum $[K^+]$ fell during the first hour of insulin infusion.

3d. What effect will intravenous administration of HCO_3^- have on the serum $[K^+]$?

3e. What is the mechanism for the polyuria in this man? What effect, if any, does the increased urine output have on his K^+ homeostasis?

		T A B L E 1		
Time	Serum [K⁺] (mEq/L)	Arterial blood pH	Serum [HCO₃⁻] (mEq/L)	Serum [glucose] (mg/dl)
2:00 AM	8.0	6.99	7	1200
3:00 AM	6.0	7.01	8	400
4:00 AM	4.5	7.10	12	100
5:00 AM	4.5	7.10	12	100
7:00 AM	3.5	7.08	11	100

3f. This man's serum $[Na^+]$ was 135 mEq/L before the initiation of therapy. By 7:00 AM it had risen to 152 mEq/L. What is the mechanism for the development of hypernatremia?

■ CASE 4

A 75-year-old woman (body weight = 60 kg) is admitted to the intensive care unit after having fallen at home 2 days earlier. For the first 4 days of her hospitalization, her urine output is approximately 400 ml/day. On physical examination she has orthostatic changes in blood pressure, tachycardia, and poor skin turgor. Her serum creatinine has risen progressively from 1 mg/dl on the day of admission to 5.9 mg/dl on Day 4. After 2 weeks in the intensive care unit, she is transferred to a medical floor, where her urine output is noted to be approximately 1 L/day and her serum [creatinine] to be stable at 1.0 mg/dl. In addition, she is found to have signs and symptoms of congestive heart failure, with decreased cardiac output. She has fractured several ribs as a result of her fall and requests medication to relieve the pain. A nonsteroidal antiinflammatory pain reliever is prescribed. By morning the patient's rib pain is better. Because she has developed some edema secondary to the congestive heart failure, she is treated with a loop diuretic. She responds well to the diuretic with resolution of her edema. Her serum creatinine is now stabilized at 1 mg/dl. A 24-hour urine collection is performed to determine her glomerular filtration rate (GFR).

Urine [creatinine] = 64.8 mg/dl
Urine volume = 1 L
Serum [creatinine] = 1.0 mg/dl

Questions

4a. How do you explain the increase of serum [creatinine] during the first 4 days of this woman's hospitalization?

4b. The nonsteroidal antiinflammatory pain reliever has inhibition of prostaglandin synthesis as its mechanism of action. What potential adverse effects could this pain reliever have on her clinical course?

4c. What effect does furosemide have on this woman's ECV?

4d. Calculate the creatinine clearance. Is the value consistent with what was expected on the basis of her serum [creatinine]?

■ CASE 5

A 70-year-old man with lung cancer develops the syndrome of inappropriate antidiuretic hormone secretion (SIADH). He is admitted to the hospital, and the following data are obtained.

Body weight = 70 kg
Serum $[Na^+]$ = 120 mEq/L
Urine osmolality = 600 mOsm/kg H_2O
Urine $[Na^+]$ = 80 mEq/L

Questions

5a. What determines the amount of Na^+ that is excreted in the urine, and is Na^+ excretion in this patient normal?

5b. Two liters of isotonic saline is administered intravenously in an effort to raise the serum $[Na^+]$. How much of the infused NaCl will be excreted in the urine? (For simplicity, assume that 1L of isotonic saline contains 150 mmol/L of NaCl.) What effect will this infusion have on the plasma $[Na^+]$?

5c. What effect would the administration of 1 L of hypertonic saline (3% NaCl solution) have on the plasma $[Na^+]$?

5d. What effect would administering a loop diuretic together with an infusion of 1 L of 3% saline have on the plasma $[Na^+]$? (Assume the loop diuretic reduces Uosm to 300 mOsm/kg H_2O.)

■ CASE 6

A 45-year-old man is brought to the hospital by his wife, who complains that he is drinking water (polydipsia) and urinating (polyuria) "all the time." On further questioning, you find that the patient urinates approximately 500 ml of urine every hour and has been drinking approximately 2 L of water 6 to 7 times/day for the past 3 weeks. He denies any previous medical problems.

Questions

6a. What are the possible causes of polyuria in this man?

6b. What simple laboratory tests could be done on the urine to help sort these causes out?

6c. What might his serum $[Na^+]$ concentration be and why?

■ CASE 7

A 55-year-old man has a cardiac arrest. Measurements of blood gases and serum electrolytes are obtained.

Arterial pH	= 7.30
Arterial P_{CO_2}	= 30 mm Hg
Serum $[Na^+]$	= 140 mEq/L
Serum $[K^+]$	= 4.1 mEq/L
Serum $[Cl^-]$	= 100 mEq/L
Serum $[HCO_3{}^-]$	= 15 mEq/L

Questions

7a. What is the acid-base disorder?

7b. Calculate the anion gap. What information does it give regarding the acid-base disorder in this man?

7c. What is the most likely cause of the acid-base disorder?

■ CASE 8

A previously healthy 28-year-old man is seen in the emergency room with right side flank pain. Shortly after arrival, he passes a small kidney stone. He denies any significant previous renal or gastrointestinal problems. There is a family history of kidney stones. The results of laboratory tests done in the emergency room include the following:

Serum $[Na^+]$	= 137 mEq/L
Serum $[K^+]$	= 3.1 mEq/L
Serum $[Cl^-]$	= 111 mEq/L
Serum $[HCO_3{}^-]$	= 13 mEq/L
Arterial pH	= 7.28
Arterial P_{CO_2}	= 28 mm Hg
Urine pH	= 6.4

Questions

8a. What is the acid-base disorder?

8b. Why do you think the serum $[K^+]$ is low in this condition?

■ CASE 9

A 50-year-old man with a history of a duodenal ulcer is admitted to the hospital after several days of intermittent vomiting. On physical examination he is noted to have orthostatic changes in his blood pressure and pulse, no visible jugular venous distension, and marked decrease in his skin turgor. Laboratory tests reveal the following:

Serum $[Na^+]$	= 138 mEq/L
Serum $[K^+]$	= 2.4 mEq/L
Serum $[Cl^-]$	= 88 mEq/L
Serum $[HCO_3{}^-]$	= 40 mEq/L
Arterial pH	= 7.52
Arterial P_{CO_2}	= 50 mm Hg
Urine $[Na^+]$	= 38 mEq/L
Urine $[K^+]$	= 60 mEq/L

Questions

9a. What is the acid-base disorder?

9b. Gastric secretions contain about 10 mEq/L of potassium. How do you account for the low serum potassium in this patient?

CASE 10

A 60-year-old man with a long-standing history of smoking and chronic obstructive pulmonary disease is admitted to the hospital because of worsening edema. On physical examination he is noted to have pitting edema of the ankles and jugular distension. He is admitted to the hospital for a salt-restricted diet and begins intravenous doses of a loop diuretic. He has a marked diuresis with a 12 kg weight loss. However, he still has significant generalized edema. The following laboratory values are shown in Table 2.

Because of the abnormalities noted on Day 3, he is given a carbonic anhydrase inhibitor. He subsequently has a diuresis with a reduction in his edema.

Questions

10a. What is the acid-base disturbance on admission?

10b. What is the acid-base disturbance on Day 3?

10c. Has there been a change in the rate of alveolar ventilation on Day 3?

10d. Why has his ventilation improved on Day 6?

	Day 1	Day 3	Day 6
Serum [Na$^+$], mEq/L	139	136	135
Serum [K$^+$], mEq/L	4.2	3.5	3.2
Serum [Cl$^-$], mEq/L	98	83	98
Serum [HCO$_3^-$], mEq/L	31	42	27
Serum [creatinine], mg/dl	1.0	1.5	1.1
Arterial pH	7.34	7.43	7.31
Arterial P_{CO_2}, mm Hg	60	65	55
Arterial O$_2$ (room air), mm Hg	48	39	52

TABLE 2

Normal Laboratory Values

	Traditional units	SI units
Arterial Blood Gases		
P_{CO_2}	33-44 mm Hg	4.4-5.9 kPa
P_{O_2}	75-105 mm Hg	10.0-14.0 kPa
pH	7.35-7.45	[H^+] 36-44 nmol/L
Serum Electrolytes*		
Na^+	135-147 mEq/L	135-147 mmol/L
Cl^-	95-105 mEq/L	95-105 mmol/L
K^+	3.5-5.0 mEq/L	3.5-5.0 mmol/L
HCO_3^-	22-28 mEq/L	22-28 mmol/L
Ca^{++}	8.4-10.0 mg/dl	2.1-2.8 mmol/L
Pi	3.0-4.5 mg/dl	1.0-1.5 mmol/L
Serum Proteins		
Total	6.0-7.8 g/dl	60-78 g/L
Albumin	3.5-5.5 g/dl	35-55 g/L
Globulin	2.3-3.5 g/dl	23-35 g/L
Other Serum Constituents		
Creatinine	0.6-1.2 mg/dl	53-106 µmol/L
Glucose (fasting)	70-110 mg/dl	3.8-6.1 mmol/L
Urea nitrogen (BUN)	7-18 mg/dl	1.2-3.0 mmol/L
Serum Osmolality	275-295 mOsm/kg H_2O	275-295 mOsm/kg H_2O
Creatinine Clearance		
Male	97-137 ml/min	97-137 ml/min
	140-197 L/day	140-197 L/day
Female	88-128 ml/min	88-128 ml/min
	127-184 L/day	127-184 L/day

*Serum is derived from clotted blood (devoid of clotting factors), whereas plasma is derived from unclotted blood (contains clotting factors). However, concentrations of most substances are the same whether determined on a sample of plasma or serum. Most clinical chemistry laboratories determine concentrations of serum samples.

Nephron Function

■ SUMMARY BY TRANSPORT PROCESS

Na⁺ and Cl⁻ reabsorption

In all tables: (+) = stimulation; (−) = inhibition

Nephron segment	Mechanism	Regulation
Proximal tubule	Na^+-H^+ antiport	Angiotensin II (+)
	Na^+-solute symport	Sympathetic nerves (+)
	Na^+-H^+/Cl^--Anion antiport	Epinephrine (+)
	Paracellular	Dopamine (−)
Henle's loop		
Descending thin limb	None	
Ascending thin limb	Paracellular	
Thick ascending limb	1Na^+-1K^+-2Cl^- symport	Aldosterone (+)
	Paracellular	Sympathetic nerves (+)
Early distal tubule	Na^+-Cl^- symport	Aldosterone (+)
		Sympathetic nerves (+)
Late distal tubule and collecting duct	Na^+ channel	Aldosterone (+)
		Sympathetic nerves (+)
		ANP (−)
		Urodilatin (−)

	TABLE C - 2	
	K$^+$ reabsorption	
Nephron segment	**Mechanism**	**Regulation**
Proximal tubule	Paracellular	
Henle's loop		
Descending thin limb	None	
Ascending thin limb	None	
Thick ascending limb	1Na$^+$-1K$^+$-2Cl$^-$ symport	
	Paracellular	
Early distal tubule	None	
Late distal tubule and collecting duct	H$^+$-K$^+$-ATPase	Dietary K$^+$ depletion (+)

(+) = stimulation; (−) = inhibition

	TABLE C - 3	
	K$^+$ secretion	
Nephron segment	**Mechanism**	**Regulation**
Proximal tubule	None	
Henle's loop		
Descending thin limb	None	
Ascending thin limb	None	
Thick ascending limb	None	
Early distal tubule	None	
Late distal tubule and collecting duct	K$^+$ channels	Plasma [K$^+$] (+)
		Aldosterone (+)
		ADH (+)
		Flow rate (+)
		Acid-base balance (+/ −)

(+) = stimulation; (−) = inhibition

TABLE C·4

H⁺ secretion (HCO₃⁻ reabsorption)

Nephron segment	Mechanism	Regulation
Proximal tubule	Na⁺-H⁺ antiport H⁺-ATPase	↑ Filtered load of HCO_3^- (+) ↓ ECV (+) ↑ P_{CO_2} (+) ↓ Plasma $[HCO_3^-]$ (+)
Henle's loop		
Descending thin limb	None	
Ascending thin limb	None	
Thick ascending limb	Na⁺-H⁺ antiport H⁺-ATPase	↑ P_{CO_2} (+) ↓ Plasma $[HCO_3^-]$ (+)
Early distal tubule	H⁺-ATPase H⁺-K⁺-ATPase	↑ P_{CO_2} (+) ↓ Plasma $[HCO_3^-]$ (+)
Late distal tubule and collecting duct	H⁺-ATPase H⁺-K⁺-ATPase	↑ Increase P_{CO_2} (+) ↓ Plasma $[HCO_3^-]$ (+) Aldosterone (+)

(+) = stimulation; (−) = inhibition

TABLE C·5

HCO₃⁻ secretion

Nephron segment	Mechanism	Regulation
Proximal tubule	None	
Henle's loop		
Descending thin limb	None	
Ascending thin limb	None	
Thick ascending limb	None	
Early distal tubule	None	
Late distal tubule and collecting duct	Cl⁻-HCO₃⁻ antiport	Metabolic alkalosis (+)

(+) = stimulation; (−) = inhibition

TABLE C-6

Water reabsorption

Nephron segment	Mechanism	Regulation
Proximal tubule	Water channels	
	Paracellular	
Henle's loop		
Descending thin limb	Water channels	
Ascending thin limb	None	
Thick ascending limb	None	
Early distal tubule	None	
Late distal tubule and collecting duct	Water channels	ADH (+)

(+) = stimulation; (−) = inhibition

TABLE C-7

Pi reabsorption

Nephron segment	Mechanism	Regulation
Proximal tubule	Na^+-Pi symport	PTH (−)
		Pi depletion (+)
		↓ ECV (+)
		Acidosis (+)
		Glucocorticoids (−)
Henle's loop		
Descending thin limb	None	
Ascending thin limb	None	
Thick ascending limb	None	
Early distal tubule	None	
Late distal tubule and collecting duct	None	

(+) = stimulation; (−) = inhibition

TABLE C-8

Ca^{++} reabsorption

Nephron segment	Mechanism	Regulation
Proximal tubule	Ca^{++} channel Paracellular	PTH ($-$) $\downarrow$ ECV (+) $\downarrow$ Plasma [Pi] (+)
Henle's loop		
Descending thin limb	None	
Ascending thin limb	None	
Thick ascending limb	Ca^{++} channel Paracellular	PTH (+) Calcitonin (+) Calcitriol (+) $\downarrow$ Plasma [Pi] (+)
Early distal tubule	Ca^{++} channel	PTH (+) Calcitonin (+) Calcitriol (+) $\downarrow$ Plasma [Pi] (+) Acidosis ($-$)
Late distal tubule and collecting duct	None	

(+) = stimulation; ($-$) = inhibition

■ SUMMARY BY NEPHRON SEGMENT

Proximal Tubule

Reabsorption

Water:	67% of filtered load
NaCl:	67% of filtered load
K^+:	67% of filtered load
Ca^{++}:	70% of filtered load
Pi:	80% of filtered load
HCO_3^-:	80% of filtered load
Protein:	100% of filtered load
Urea:	67% of the filtered load

Secretion

NH_4^+
Organic anions
Organic cations

Henle's Loop (Thick Ascending Limb)

Reabsorption

Water:	15% of filtered load (thin descending limb only)
NaCl:	25% of filtered load
K^+:	20% of filtered load
Ca^{++}:	20% of filtered load
HCO_3^-:	15% of filtered load
NH_4^+	

Secretion

Urea   (thin descending and thin ascending limbs only)

Early Distal Tubule

Reabsorption

NaCl:	4% of the filtered load
Ca^{++}:	9% of the filtered load
HCO_3^-:	3% of the filtered load
Pi:	10% of the filtered load

Late Distal Tubule and Collecting Duct

Reabsorption

Water:	8-17% depending on ADH levels
NaCl:	3% of the filtered load
K^+:	normally zero
Ca^{++}:	<1% of the filtered load
HCO_3^-:	2% of the filtered load
Urea	(medullary collecting duct only)

Secretion

K^+:	0% to 70% of the filtered load
NH_4^+	
Urea	(medullary portion only)

Answers to Self-Study Problems

■ CHAPTER 1

1.

	Molarity (mmol/L)	Osmolality (mOsm/kg H_2O)
9 g NaCl	154	308
72 g Glucose	400	400
22.2 g $CaCl_2$	200	600
3 g Urea	50	50
8.4 g $NaHCO_3$	100	200

2. The cell will swell when placed in the solution because the solute is only a partially effective osmole (i.e., this is a hypotonic solution). Because the reflection coefficient (σ) is 0.5, the effective osmolality of the solution is only 150 mOsm/kg H_2O. The solution would have to contain 600 mmol/L of this solute to be isotonic.

3. Na^+, with its anions Cl^- and HCO_3^-, constitutes the majority of particles in the ECF and is therefore the major determinant of plasma osmolality. Consequently, plasma osmolality can be estimated by simply doubling the plasma $[Na^+]$. Thus, the estimated plasma osmolality in this individual is as follows:

$$P_{osm} = 2(130) = 260 \text{ mOsm/kg } H_2O$$

This value is well below the normal range of 275 to 295 mOsm/kg H_2O and will result in movement of water from the ECF into the ICF. Because ions move freely across the capillary wall, the $[Na^+]$ (and osmolality) in the plasma and interstitial fluid will be the same. Therefore water movement across the capillary endothelium will not be affected.

4. The increase in venous pressure causes increased movement of fluid out of the capillary. As a result, fluid accumulates in the interstitial space. Some of this fluid will be taken up by the lymphatics, and lymphatic flow will increase. However, when the capacity of the lymphatics to remove this fluid is reached, the volume of the interstitial space increases, and edema forms (see Chapter 6). See p. D-2.

5. The initial volumes of the body fluid compartments and the osmoles in these compartments are calculated as follows (osmolality is estimated as $2 \times [Na^+]$):

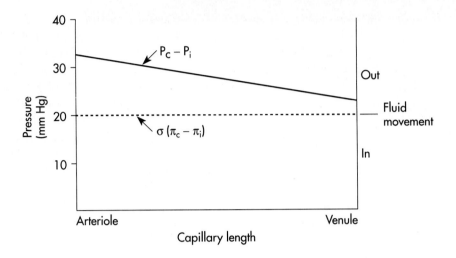

Initial total body water = 0.6 × (60 kg) = 36 L
Initial ICF volume   = 0.4 × (60 kg) = 24 L
Initial ECF volume   = 0.2 × (60 kg) = 12 L
Initial total body   = (Total body water)(body
  osmoles   fluid osmolality)
                         = (36 L)(280 mOsm/kg
                           H_2O) = 10,080 mOsm
Initial ICF osmoles   = (ICF volume)(body fluid
                           osmolality)
                         = (24 L)(280 mOsm/kg
                           H_2O) = 6720 mOsm
Initial ECF osmoles   = Total body osmoles −
                           ICF osmoles
                         = 10,080 mOsm − 6720
                           mOsm = 3360 mOsm

Four kilograms of body weight is lost. It is assumed that this entire weight reduction reflects fluids lost through vomiting and diarrhea. Thus, 4 L of fluid is lost. Because the
plasma [Na^+] is unchanged, a proportional
amount of solute was also lost (isotonic loss
of fluid). No fluid shifts occur between the
ECF and ICF because of the absence of an osmotic gradient between these compartments.
Therefore the ECF loses 4 L of volume, and
4 × 280 = 1120 mOsm of solute.

New total body water = 36 L − 4 L = 32 L
New ICF volume   = 24 L (unchanged)
New ECF volume   = 12 L − 4 L = 8 L
New total body   = 10,080 mOsm − 1120
  osmoles   mOsm = 8960 mOsm
New ICF osmoles   = 6720 mOsm
                       (unchanged)
New ECF osmoles   = 3360 mOsm − 1120
                       mOsm = 2240 mOsm

6. The initial volumes of the body fluid compartments and the osmoles in these compartments are calculated as in Problem 5:

Initial total body water = 0.6 × (50 kg) = 30 L
Initial ICF volume   = 0.4 × (50 kg) = 20 L
Initial ECF volume   = 0.2 × (50 kg) = 10 L
Initial total body   = (Total body water)(body
  osmoles   fluid osmolality)
                         = (30 L)(290 mOsm/kg
                           H_2O) = 8700 mOsm
Initial ICF osmoles   = (ICF volume)(body fluid
                           osmolality)
                         = (20 L)(290 mOsm/kg
                           H_2O) = 5800 mOsm
Initial ECF osmoles   = Total body osmoles −
                           ICF osmoles
                         = 8700 mOsm − 5800
                           mOsm = 2900 mOsm

The total amount of mannitol infused must be calculated to determine its effect on body fluids. At 5 g/kg, a total of 250 g was infused (1.374 moles of mannitol). Because mannitol is a single particle in solution, this adds 1374 mOsm to the ECF. The mannitol will raise ECF osmolality and result in the shift of fluid from the ICF into the ECF.

New total body water = 30 L (unchanged)
New total body osmoles = 8700 mOsm + 1374 mOsm = 10,074 mOsm
New ICF osmoles = 5800 mOsm (unchanged)
New ECF osmoles = 2900 mOsm + 1374 mOsm = 4274 mOsm

$$\text{New plasma osmolality} = \frac{\text{New total osmoles}}{\text{Total body water}}$$
$$= \frac{10,074 \text{ mOsm}}{30 \text{ L}} = 336 \text{ mOsm/kg } H_2O$$

$$\text{New ICF volume} = \frac{\text{ICF osmoles}}{\text{New } p_{osm}} =$$
$$\frac{5800 \text{ mOsm}}{336 \text{ mOsm/kg } H_2O} = 17.3 \text{ L}$$

New ECF volume = Total body water − ICF volume
= 30 L − 17.3 = 12.7 L

Because mannitol increases the osmolality of the ECF, 2.7 L of fluid shifts from the ICF into the ECF. To calculate the new plasma [Na+], assume that the amount of Na+ in the ECF is unchanged after mannitol infusion. Originally, there were 2900 mOsm due to Na+ (2 × [Na+] × ECF volume) in the ECF. Because the Na+ osmoles are unchanged but are now present in a larger volume, the new plasma [Na+] is calculated as follows:

$$\text{New plasma Na}^+ \text{ osmoles} = \frac{2900 \text{ mOsm due to Na}^+}{12.7 \text{ L}}$$
$$= 228 \text{ mOsm/L}$$

$$\text{New plasma [Na}^+] = \frac{\text{Na}^+ \text{ osmoles}}{2} = \frac{228 \text{ mOsm}}{2}$$
$$= 114 \text{ mEq/L}$$

7. Because dextrose is an effective osmole, the 5% solution is isotonic. Immediately after infusion it will therefore remain in the ECF and increase the volume of this compartment by 2 L. The osmolality of the ECF and ICF will not change. However, over time the dextrose is metabolized to CO_2 and H_2O, essentially converting the entire 2 L to H_2O. The 2 L of H_2O will distribute throughout the ECF and ICF, increasing the volume of these compartments by 0.67 and 1.33 L, respectively, and reducing the osmolality of both fluid compartments.

8. Both individuals have lost water and solute from the body. Individual A lost 1 L of water and 1200 mOsm of solute, whereas Individual B lost 3 L of water and 900 mOsm of solute. Both have the same initial total body water (0.6 × 70 kg = 42 L) and total body osmoles (290 mOsm/kg H_2O × 42 L = 12,180 mOsm). Their new P_{osm} values are calculated as follows:

$$P_{osm} (A) = \frac{12,180 \text{ mOsm} - 1200 \text{ mOsm}}{42L - 1L}$$
$$= 268 \text{ mOsm/kg } H_2O$$

$$P_{osm} (B) = \frac{12,180 \text{ mOsm} - 900 \text{ mOsm}}{42L - 3L}$$
$$= 289 \text{ mOsm/kg } H_2O$$

■ CHAPTER 2

1. The glomerular capillaries have a fenestrated endothelium that prevents the filtration of cells. The capillaries are surrounded by a basement membrane composed of three layers: lamina rara interna, lamina densa, and lamina rara externa. The basement membrane is an important filtration barrier to plasma proteins. Filtration slits of the podocytes, which encircle the glomerular capillaries, are also a filtration barrier for proteins.

2. Structures that compose the juxtaglomerular apparatus include the macula densa of the thick ascending limb, extraglomerular mesan-

gial cells, and the renin-producing cells of the afferent and efferent arterioles. The juxtaglomerular apparatus is one component of a feedback mechanism that regulates renal blood flow and glomerular filtration rate. Details of this mechanism are provided in Chapter 3.

3. Micturition is the process of emptying the urinary bladder. Filling of the bladder stretches the wall, which activates sensory nerves. These nerves send impulses from the bladder to the spinal cord via the pelvic nerves. Stretch stimulates the parasympathetic nerves, which causes intense contraction of the detrusor. This contraction, coupled with the voluntary relaxation of the external sphincter, allows urine to flow through the external meatus. Voluntary elimination of urine requires intact parasympathetic nerves and conscious control of the external sphincter.

4. A spinal cord injury at the level of the 12th thoracic vertebra interrupts the ascending sensory fibers. Thus, there is no sensation of bladder fullness. The descending fibers that control the muscle of the external sphincter are also interrupted, as are descending fibers that modulate the micturition reflex. Voluntary control of the external sphincter is lost, resulting in the inability to control micturition (i.e., incontinence). The micturition reflex is intact because the centers involved in this reflex arc are located in the sacral part of the spinal cord (below the injury to the spinal cord). The bladder shows spontaneous contractions as it fills (i.e., spasticity). These spontaneous contractions are normal, but they are usually inhibited by descending fibers from the brain. This inhibitory influence allows the bladder to fill to capacity before voiding. However, in this situation the inhibitory input is lost, and small volumes of urine are voided frequently.

■ CHAPTER 3

1. **Before pflorizin**

Serum [inulin]:	1 mg/ml
Serum [glucose]:	1 mg/ml
Inulin excretion rate:	100 mg/min
Glucose excretion rate:	0 mg/min
Inulin clearance:	100 ml/min
Glucose clearance:	0 ml/min

After pflorizin

Serum [inulin]:	1 mg/ml
Serum [glucose]:	1 mg/ml
Inulin excretion rate:	100 mg/min
Glucose excretion rate:	10 mg/min
Inulin clearance:	100 ml/min
Glucose clearance:	100 ml/min

Before treatment with pflorizin the filtered load of glucose (GFR × [glucose]) is 100 mg/min (GFR calculated from inulin clearance). With this filtered load of glucose, all the glucose is reabsorbed and none is excreted. Thus, the clearance of glucose is zero. After pflorizin the filtered load is unchanged, but there is no glucose reabsorption. Therefore all the glucose that is filtered is excreted, and the clearance of glucose equals that of inulin.

2. a: Although the appearance of red cells in the urine can result from damage to the glomerular filtration barrier, red cells can also appear in the urine for other reasons. For example, they can appear as a result of bleeding in any part of the lower urinary tract. Such bleeding is seen with kidney stones and occasionally as a result of a bacterial infection of the lower urinary tract, which causes bleeding. Thus, the appearance of blood in the urine does not necessarily mean the glomerular filtration barrier is damaged.

b: Because glucose is filtered and completely reabsorbed by the proximal tubule, it is not normally found in the urine. Its presence in the urine indicates an elevated plasma glucose level such that the filtered load (i.e., GFR × [glucose]) is greater than the ability of the proximal tubule to reabsorb glucose. Because glucose is freely filterd by the normal glomerulus, damage to the ultrafiltration barrier would not increase its filtration.

c: In healthy individuals, Na^+ normally appears in the urine. Like glucose, Na^+ is freely filtered by the normal glomerulus. Therefore damage to the filtration barrier does not increase the rate of Na^+ excretion.

d: This is the correct answer. Normally the urine contains essentially no protein. The glomerulus prevents the filtration of plasma proteins. However, when the glomerulus is damaged, large amounts of plasma proteins are filtered. If the amount filtered overwhelms the reabsorptive capacity of the proximal tubule, protein appears in the urine (proteinuria).

3. The equation for blood flow through an organ is Q = ΔP/R. Sympathetic agonists, angiotensin II, and prostaglandins change blood flow by altering the resistance (R). Whereas sympathetic agonists and angiotensin II increase R and thereby decrease RBF, prostaglandins decrease R and thereby increase RBF.

4. Normally, renal prostaglandin production is low, and nonsteroidal antiinflammatory drugs (NSAIDs) do not have an appreciable effect on prostaglandin production. However, during reductions in GFR and RBF, elevated prostaglandin levels cause vasodilatation of the afferent and efferent arterioles. This effect prevents excessive decreases in RBF and GFR. Administration of NSAIDs to patients with low GFR and RBF inhibits prostaglandin production and further reduces GFR and RBF.

■ CHAPTER 4

1. The glomeruli filter 25,200 mEq of Na^+ and 18,000 mEq of Cl^- each day, and over 99% is reabsorbed by the nephrons, with less than 1% appearing in the urine. Although Na^+ and Cl^- uptake into cells across the apical membrane and NaCl reabsorption across the paracellular pathway are passive processes (i.e., they do not require the direct input of ATP), they ultimately depend on the operation of the Na^+-K^+-ATPase. Accordingly, reabsorption of NaCl requires a considerable quantity of ATP, the synthesis of which by kidney cells requires large amounts of oxygen and, hence, a high blood flow.

2. "Normal" or "average" urine composition does not actually exist because of the variability in the volume excreted, as well as variations in the intake of solutes in the diet. Consider Table D-1 (see p. D-6):
Urine was collected on three different days from a subject who ate a consistent diet but ingested different amounts of water each day. Although the amount of each solute excreted was similar each day (see Table D-2), the concentration of each solute in the urine was different because the volume of urine varied each day. This question demonstrates that the amount (or rate) of a solute excreted, not the concentration of the solute in the urine, is important in the clinical evaluation of urine.

3. Passive transport always occurs down an electrochemical gradient. Diffusion of a gas (e.g., O_2) through the lipid portion of the plasma membrane occurs passively. For coupled transporters (antiport and symport) the movement of one molecule moving down its electrochemical gradient can drive uphill movement of the coupled molecule. When this occurs, the uphill movement is termed *secondary active* transport because the trans-

	TABLE D-1		
	Urine flow rate		
	0.5 L/day	1 L/day	2 L/day
Na$^+$, mEq/L	300	150	75
K$^+$, mEq/L	200	100	50
Cl$^-$, mEq/L	300	150	75
HCO$_3^-$, mEq/L	≈4	≈2	≈1
Ca^{++}, mg/dl	40	20	10
NH$_4^+$, mEq/L	100	50	25
Creatinine, mg/L	2000	1000	500
Glucose, mmol/L	1.0	0.5	0.25
Urea, mmol/L	600	300	150
Urea, mg/L	14,000	7000	3500
pH	5.0	to	7.0
Osmolality, mOsm/kg H$_2$O	1600	800	400

(Modified from Valtin HV: *Renal function*, ed 2, Boston, 1983, Little, Brown. Lab values from DSM [1989])

TABLE D-2	
Solute	Solute excretion/day
Na$^+$, mEq	150
K$^+$, mEq	100
Cl$^-$, mEq	150
HCO$_3^-$, mEq	≈2
Ca^{++}, mg	200
NH$_4^+$, mEq	50
Creatinine, mg	1000
Glucose, mmol	0.5
Urea, mmol	300
Urea, mg/L	7000
Osmolytes, mOsm	800

porter is not coupled directly to the hydrolysis of ATP. Active transport occurs against an electrochemical gradient and requires the direct input of energy (i.e., ATP). Some authors refer to such transport as *primary active* to emphasize the direct coupling to ATP.

4. Because the Na$^+$-K$^+$-ATPase is ultimately responsible for the reabsorption and secretion of all solutes (except H$^+$) and water by the nephron, complete inhibition of this transport protein would block all solute and water transport (both cellular and paracellular). Hence, in this hypothetical example, each day the kidneys would excrete 180 L of fluid that would be similar in composition to the glomerular ultrafiltrate.

5. In the first phase of proximal reabsorption, Na$^+$ enters the cell across the apical membrane by several symport and antiport mechanisms (e.g., Na$^+$-glucose symport, Na$^+$-amino acid symport, and Na$^+$-H$^+$ antiport). Na$^+$ exits from the cell into the blood via the Na$^+$-K$^+$-ATPase. Therefore Na$^+$ is reabsorbed across the cell with glucose, amino acids, and HCO$_3^-$. When tubular fluid reaches the second half of the proximal tubule, the concentrations of glucose, amino acids, and HCO$_3^-$ are greatly reduced. As a result, the tubular

fluid at this point is primarily NaCl. In the second phase of proximal tubule reabsorption, NaCl uptake across the apical membrane occurs by the parallel operation of Na^+-H^+ and Cl^--anion antiporters. Na^+ efflux from the cell occurs via the Na^+-K^+-ATPase, and Cl^- exit via KCl symport. Paracellular NaCl reabsorption also occurs. Paracellular Cl^- reabsorption, in the second half of the proximal tubule, is driven by the Cl^- concentration gradient across the proximal tubule, which develops because relatively little Cl^- is reabsorbed in the first half of the proximal tubule (i.e., Na^+ is reabsorbed with other solutes). Because the amount of water reabsorbed is proportionally more than the amount of Cl^- reabsorbed in the first half of the proximal tubule, the $[Cl^-]$ in tubular fluid increases, which provides the driving force for Cl^- diffusion across the tight junctions. Cl^- diffusion also renders the transepithelial voltage lumen-positive, which in turn provides the driving force for the passive, paracellular diffusion of Na^+. The transport of solutes (NaCl) across the cellular and paracellular pathways lowers the osmolality of the tubular fluid and increases the osmolality of the interstitial fluid, which establishes a driving force for water reabsorption across the proximal tubule. Some solutes are reabsorbed with this water by the process of solvent drag. Starling forces across the wall of the peritubular capillary are important for the uptake of this interstitial fluid and can regulate the rate of solute and water backflux across the tight junctions and thereby modulate net solute and water reabsorption.

6. NaCl is reabsorbed across the thick ascending limb by two mechanisms. First, transcellular transport involves Na^+ and Cl^- entry into the cell across the apical membrane via the $1Na^+$-$1K^+$-$2Cl^-$ (some Na^+ is also reabsorbed by the apical membrane Na^+-H^+ antiporter) and exit across the basolateral membrane via the Na^+-

K^+-ATPase (for Na^+) and via a KCl symporter and Cl^- channel (for Cl^-; mechanism not shown in Figure 4-8). Second, Na^+ is also reabsorbed across the paracellular pathway, owing to the lumen-positive transepithelial voltage. Furosemide would have no effect on water reabsorption in the thick ascending limb because this segment of the nephron is relatively impermeable to water and water is not reabsorbed even when NaCl reabsorptive rates are high. Furosemide increases water excretion by reducing the osmolality of the medullary interstitial fluid, which in turn reduces water reabsorption from the descending thin limb of Henle's loop.

7. Glomerulotubular balance describes the phenomenon whereby an increase in the filtered load of water and NaCl is accompanied by a parallel increase in water and NaCl reabsorption by the proximal tubule. If a constant amount of NaCl and water was reabsorbed by the proximal tubule, increases in GFR and the filtered load of NaCl and water would result in an increased delivery to more distal segments. If these segments were not able to reabsorb the excess NaCl and water, large amounts could be lost in the urine. If such an increase in excretion were not accompanied by a corresponding rise in dietary intake, the organism would develop negative NaCl and water balance. Hence, glomerulotubular balance helps to maintain NaCl and water homeostasis despite changes in GFR and the filtered load of water and NaCl.

8. See Table 4-7.

■ **CHAPTER 5**

1. This problem illustrates the importance of effective versus ineffective osmoles in regulating ADH secretion. Although plasma osmolality is elevated, the increased osmolality is due to urea. Because urea is an ineffective osmole with regard to ADH secretion, it is necessary

to estimate the osmolality of plasma that is due to effective osmoles (Na^+ and its anions). The effective osmolality of the plasma is estimated by doubling the plasma $[Na^+]$, which yields a value of 270 mOsm/kg H_2O. Because the effective osmolality is reduced, ADH secretion is suppressed and plasma levels reduced.

2. See Table D-3.

Regardless of the presence of ADH, tubular fluid osmolality is the same in all segments except the collecting duct. When ADH is present, the tubular fluid within the lumen of the collecting duct comes to osmotic equilibrium with the surrounding interstitial fluid (300 mOsm/kg H_2O in the cortex and 1200 mOsm/kg H_2O in the medulla). In the absence of ADH, solute reabsorption along the collecting duct leads to further dilution of the tubular fluid.

3. a: The first step in calculating the free-water clearance is to calculate the osmolar clearance (C_{osm}):

$$C_{osm} = \frac{U_{osm} \times \dot{V}}{P_{osm}}$$

$$= \frac{70 \text{ mOsm/kg } H_2O \times 3 \text{ ml/min}}{295 \text{ mOsm/kg } H_2O}$$

$$= 0.7 \text{ ml/min}$$

C_{H_2O} is then calculated as follows:

$$C_{H_2O} = \dot{V} - C_{osm} = 3 \text{ ml/min} - 0.7 \text{ ml/min}$$
$$= 2.3 \text{ ml/min}$$

b: In this example the following equation is used:

$$C_{osm} = \frac{U_{osm} \times \dot{V}}{P_{osm}} =$$

$$\frac{1100 \text{ mOsm/kg } H_2O \times 0.4 \text{ ml/min}}{295 \text{ mOsm/kg } H_2O} = 1.5 \text{ ml/min}$$

C_{H_2O} is then calculated as follows:

$$C_{H_2O} = \dot{V} - C_{osm} = 0.4 \text{ ml/min} - 1.5 \text{ ml/min}$$
$$= -1.1 \text{ ml/min} (T^c_{H_2O})$$

4. a. **Decreased renal perfusion:** With a decrease in renal perfusion as would occur with contraction of the effective circulating volume, delivery of solute and water to Henle's loop is reduced (GFR is decreased, and therefore filtered load is decreased and proximal tubule fractional reabsorption is enhanced). As a result, there will be less separation of solute and water and a reduction in $T^c_{H_2O}$.

b. **Inhibition of thick ascending limb transport:** Inhibition of thick ascending limb NaCl transport decreases the separation of solute and water that occurs at this

---

T A B L E D - 3		

Osmolality of tubular fluid

Nephron site	0-ADH	Max. ADH
Proximal tubule	300	300
Beginning of thin descending limb	300	300
Beginning of thin ascending limb	1200	1200
End of thick ascending limb	≈100	≈100
End of cortical collecting duct	<100	300
Urine	≈50	1200

site. Because transport by the thick ascending limb is necessary for the generation of the medullary interstitial osmotic gradient, the osmolality of the interstitium falls. This impairs the reabsorption of water from the medullary collecting duct. As a result, $T^c_{H_2O}$ is reduced. The urine osmolality will approach 300 mOsm/kg H_2O, reflecting the fact that fluid entering Henle's loop from the proximal tubule has an osmolality of this value, and separation of solute and water is impaired.

c. **Nephrogenic diabetes insipidus:** In nephrogenic diabetes insipidus the collecting duct does not respond to ADH. As a result, water cannot cross. This obviously impairs the ability of the kidneys to concentrate the urine and reabsorb solute-free water ($T^c_{H_2O}$).

5. If daily solute excretion is 800 mOsm and the individual can produce concentrated urine that only has an osmolality of 400 mOsm/kg H_2O, the minimum volume of urine required for this solute excretion is as follows:

$$\frac{800 \text{ mOsm}}{400 \text{ mOsm/kg } H_2O} = 2 \text{ L}$$

If insensible loss is 1 L, this individual must drink at least 3 L of water (or other dilute beverage) in that 24-hour period to prevent the development of hyperosmolality. This is slightly more than the average daily intake of most individuals. For the second individual the daily water requirement is much less because of the ability to excrete a more concentrated urine. Minimum urine volume required in this individual is as follows:

$$\frac{800 \text{ mOsm}}{1200 \text{ mOsm/kg } H_2O} = 0.67 \text{ L}$$

With insensible loss of 1 L, daily water intake could be less than 2 L, and body fluid osmolality would be maintained. A corollary to these examples is that solute excretion also places constraints on the maximum volume of water that can be ingested. For example, if an individual who can dilute urine to 100 mOsm/kg H_2O excretes 800 mOsm of solute, this person could drink as much as 8 L of water without reducing body fluid osmolality. If, however, the individual excretes more solute (e.g., 1200 mOsm), 12 L of water could be ingested. Indeed, a decline in body fluid osmolality can be seen in individuals who drink large quantities of water without sufficient solute intake.

■ CHAPTER 6

1. It is assumed that the 3 kg weight loss reflects only the loss of ECF. Because the plasma [Na^+] is unchanged, this represents a loss of isotonic fluid (3 L) from the ECF.

   Plasma osmolality: Because the plasma [Na^+] is unchanged, the plasma osmolality is unchanged.

   Effective circulating volume (ECV): The loss of fluid from the ECF decreases the effective circulating volume.

   ADH secretion: The decrease in ECV through the vascular baroreceptors stimulates ADH secretion.

   Urine osmolality: The increased levels of ADH lead to water conservation by the kidneys and excretion of a concentrated urine.

   Sensation of thirst: Again, the decrease in ECV through the vascular baroreceptors leads to an enhanced sensation of thirst.

2. The individual is euvolemic. To maintain Na^+ balance, the amount of Na^+ ingested in the diet must equal the amount excreted from the body. Because the kidneys are the primary route for Na^+ excretion, the amount of Na^+ excreted daily is very nearly equal to the amount ingested in the diet (small amounts of Na^+ are lost in perspiration and feces). Therefore the Na^+ excretion rate in this individual is approximately 200 mEq/day.

T A B L E D - 4		
Changes in ECV		
Regulatory factor	Increased ECV	Decreased ECV
Renal sympathetic nerves	↓	↑
ANP	↑	↓
Renin-angiotensin	↓	↑
Aldosterone	↓	↑
ADH	↓	↑

3. Table D-4.

4. This individual has gained 4 kg. This represents the accumulation of 4 L of fluid (1 kg = 1 L) in the ECF, a portion of which will accumulate in the interstitial fluid compartment as edema. The composition of this fluid is the same as that of plasma and has an $[Na^+]$ of 140 mEq/L. Recall that the accumulation of the fluid requires Na^+ retention by the kidneys. Therefore the amount of Na^+ retained by the kidneys must be equal to the amount contained in 4 L of fluid having a $[Na^+]$ of 140 mEq/L or 560 mEq of Na^+.

5. Aldosterone stimulates Na^+ reabsorption primarily in the collecting duct, which explains the reduction in Na^+ excretion seen during the beginning of aldosterone treatment. As a result of the positive Na^+ balance, the effective circulating volume is increased. This in turn increases GFR (i.e., increases the filtered load of Na^+), reduces proximal tubule reabsorption, and thereby enhances delivery of Na^+ to the collecting duct. Additionally, ANP and urodilatin levels are increased, and their action on the collecting duct to inhibit Na^+ reabsorption, together with increased Na^+ delivery to this site, results in the return of Na^+ excretion to its previous level. A new steady state is reached in which ECV is expanded and body weight is increased, reflecting the increased volume of the ECF compartment.

With cessation of aldosterone treatment the Na^+ reabsorptive rate of the collecting duct decreases. Because of the increased ECV and therefore enhanced Na^+ delivery to the collecting duct, the reabsorptive capacity of the collecting duct is overwhelmed, and Na^+ excretion increases. After a period of negative Na^+ balance the ECV decreases back to normal. A new steady state is reached, and the body weight returns to its original value as the ECF volume decreases.

■ CHAPTER 7

1. Intravenous infusion of K^+ into a subject with a combination of sympathetic blockade (i.e., no catecholamine release) and insulin deficiency would result in significant hyperkalemia compared with a similar infusion of K^+ in a normal subject. Although aldosterone secretion would be stimulated by the hyperkalemia, this hormone stimulates cell K^+ uptake after a 1-hour lag period. In the first hour following K^+ infusion, less than 50% of the infused K^+ is excreted by the kidneys, and because sympathetic activity and insulin release are suppressed, most of the K^+ remaining in the body is retained in the extracellular fluid.

2. Aldosterone deficiency would initially reduce urinary potassium excretion, and K^+ would be retained in the body (i.e., dietary intake would exceed excretion). This would lead to hyper-

kalemia, which is a potent stimulus of K$^+$ excretion. Because the individual is initially in positive K$^+$ balance, plasma K$^+$ rises until urinary K$^+$ excretion becomes equal to dietary K$^+$ intake. In the new steady state, K$^+$ intake would equal K$^+$ excretion; however, the subject has hyperkalemia. Thus, it is possible to match dietary K$^+$ intake with excretion in the absence of aldosterone, although this occurs at an elevated plasma [K$^+$].

3. In the first hour after a meal, the rise in plasma K$^+$ is blunted by the rapid (minutes) uptake of K$^+$ into skeletal muscle, liver, bone, and red blood cells. Some K$^+$ is excreted by the kidneys, but in the first hour following the meal most K$^+$ is sequestered in the intracellular fluid. In the ensuing hours, K$^+$ slowly leaves the cells and is excreted by the kidneys, thereby maintaining K$^+$ balance and plasma [K$^+$].

4. Normally, K$^+$ excretion is determined primarily by the rate of K$^+$ secretion by the distal tubule and collecting duct and is largely independent of the GFR and the filtered load of K$^+$. When 50% of the nephrons are lost, the distal tubules and collecting ducts in the remaining functioning nephrons secrete more K$^+$ so that K$^+$ excretion and plasma [K$^+$] are maintained at normal levels. However, if 80% to 85% of the nephrons are lost and GFR falls below 15% to 20% of normal, K$^+$ secretion by the distal tubule and collecting duct cannot increase enough to maintain constant urinary K$^+$ excretion, and hyperkalemia ensues. Consult Chapter 11 for more details on the function of remnant nephrons.

■ CHAPTER 8

1. If urinary buffers were not available, the 70 mEq of acid needed to be excreted by the kidneys to maintain acid-base balance (net acid excretion = nonvolatile acid production) would have to be excreted as free H$^+$. If the minimum urine pH equals 4.0, this represents only 0.1 mEq/L of H$^+$. Thus, for 70 mEq of H$^+$ to be excreted, the daily urine output would need to be as follows:

$$\frac{70 \text{ mEq/day}}{0.1 \text{ mEq/L}} = 700 \text{ L/day}$$

This exceeds the daily GFR (180 L/day). Thus, the urinary buffers are essential for the kidneys' ability to excrete sufficient quantities of H$^+$ and maintain acid-base balance.

2. See Table D-5 below.
   The first six disorders are simple acid-base dis-

TABLE D-5

Acid-base disorders

pH	[HCO$_3$$^-$] mEq/L	P$_{CO_2}$ mm Hg	Disorder	Compensation
7.34	15	29	Metabolic acidosis	Buffering & respiratory
7.49	35	48	Metabolic alkalosis	Buffering & respiratory
7.47	14	20	Chronic respiratory alkalosis	Buffering & renal
7.34	31	60	Chronic respiratory acidosis	Buffering & renal
7.26	26	60	Acute respiratory acidosis	Buffering
7.62	20	20	Acute respiratory alkalosis	Buffering
7.09	15	50	Metabolic + respiratory acidosis	Buffering
7.40	15	25	Metabolic acidosis + respiratory alkalosis	Buffering

orders. The last two represent mixed disorders. Mixed metabolic and respiratory acidosis is seen during cardiopulmonary arrest. With cessation of cardiac function the tissues are inadequately perfused and resort to anaerobic metabolism (production of lactic acid). With cessation of respiration, CO_2 retention also occurs. In the example of mixed metabolic acidosis and respiratory alkalosis, pH is normal but both the $[HCO_3^-]$ and P_{CO_2} are abnormal. An example of a clinical condition producing such a disorder is an overdose of aspirin. The metabolic acidosis is the result of the salicylic acid (active ingredient of aspirin), and the respiratory alkalosis is the result of hyperventilation secondary to salicylic-acid stimulation of the respiratory centers.

3. The initial set of laboratory data indicates the presence of a metabolic alkalosis with appropriate respiratory compensation. Given the individual's history, the most likely cause of this simple acid-base disorder is the loss of gastric acid by vomiting. The second set of laboratory data continues to show the presence of a metabolic alkalosis with respiratory compensation. In addition, there is evidence for fluid loss (decrease in body weight by 2 kg) and a resultant decrease in ECV (decrease in blood pressure). Given the worsening of this individual's metabolic alkalosis, it is somewhat surprising that the urine pH is so acidic. The appropriate renal response should be an increase in HCO_3^- excretion to correct the alkalosis. However, by decreasing the filtered load of HCO_3^- (decreased GFR) and stimulating proximal Na^+ reabsorption, the decreased ECV prevents the excretion of HCO_3^- (HCO_3^- reabsorption is linked to Na^+). In addition, the decreased ECV stimulates aldosterone secretion, which increases H^+ secretion by the intercalated cells of the

collecting duct. Therefore the urine is more acidic than expected for the degree of alkalosis. The ECV must be restored to its normal value to correct this situation. Infusion of isotonic NaCl would accomplish this and also allow the kidneys to excrete the excess HCO_3^-, thereby restoring acid-base balance.

4. Carbonic anhydrase plays a critical role in the reabsorption of HCO_3^- by the cells of the proximal tubule and by intercalated cells of the collecting duct. Inhibition of this enzyme would therefore inhibit the reabsorption of HCO_3^- at these nephron sites. Because of the large fraction of the filterd load of HCO_3^- reabsorbed by the proximal tubule, the effect at this site is quantitatively more important. With decreased reabsorption, more HCO_3^- would be excreted in the urine, and urine pH would become alkaline. This loss of HCO_3^- from the body would result in the development of a metabolic acidosis.

■ CHAPTER 9

1. Approximately two-thirds of Ca^{++} reabsorption across the proximal tubule occurs by solvent drag, a process that depends on Na^+ reabsorption. Mannitol would inhibit Ca^{++} reabsorption by blocking solvent drag in the proximal tubule and thereby increase urinary Ca^{++} excretion.

2. Furosemide would inhibit the $1Na^+$-$1K^+$-$2Cl^-$ symporter and reduce the lumen-positive transepithelial voltage to 0. This, in turn would inhibit passive Ca^{++} reabsorption via the paracellular pathway.

3. A rise in plasma [Pi] increases the amount of Pi filtered by the glomeruli. Because the amount of Pi normally filtered is equal to the reabsorptive capacity of the kidneys, an increase in the amount of Pi filtered will increase urinary Pi excretion and reduce plasma [Pi].

■ CHAPTER 10

1. See Table D-6.

To determine the type of diuretic, its effect on both C_{H_2O} and $T^c_{H_2O}$ must be determined.

Diuretic A: Diuretic A increases both C_{H_2O} and $T^c_{H_2O}$. This diuretic must be acting proximal to the thick ascending limb of Henle's loop. The delivery of solute and water to this segment will be increased by inhibiting Na^+ transport at a site proximal to the thick ascending limb. With increased delivery there will be increased separation of solute and water, which increases both C_{H_2O} and $T^c_{H_2O}$. Diuretic A could be either an osmotic diuretic or a carbonic anhydrase inhibitor.

Diuretic B: Diuretic B inhibits C_{H_2O} and $T^c_{H_2O}$. Therefore it must be acting on a nephron site that separates solute from water. In addition, at least a portion of this nephron segment must be in the medulla in order to account for the decrease in $T^c_{H_2O}$. This nephron site is the thick ascending limb of Henle's loop. Separating solute from water at this site contributes to the generation of C_{H_2O}. It also contributes to the maintenance of the medullary interstitial osmotic gradient and thus $T^c_{H_2O}$. Diuretic B is a loop diuretic (e.g., furosemide, ethacrynic acid, bumetanide).

Diuretic C: Diuretic C inhibits C_{H_2O} but has no effect on $T^c_{H_2O}$. This diuretic must be acting in the cortex to inhibit the separation of solute and water. Both thiazide diuretics and K^+-sparing diuretics act in the cortex. However, the K^+-sparing diuretics do not have an appreciable effect on C_{H_2O} (the magnitude of Na^+ transport inhibited by the K^+-sparing diuretics is too small). Therefore Diuretic C must be a thiazide diuretic (e.g., chlorothiazide, metolazone).

TABLE D-6

Classes of diuretics

Condition	P_{osm} (mOsm/kg H_2O)	U_{osm} (mOsm/kg H_2O)	$\dot{V}$ (ml/min)	C_{H_2O} (ml/min)	$T^c_{H_2O}$ (ml/min)
Water Diuresis					
Before Diuretic A	285	70	10	7.54	
After Diuretic A	284	125	16	8.96	
Before Diuretic B	286	65	12	9.27	
After Diuretic B	286	200	19	5.71	
Before Diuretic C	284	70	11	8.29	
After Diuretic C	285	195	15	4.74	
Antidiuresis					
Before Diuretic A	288	1200	0.6		1.90
After Diuretic A	289	450	12		6.69
Before Diuretic B	290	1100	0.7		1.96
After Diuretic B	288	300	13		0.54
Before Diuretic C	287	1200	0.7		2.23
After Diuretic C	290	355	10		2.24

2. Nephrogenic diabetes insipidus is a condition in which the collecting duct does not respond to ADH. As a result, water cannot be reabsorbed, and large volumes of dilute urine are excreted. The key to understanding how long-term thiazide diuretic therapy can lead to a reduction in urine excretion with this condition is the fact that this therapy leads to a reduction in the ECV. With this decrease in ECV, reabsorption of solute and water by the proximal tubule is enhanced. As a result, less fluid is delivered to Henle's loop and therefore into the collecting duct, which water cannot penetrate. With this decreased distal delivery of fluid, urine volume is reduced, even though the collecting duct cannot reabsorb water. The thiazide diuretic does not correct the underlying cause of nephrogenic diabetes insipidus, but it does provide symptomatic relief from the polyuria. The beneficial effect of the thiazide diuretic can be negated if the ECV is allowed to reexpand (e.g., by the ingestion of large quantities of Na^+).

3. a. The long-term effect of diuretic therapy is the reduction of the ECV. With such a decrease the blood volume and thus cardiac output are reduced. Because blood pressure is equal to cardiac output multiplied by the total peripheral vascular resistance, a decrease in cardiac output reduces blood pressure. Additionally, diuretics may cause some degree of vascular smooth muscle vasodilatation, although the mechanism by which this occurs is not fully understood. This vasodilatation reduces total peripheral vascular resistance, thereby decreasing blood pressure.

   b. Hypokalemia is a side effect of all diuretics acting proximal to the K^+ secretory site (distal tubule and the cortical collecting duct). The most common diuretics given for the treatment of hypertension are thiazides. However, the loop diuretics, osmotic diuretics, and carbonic anhydrase inhibitors can also lead to hypokalemia. By their action, tubular fluid flow rate to the K^+ secretory site is enhanced, which in turn stimulates K^+ secretion. Additionally, the diuretic-induced decrease in ECV leads to stimulation of aldosterone secretion by the adrenal cortex via the renin-angiotensin system. Aldosterone also directly stimulates K^+ secretion by the distal tubule and cortical collecting duct.

   c. Treatment of the hypokalemia could involve supplementation of the diet with foods containing high levels of K^+ or with KCl tablets. Alternatively, a K^+-sparing diuretic could be given in combination with the thiazide diuretic.

4. Thiazide diuretics are secreted into the lumen of the proximal tubule by the same organic anion transport system that secretes penicillin. Competitive inhibition of secretion of the thiazide could decrease the effective concentration of the diuretic in the tubular field. Since thiazides act from the lumen, a reduction in their concentration at this site could reduce their effectiveness.

■ CHAPTER 11

1.

	Single nephron	Whole kidney
GFR	↑	↓
Fractional Na^+ excretion	↑	↑
C_{H_2O}	↑	↓
$T^c_{H_2O}$	↑	↓
Pi excretion	↑	↓
Ammonium excretion	↑	↓

2. a. Na^+ excretion rate:

   Individual A = 150 mEq/day
   Individual B = 150 mEq/day

   b. Fraction Na^+ excretion (FE_{Na}):

   Individual A = 0.6%
   Individual B = 2.1%

This problem illustrates the fact that steady state balance for Na$^+$ can be maintained (excretion rate equal to intake) for both individuals. However, the individual with renal disease must excrete a larger percentage of the filtered load of Na$^+$ to maintain the needed excretion rate.

3. For the maintenance of water balance the amount of water ingested each day cannot be less than or in excess of the range for water excretion by the kidney. The decreased ability to dilute (minimum urine osmolality = 200 mOsm/kg H$_2$O) and concentrate (maximum urine osmolality = 400 mOsm/kg H$_2$O) the urine reduces this excretory range. Therefore

Minimum water ingestion = 1.25 L/day
Maximum water ingestion = 2.5 L/day

If water intake was less than 1.25 L/day, negative balance would exist and body fluid osmolality would increase. Conversely, if water intake exceeded 2.5 L/day, positive balance would occur and body fluid osmolality would decrease. This example clearly illustrates the need for individuals with renal disease to monitor and regulate their intake of water.

Answers to Integrative Case Studies

■ CASE 1

1a. The ECF volume of this man is above normal. The presence of edema, distension of the neck veins, and rales (sounds caused by fluid in the lungs) is evidence of this increased volume. Additional evidence could be obtained by measuring weight gain, because accumulation of each liter of ECF would increase body weight by 1 kg.

1b. The ECV in this man would be decreased from normal. With damage to the myocardium, cardiac output and therefore tissue perfusion would be reduced and sensed by the body as a decrease in the ECV. The ECV cannot be measured directly. Therefore measurements would have to be made of parameters that change in response to alterations in the ECV to determine if the ECV is reduced. For example, the kidneys reduce Na^+ excretion in response to a decrease in the ECV. Measurement of fractional Na^+ excretion could confirm the existence of a reduced effective circulating volume (fraction Na^+ excretion below 1%). However, in this man fractional excretion may not be this low because of the use of a thiazide diuretic. Alternatively, measurements could be made of plasma renin activity, catecholamines, and ADH because these would be elevated with the decreased ECV.

1c. The kidneys would be avidly retaining Na^+. With a decrease in ECV, sensors in the low-pressure (cardiac atria and pulmonary vasculature) and high-pressure (juxtaglomerular apparatus, aortic arch, and carotid sinus) sides of the circulation would be activated, and signals sent to the kidneys to retain Na^+.

- Sympathetic nerves innervating the afferent and efferent arterioles of the glomeruli would cause vasoconstriction. The net result would be to reduce the GFR. This in turn would reduce the filtered load of Na^+.
- Sympathetic innervation of the proximal tubule, thick ascending limb of Henle's loop, and collecting duct also increases Na^+ reabsorption at these sites.
- Increased sympathetic nerve activity, together with decreased perfusion pressure at the afferent arteriole, results in the secretion of renin. This activation of the renin-angiotensin-aldosterone system further stimulates Na^+ reabsorption, because

angiotensin II increases proximal tubule Na$^+$ reabsorption and aldosterone increases Na$^+$ reabsorption in the distal tubule and collecting duct. With the increase in the ECF, atrial natriuretic peptide (ANP) levels are elevated. However, the effect of ANP (inhibition of renin secretion and natriuresis) appears to be blunted by the effect of the other factors, all of which act to reduce Na$^+$ excretion. The net effect of these responses is retention of Na$^+$ by the kidneys. As a result of this Na$^+$ retention (positive Na$^+$ balance), the ECF volume increases, leading to the formation of edema as seen during the physical examination of this man.

1d. The development of hyponatremia indicates that this man is in positive water balance. In this case the ingestion of water has exceeded the capacity of the kidneys to excrete solute-free water. There are several reasons that solute-free water excretion is impaired in this man.

- ADH secretion is stimulated because of the decreased ECV. As a consequence, solute-free water is reabsorbed by the collecting duct.
- The decreased ECV results in a decrease in the filtered load of solute (NaCl) and water and an increase in fractional reabsorption by the proximal tubule. As a result, the delivery of solute and water to the thick ascending limb, the primary site where solute-free waer is generated, is decreased.
- The thiazide diuretic inhibits NaCl reabsorption in the distal tubule. This portion of the nephron also participates in the generation of solute-free water. With impaired NaCl reabsorption, less solute-free water can be generated.

1e. Increased renal K$^+$ excretion causes the hypokalemia in this man. Two factors contribute to enhanced K$^+$ excretion. The first is related to the administration of the thiazide diuretic. Thiazide diuretics act on the distal tubule to inhibit NaCl reabsorption. Inhibition of NaCl reabsorption in the distal tubule results in the delivery of increased quantities of fluid to the portion of the nephron responsible for K$^+$ secretion (distal tubule and cortical collecting duct). This increased delivery stimulates K$^+$ secretion by the principal cells in this part of the nephron. Second, the ECV is decreased in this man, which in turn stimulates the renin-angiotensin-aldosterone system. Aldosterone then acts on the collecting duct to stimulate K$^+$ secretion. The enhanced secretion of K$^+$ by the distal tubule and cortical collecting duct results in increased K$^+$ excretion and the development of hypokalemia. Extrarenal factors also contribute to the development of hypokalemia because both alkalosis and aldosterone cause K$^+$ to move into cells.

1f. Although an arterial blood sample was not obtained, the plasma [HCO$_3$$^-$] is elevated, suggesting the presence of a metabolic alkalosis. The development of a metabolic alkalosis could reflect enhanced renal HCO$_3$$^-$ reabsorption and H$^+$ excretion. HCO$_3$$^-$ reabsorption by the proximal tubule would be stimulated because proximal tubule reabsorption is enhanced when the ECV is decreased (see Question 1c). Virtually all of the filtered load of HCO$_3$$^-$ will be reabsorbed by the time the tubular fluid reaches the distal tubule and collecting duct. H$^+$ secretion at these sites will titrate urinary buffers and lead to the generation of "new HCO$_3$$^-$." Because of the decreased ECV, aldosterone levels are elevated. Because aldosterone stimulates H$^+$ secretion in the distal tubule and collecting duct, "new HCO$_3$$^-$" generation will be increased and metabolic alkalosis will develop.

1g. Creatinine is excreted from the body primarily by glomerular filtration (10% is excreted as a result of secretion by the proximal tubule). Therefore the amount of creatinine excreted is determined primarily by its filtered load. With a reduction in the ECV the GFR is reduced (see Question 3). The reduced filtration rate decreases the filtered load of creatinine and thus its excretion. As a result, the serum [creatinine] increases. The serum [creatinine] should decline when the ECV is restored to its normal value.

1h. A loop diuretic acts on the thick ascending limb of Henle's loop to inhibit NaCl reabsorption and increase Na^+ excretion. This enhanced excretion of Na^+ results in a further decrease in the ECV. The loop diuretic has the potential to cause further reductions in the serum Na^+ and K^+ concentrations, to make the metabolic alkalosis worse, and to further increase the serum [creatinine] for the following reasons:

- The thick ascending limb of Henle's loop is the primary site where tubular fluid is diluted. The loop diuretic will inhibit the separation of solute (NaCl) and water at this site and futher impair the generation of solute-free water. If water ingestion is not reduced, hyponatremia could become more severe.

- The thick ascending limb of Henle's loop reabsorbs approximately 20% of the filtered load of K^+. This process is inhibited by loop diuretics. Also, the loop diuretic will cause increased delivery of Na^+ and fluid to the distal tubule and cortical collecting duct. Together, these effects will further enhance K^+ secretion and thus renal K^+ excretion, leading to a worsening of the hypokalemia.

- Because the loop diuretic leads to a further reduction in the ECV, the stimuli for enhancing both proximal tubule HCO_3^- reabsorption and distal tubule and collecting duct H^+ secretion are increased. As a result, the metabolic alkalosis may become more severe.

- With the added decrement in the ECV caused by the loop diuretic, the glomerular filtration rate will fall further and thereby cause the serum [creatinine] to increase.

The abnormalities in serum electrolytes seen in this man are caused primarily by the decreased ECV caused by his myocardial infarction (i.e., decreased cardiac output). The diuretic therapy is directed at preventing the kidneys from responding to the decreased ECV. Although the diuretics reduce Na^+ retention by the kidneys and help alleviate edema formation, they decrease the ECV further and thus have the potential to produce the water, Na^+, K^+, and acid-base abnormalities seen in this man.

■ CASE 2

2a. These symptoms and electrolyte disturbances are most characteristic of decreased levels of adrenal cortical steroids and especially the mineralocorticoid hormone aldosterone. This patient has Addison's disease. The presence of hyperpigmentation suggests that the problem is at the level of the adrenal gland (i.e., nonresponsive to ACTH). ACTH levels are elevated in response to the decreased circulating levels of adrenal cortical steroids. These elevated levels of ACTH stimulate melanocytes, leading to the hyperpigmentation of the gums and skin.

2b. The hypotension is a result of the negative Na^+ balance present in this woman, which in turn reflects the decreased circulating levels of aldosterone. With hypoaldosteronism, Na^+ reabsorption by the thick ascending limb of Henle's loop and the collecting duct is reduced, and negative Na^+ balance develops (Na^+ excretion exceeds Na^+ intake). Because ECF volume reflects Na^+ balance, ECF volume is decreased. Because plasma is a component of the ECF, vascular volume and therefore blood pressure are decreased. This in turn reduces the ECV.

2c. Hyponatremia indicates a problem in water metabolism. Thus, the ability of this woman's kidneys to excrete solute-free water is impaired, and she is in positive water balance (solute-free water ingestion exceeds solute-free water excretion). Excretion of solute-free water is impaired for two primary reasons, both of which relate to a decreased ECV. With the decreased ECV the GFR is reduced, which reduces the filtered load of solute (NaCl) and water. Also, the proximal tubule reabsorbs a greater fraction of the filtered load of NaCl. Together, these effects reduce the delivery of solute and water to the thick ascending limb of Henle's loop, the portion of the nephron where solute-free water is generated. In addition, the decreased ECV causes the secretion of ADH. With ADH present the collecting duct reabsorbs water, thereby reducing its excretion.

2d. Urinary K^+ excretion is largely determined by the amount of K^+ secreted into tubular fluid by the distal tubule and cortical collecting duct. K^+ secretion at these nephron sites is reduced by the low levels of plasma aldosterone. Therefore K^+ excretion by the distal tubule and cortical collecting duct will be reduced in this woman, and she will be in positive K^+ balance (intake exceeds excretion). In addition, aldosterone causes the uptake of K^+ into cells (e.g., skeletal muscle). In the absence of aldosterone there is less cellular uptake. This contributes to the development of hyperkalemia.

2e. This woman's acid-base disturbance is likely to be a metabolic acidosis secondary to reduced net acid excretion by the kidneys. Although arterial blood pH is not reported, the reduced plasma $[HCO_3^-]$ is consistent with a metabolic acidosis. Net acid excretion by the kidneys is impaired for two reasons. First, aldosterone stimulates H^+ secretion by the intercalated cells of the collecting duct. In the absence of aldosterone, H^+ secretion at this site is diminished and less H^+ is excreted. Second, hyperkalemia inhibits ammoniagenesis by cells of the proximal tubule. Because ammonium production is an important source of "new HCO_3^-," a reduction in this process contributes to the impairment of net acid excretion.

■ CASE 3

3a. The acid-base disorder of this man is a metabolic acidosis. In the absence of insulin the metabolism of fats and carbohydrates is altered so that nonvolatile acids (keto acids) are produced. The nonvolatile acids are rapidly buffered by cellular and extracellular buffers. Buffering in the ECF results in a decrease in the plasma $[HCO_3^-]$. The deep, rapid breathing reflects the respiratory compensation (P_{CO_2} is lowered). Although the anion gap was not measured in this man, it would be increased because of the accumulation of the anions of the keto acids.

3b. Hyperkalemia in this man results from a shift of K^+ out of cells (e.g., skeletal muscle) into the ECF. This shift occurs because of the lack of insulin and the hypertonicity of the ECF secondary to the elevated [glucose]. The acidosis is probably not a major contributing factor to the development of hyperkalemia in this situation. When acidosis is induced by mineral acids (e.g., HCl), movement of H^+ into cells during the process of intracellular buffering results in a shift of K^+ out of the cell into the ECF. However, with organic acidosis, as occurs in this situation, the cellular buffering of the organic acids does not result in a significant shift of K^+ out of the cell.

3c. Insulin causes K^+ to move into cells. The mechanism responsible for this effect of insulin appears to be related to stimulation of the Na^+-K^+-ATPase. With increased activity of the Na^+-K^+-ATPase, K^+ uptake into the cell is enhanced. In addition, insulin's effect on glucose metabolism will lower the serum [glucose]. As a consequence, the osmolality of the ECF will decrease and cause additional K^+ to move into cells.

3d. The administration of HCO_3^- would increase the blood pH and shift some K^+ into cells. The HCO_3^--containing intravenous fluid would also increase the volume of the ECF and decrease the $[K^+]$ in this compartment. Experimental animal studies have shown that the dilution of K^+ by expansion of the ECF is the primary mechanism by which the infusion of a HCO_3^--containing solution decreases the serum $[K^+]$.

3e. The polyuria results from an osmotic diuresis induced by glucose. Normally all of the filtered load of glucose is reabsorbed by the proximal tubule. However, in this man the filtered load of glucose exceeds the reabsorptive capacity of the proximal tubule. Consequently, the glucose that is not reabsorbed will remain in the lumen of the proximal tubule, where it will act as an osmotically active particle. As NaCl and water are reabsorbed by the proximal tubule, the concentration of the nonreabsorbed glucose will increase. With this increase in glucose concentration, an osmotic gradient opposite to that generated by the NaCl reabsorptive process is developed. Because reabsorption of water by the proximal tubule depends on an osmotic pressure gradient, the presence of glucose in the tubular fluid will reduce the osmotic gradient and thereby water reabsorption. The glucose-induced osmotic diuresis will increase the delivery of NaCl and water to the distal tubule and cortical collecting duct, which stimulates K^+ secretion at these sites. As a result, K^+ excretion from the body will be increased. Increased K^+ excretion, together with the shift of K^+ from the ICF to the ECF secondary to the insulin deficiency and hyperosmolality, will lead to progressive whole-body K^+ depletion. Accordingly, an increase in serum $[K^+]$ does not always indicate positive K^+ balance. This man is in negative K^+ balance and is at risk for the development of hypokalemia when insulin is administered and the metabolic abnormalities are corrected.

3f. The glucose-induced osmotic diuresis causes a loss of water from the body in excess of solute. This would lead to the development of hypernatremia. However, the hyperglycemia causes a shift of water from the ICF to the ECF, which tends to decrease the ECF $[Na^+]$. As therapy is initiated and the hyperglycemia corrected, water will move back into the ICF, leading to the development of hypernatremia.

■ CASE 4

4a. This woman has signs and symptoms of a reduced effective circulating volume (i.e., orthostatic changes in blood pressure, tachycardia, and poor skin turgor). As a result of her decreased ECV, GFR is reduced and clearance of creatinine is decreased. The reduced clearance of creatinine will cause the serum [creatinine] to increase. During the first 4 days in the hospital, and based on the serum [creatinine] alone, it is not possible to determine whether renal function is normal and creatinine excretion is reduced because of the decreased GFR or whether this woman also has some underlying renal disease.

4b. The decreased cardiac output in this woman will be sensed by the low- and high-pressure baroreceptors as decreased ECV. As a result, the renin-angiotensin-aldosterone system will be activated, as well as the sympathetic nervous system. These systems tend to reduce the GFR because of their vasoconstrictor effects on the afferent arterioles. The effects of these vasoconstrictors are balanced somewhat by intrarenal prostaglandins, which vasodilate the afferent arterioles. Administration of a nonsteroidal antiinflammatory agent that inhibits prostaglandin production could therefore result in further vasoconstriction and reduction of GFR.

4c. The loop diuretic is used to prevent the kidneys from avidly reabsorbing Na^+ in response to the perceived decrease in ECV. (ECV is reduced because of the low cardiac output.) The Na^+ retention by the kidney is responsible for the development of this woman's edema. Thus, the diuretic will help reduce the edema, but its action to increase renal Na^+ excretion will further decrease the ECV.

4d. The creatine clearance (C_{cr}) is calculated as follows:

$$C_{cr} = \frac{64.8 \text{ mg/dl} \times 0.69 \text{ ml/min}^*}{1 \text{ mg/dl}} = 44.7 \text{ ml/min}$$

This is a normal GFR for a 75-year-old woman. Given her age and the fact that muscle mass usually decreases in the elderly, the plasma [creatinine] of 1 mg/dl is consistent with a GFR of 45 ml/min. By contrast, a plasma [creatinine] of this level in a 40-year-old woman with normal muscle mass would reflect a GFR in the range of 100 ml/min or more. It is important to remember that creatinine production is proportional to muscle mass. Therefore the same plasma [creatinine] in two individuals does not necessarily mean they will have the same GFR. Doing a creatinine clearance requires proper collection of urine. If the urine was collected for less than

_____
*1000 ml/day = 0.69 ml/min.

a 24-hour period or some of the urine was lost, the calculated GFR would be artificially low. The total amount of creatinine excreted should be determined to check if the collection was complete. Because in the steady state the amount excreted must equal the amount produced by muscle metabolism, this number can be compared to expected creatinine production rates. For example, in males under the age of 60, creatinine production is in the range of 20 to 25 mg/kg of body weight. The production rate in females is slightly lower (15 to 20 mg/kg of body weight). In people over 60 years of age, these production rates are approximately 50% less, reflecting the decrease in muscle mass. In this woman, creatinine production is 648 mg (excretion rate = production rate in the steady state). Based on her weight, the expected excretion rate is approximately 450 to 600 mg/day. This is therefore an accurate collection and a reasonable measure of her GFR.

■ CASE 5

5a. Na^+ excretion is determined by diet and the ECV. In a euvolemic individual the amount of Na^+ excreted each day equals the amount ingested in the diet. Measurement of the [Na^+] in a single urine sample cannot indicate whether Na^+ excretion is normal. Also, the plasma [Na^+] does not reflect Na^+ balance; instead, it reflects water balance. The hyponatremia in this man indicates he is in positive water balance (i.e., intake exceeds excretion).

5b. Infusion of 2 L of isotonic saline will add 600 mOsm of NaCl (300 mmol NaCl = 600 mOsm) to his ECF, together with 2 L of water. The entire amount of NaCl will be excreted because he is in steady state Na^+ balance (excretion = intake). However, because of the inappropriate secretion of ADH, he will not be able to excrete the water. With a U_{osm} of 600 mOsm/kg H_2O, he will excrete the infused NaCl (600 mOsm) in 1 L of urine. Thus, 1 L of solute-free water will be added to the body, and the plasma [Na^+] will decrease. For this man the addition of 1 L of solute-free water to his body fluid will reduce the plasma [Na^+] to 117 mEq/L.

Total body osmoles (unchanged) = 10,080 mOsm
New total body water = 42 L + 1 L = 43 L
New plasma osmolality = $\dfrac{10{,}080 \text{ mOsm}}{43 \text{ L}}$
$\qquad\qquad\qquad = 234 \text{ mOsm/kg } H_2O$
New plasma [Na^+] = $\dfrac{234 \text{ mOsm/kg } H_2O}{2}$
$\qquad\qquad\qquad = 117 \text{ mEq/L}$

5c. A 3% saline solution contains 513 mmol/L of NaCl (1026 mOsm/L). Thus, 1L of fluid and 1026 mOsm of solute are added to the body fluids. With the establishment of a new steady state, the infused NaCl will be excreted with 1.7 L of urine.

$$\frac{1026 \text{ mOsm}}{600 \text{ mOsm/kg } H_2O} = 1.7 \text{ L}$$

(U_{osm} = 600 mOsm/kg H_2O because of the unregulated secretion of ADH. Therefore, 1 liter of infused water is excreted with an additional 0.7 L of solute-free water. This will result in a new plasma [Na^+] of 122 mEq/L.

Total body osmoles (unchanged) = 10,080 mOsm
New total body water = 42 L − 0.7 L = 41.3 L
New plasma osmolality = $\dfrac{10{,}080 \text{ mOsm}}{41.3 \text{ L}}$
$\qquad\qquad\qquad = 244 \text{ mOsm/kg } H_2O$
New plasma [Na^+] = $\dfrac{244 \text{ mOsm/kg } H_2O}{2}$
$\qquad\qquad\qquad = 122 \text{ mEq/L}$

5d. The loop diuretic will inhibit the 1Na^+-1K^+-2Cl^- symporter in the thick ascending limb of Henle's loop and thereby inhibit the reabsorption of NaCl. Because NaCl reabsorption at this nephron site is responsible for

maintaining a hyperosmotic medullary interstitium, the osmolality of this interstitial fluid will decrease. Thus, even in the presence of ADH, there will be less water reabsorbed from the collecting duct (i.e., more water will be excreted). In this example, U_{osm} = 300 mOsm/kg H_2O. Therefore the excretion of the infused NaCl (1026 mOsm) will occur with 3.4 L of urine.

$$\frac{1026 \text{ mOsm}}{300 \text{ mOsm/kg } H_2O} = 3.4 \text{ L}$$

The net effect of this maneuver will be to lose 2.4 L of solute-free water from the body (3.4 L of urine = 1 L of infused volume + 2.4 L of solute-free body fluid water). This will then raise the plasma [Na^+] to 127 mEq/L.

Total body osmoles (unchanged) = 10,080 mOsm
New total body water = 42 L − 2.4 L = 39.6 L
New plasma osmolality = $\dfrac{10{,}080 \text{ mOsm}}{39.6 \text{ L}}$
$\qquad\qquad\qquad = 254 \text{ mOsm/kg } H_2O$
New plasma [Na^+] = $\dfrac{254 \text{ mOsm/kg } H_2O}{2}$
$\qquad\qquad\qquad = 127 \text{ mEq/L}$

■ CASE 6

6a. Polyuria can result from a water diuresis such as that which occurs in primary polydipsia (i.e., ingestion of large volumes of water, which the kidneys excrete). Polyuria can also result from a defect in the ability of the kidneys to conserve water (polydipsia is driven by thirst). The kidneys may be unable to conserve water because ADH is absent (central diabetes insipidus), the collecting duct does not respond to ADH (nephrogenic diabetes insipidus), or water is lost with solute (solute diuresis). Diabetes mellitus and the increased excretion of glucose that occurs in this disease are a common cause of osmotic diuresis in adults and children.

6b. With careful observation, one could sort out whether primary polydipsia was the cause of the polyuria, because urine output would decrease shortly after oral intake was curtailed. A measurement of urine osmolality will help determine if the polyuria relates to problems with ADH or is secondary to a solute diuresis. The urine will be maximally dilute if there is a problem with ADH (secretion or action) but will have an osmolality near that of plasma if there is a solute diuresis. Central and nephrogenic diabetes insipidus can be distinguished by the effect of exogenously administered ADH. Administration of ADH to an individual with central diabetes insipidus results in a decrease in urine output and a concomitant increase in U_{osm}. Exogenously administered ADH has little effect on urine flow and U_{osm} in an individual with nephrogenic diabetes insipidus.

6c. Serum $[Na^+]$ would be normal if this man's water intake did not exceed the ability of his kidneys to excrete solute-free water. Serum $[Na^+]$ would be reduced if his water intake exceeded the ability of his kidneys to excrete solute-free water, and it would be increased if his water intake was less than the excretion of solute-free water.

■ CASE 7

7a. The acid-base disorder is a metabolic acidosis. The serum $[HCO_3^-]$ is reduced, and the P_{CO_2} is reduced, reflecting compensation. The 9 mEq/L decrease in serum $[HCO_3^-]$ should result in an approximate 10 mm Hg decrease in P_{CO_2} if respiratory compensation occurs.

7b. The anion gap is calculated as follows:

$$\text{Anion gap} = [Na^+] + ([Cl^-] - [HCO_3^-])$$
$$= 25 \text{ mEq/L}$$

This anion gap is elevated (normal = 8-16 mEq/L), indicating that the anion associated with the nonvolatile acid is unmeasured.

7c. Given the patient's history and the presence of an anion gap, the most likely cause of the acid-base disorder is lactic acidosis from decreased tissue perfusion secondary to cardiac arrest. Under conditions of decreased tissue perfusion the cells of the body resort to anaerobic glycolysis for energy metabolism.

■ CASE 8

8a. This is a metabolic acidosis with no anion gap. The two most frequent causes for non-anion gap acidoses are defects in renal acid excretion (renal tubular acidosis) and loss of HCO_3^- from the body (e.g., diarrhea). In this case, the relatively alkaline urine pH in the presence of systemic acidosis suggests a defect in renal acid excretion. Normally the urine should be maximally acidic with this degree of systemic acidosis. The most likely diagnosis is distal renal tubular acidosis (i.e., a defect in H^+ secretion or H^+ permeability of the distal tubule and collecting duct). The renal stone that brought this man to the physician probably contains calcium because the solubility of calcium is reduced in alkaline urine.

8b. The serum $[K^+]$ is low because excess K^+ is being lost in the urine. Several mechanisms may contribute to increased excretion of K^+. (1) The defect in distal tubule and collecting duct H^+ secretion may cause the transepithelial voltage to increase in magnitude. Normally this voltage is oriented with the lumen negative with respect to blood secondary to Na^+ reabsorption. If H^+ secretion is reduced, the magnitude of this voltage will increase. An increase in the magnitude of this voltage will then result in increased K^+ secretion. (2)

The H$^+$ secretion defect might involve the H$^+$-K$^+$-ATPase by decreasing its activity. If this happens, K$^+$ excretion will increase. (3) Metabolic acidosis decreases proximal tubule solute and water reabsorption. This will increase tubular fluid flow to the distal tubule and cortical collecting duct, which will stimulate K$^+$ secretion at these sites.

■ CASE 9

9a. This represents a simple metabolic alkalosis caused by vomiting.

9b. The low serum [K$^+$] reflects increased excretion by the kidneys and not loss in the vomitus. The increased K$^+$ excretion results from increased secretion by the distal tubule and cortical collecting duct. Secretion is stimulated at these sites by aldosterone, the levels of which are elevated because of a decreased ECV (e.g., manifested as orthostatic changes in blood pressure and pulse, no jugular venous pressure, and poor skin turgor). The decreased ECV will also prevent the kidneys from excreting HCO$_3^-$, thereby maintaining the metabolic alkalosis. HCO$_3^-$ excretion is impaired in this situation because proximal tubule Na$^+$ reabsorption is stimulated in response to the decreased ECV.

This obligates HCO$_3^-$ reabsorption because Na$^+$ reabsorption is linked to H$^+$ secretion via the Na$^+$-H$^+$ antiporter. In addition, H$^+$ secretion by intercalated cells of the distal tubule and collecting duct is stimulated by the increased levels of aldosterone.

■ CASE 10

10a. The initial acid-base disturbance represents a simple respiratory acidosis secondary to his pulmonary disease.

10b. On Day 3 a mixed acid-base disorder has developed, which has components of both respiratory acidosis and metabolic alkalosis. The metabolic alkalosis reflects the diuretic-induced decrease in his ECV. As described in Case 9, the kidney retains HCO$_3^-$ when the ECV is decreased.

10c. The patient has decreased alveolar ventilation as reflected in the increased P$_{CO_2}$.

10d. The decrease in P$_{CO_2}$ on Day 6 indicates that alveolar ventilation has in fact improved. The hypoxia associated with his lung disease, together with the decreased ventilation on Day 3, is probably the major stimulus for the increased ventilatory rate.

Review Examination

1. The daily excretion rate of total osmoles for an individual is 900 mOsm. If this individual has a urine-concentrating defect and can produce urine having a maximum osmolality of only 300 mOsm/kg H_2O, what is the minimum volume of water that must be ingested in order to prevent a rise in the osmolality of the body fluids? (Assume that insensible water loss is 1.5 L/day.)
   a. 1.5 L/day
   b. 3.0 L/day
   c. 4.5 L/day
   d. 6.0 L/day
   e. 7.5 L/day

2. Three individuals, each weighing 55 kg and each having a plasma $[Na^+]$ of 145 mEq/L, are infused with different solutions. Individual A is infused with 1 L of isotonic NaCl (290 mOsm/kg H_2O); Individual B is infused with 1 L of a mannitol solution (290 mOsm/kg H_2O; and Individual C is infused with 1 L of a D_5W (5% dextrose) solution (290 mOsm/kg H_2O). Assuming that there is no urine output, and after complete equilibration of the ECF and ICF, which of these individuals will have a lower plasma $[Na^+]$?
   a. Individual A (NaCl infusion)
   b. Individual B (mannitol infusion)
   c. Individual C (D_5W infusion)
   d. Individuals A, B, and C will have the same plasma $[Na^+]$

3. Intravenous infusion of 2 L of which of the following solutions will lead to the largest increase in ICF volume?
   a. D_5W
   b. Isotonic NaCl
   c. Hypotonic NaCl
   d. Hypertonic NaCl

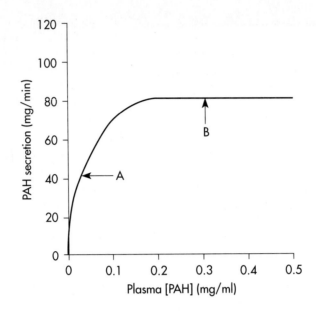

For questions 4 through 6, consider the above graph, which shows the relationship between plasma [PAH] and PAH secretion.

4. The amount of PAH filtered at the glomerulus is
   a. greater at point A than at point B.
   b. less at point A than at point B.
   c. the same at points A and B.

5. The amount of PAH excreted in the urine is
   a. greater at point A than at point B.
   b. less at point A than at point B.
   c. the same at points A and B.

6. The clearance of PAH is
   a. greater at point A than at point B.
   b. less at point A than at point B.
   c. the same at points A and B.

7. Proximal tubule HCO_3^- reabsorption is inhibited by which of the following?
   a. Increased P_{CO_2}
   b. Expansion of the ECV
   c. Systemic acidosis
   d. Decreased levels of aldosterone
   e. Hypokalemia

For Questions 8 through 11, match the appropriate diuretic with the statement.
   a. Carbonic anhydrase inhibitor
   b. Loop diuretic
   c. Thiazide diuretic
   d. K^+-sparing diuretic

8. Administration of this diuretic leads to an increase in the kidneys' ability to excrete solute-free water (C_{H_2O}).

9. Administration of this diuretic may lead to the development of hyperkalemia.

10. Administration of this diuretic impairs the ability of the kidneys to reabsorb solute-free water ($T^c_{H_2O}$).

11. Administration of this diuretic results in a decrease in renal Ca^{++} excretion.

12. An individual is stricken with an illness characterized by nausea, vomiting, and diarrhea. Over a 2-day period, this individual experiences a 3 kg loss in weight, without a change in the plasma [Na$^+$]. What can be concluded about body fluid volumes and composition in this individual?
    a. The volume of ICF is increased.
    b. The volume of the ECF is reduced.
    c. The total body osmoles increased.
    d. The plasma osmolality is reduced.

13. An individual weighs 60 kg and ingests a diet containing 100 mEq/day of Na$^+$. This individual is placed on a thiazide diuretic. After 2 months on this diuretic, and with no change in diet, what can be concluded about Na$^+$ balance in this individual?
    a. Total body Na$^+$ content is increased.
    b. Urine Na$^+$ excretion is greater than 100 mEq/day.
    c. Na$^+$ content of the ECF is reduced.
    d. The plasma [Na$^+$] is increased.
    e. The Na$^+$ content of the ICF is increased.

Match the acid-base disturbance with the clinical scenario and arterial blood gases described in Questions 14 through 18.
    a. Metabolic acidosis with respiratory compensation
    b. Metabolic alkalosis with respiratory compensation
    c. Respiratory acidosis with renal compensation (chronic respiratory acidosis)
    d. Respiratory acidosis without renal compensation (acute respiratory acidosis)
    e. Metabolic acidosis and respiratory acidosis

14. An individual with an asthma attack
    pH = 7.32; [HCO$_3$$^-$] = 25 mEq/L; P$CO_2$ = 50 mm Hg.

15. An individual with diabetes mellitus, who forgets to take insulin
    pH = 7.29; [HCO$_3$$^-$] = 12 mEq/L; P$CO_2$ = 26 mm Hg.

16. An individual with cardiopulmonary arrest
    pH = 6.85; [HCO$_3$$^-$] = 10 mEq/L; P$CO_2$ = 60 mm Hg.

17. An individual with a gastric ulcer who ingests large quantities of antacids
    pH = 7.45; [HCO$_3$$^-$] = 30 mEq/L; P$CO_2$ = 45 mm Hg.

18. An individual with a 20-year history of smoking 3 packs/day who has emphysema:
    pH = 7.37; [HCO$_3$$^-$] = 28 mEq/L; P$CO_2$ = 50 mm Hg.

19. An individual is treated with a thiazide diuretic for mild hypertension. After three months of therapy the plasma [Na$^+$] has decreased from 143 mEq/L to 135 mEq/L. Which of the following factors plays a role in the development of hyponatremia in this individual?
    a. Enhanced reabsorption of solute-free water by the early distal tubule
    b. Reduced excretion of solute-free water
    c. Shift of water from the ICF to the ECF
    d. Diuretic-induced stimulation of the thirst center
    e. Reduced effect of ADH on the collecting duct

20. An individual has a tumor of the adrenal gland that secretes aldosterone. What effect would the high levels of aldosterone have on renal electrolyte handling in this individual?
    a. Stimulation of Na$^+$ reabsorption by the principal cell of the collecting duct.
    b. Reduced K$^+$ secretion by the principal cells of the collecting duct.
    c. Stimulation of proximal tubule Na$^+$ reabsorption.
    d. Reduced secretion of H$^+$ by the intercalated cells of the collecting duct.
    e. Reduced reabsorption of Ca^{++} by the early distal tubule.

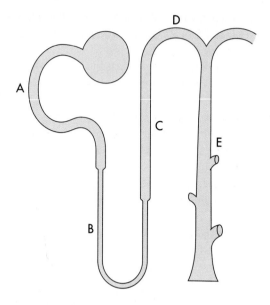

Match the portion of the nephron to the function described in Questions 21 through 24.

21. Major site of ammonium production
22. Site where calcitriol is synthesized
23. Site where PTH stimulates Ca^{++} reabsorption
24. Site where ANP and urodilatin inhibit NaCl reabsorption
25. Which of the following maneuvers would be expected to stimulate ADH secretion?
    a. Infusion of 1 L hypertonic NaCl
    b. Infusion of 1 L of an isoosmotic urea solution
    c. Expansion of the ECV
    d. Infusion of 1 L of D$_5$W
    e. An acute increase in blood pressure
26. A portion of Na$^+$ reabsorption in the late portion of the proximal tubule is passive through the paracellular pathway. What is the primary driving force for this passive reabsorption of Na$^+$?
    a. A higher luminal than peritubular hydrostatic pressure
    b. A higher luminal than peritubular [Na$^+$]
    c. A lumen-positive transepithelial voltage
    d. A lower interstitial fluid than luminal fluid oncotic pressure.

27. During a 24-hour period an individual excretes in the urine 60 mmol of NH$_4$$^+$, 40 mmol of titratable acid, and 10 mmol of HCO$_3$$^-$. If this individual is in acid-base balance, how much nonvolatile acid was produced from metabolism?
    a. 80 mmol/day
    b. 90 mmol/day
    c. 100 mmol/day
    d. 110 mmol/day
    e. 120 mmol/day
28. According to the tubuloglomerular feedback theory, an increase in the flow of tubular fluid to the macula densa will result in which of the following?
    a. A decrease in the glomerular filtration rate of the same nephron
    b. An increase in renal blood flow to the glomerulus of the same nephron
    c. Activation of the renal sympathetic nerves
    d. An increase in proximal tubule solute and water reabsorption
    e. An increase in renin secretion

Questions 29 through 31: The following graph depicts the change in tubular fluid concentration of various substances along the length of the proximal tubule plotted as the tubular fluid-to-plasma concentration ratio (TF/P). Thus, the TF/P = 1 for a substance that is at the same concentration in the tubular fluid and plasma (all substances that are freely filtered have a TF/P equal to 1 at the glomerulus).

Match the following substances to the appropriate TF/P curve.

29. Na$^+$
30. Inulin
31. Amino acids

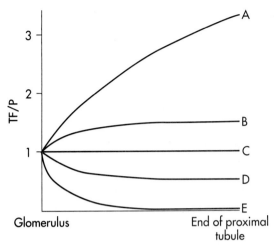

TF/P

3

2

1

A

B

C

D

E

Glomerulus   End of proximal
tubule

Proximal tubule length

32. An individual has no urine output over a 2-day period. During this time the body weight increases by 2 kg. Plasma [Na⁺] is unchanged. What can be concluded about the volumes and composition of the body fluids?
   a. The volume of the ICF is decreased.
   b. The volume of the ECF is increased.
   c. The total body water is normal.
   d. The plasma osmolality is decreased.

33. Na⁺ reabsorption by the thick ascending limb of Henle's loop is
   a. inhibited by a decrease in peritubular capillary hydrostatic pressure.
   b. inhibited by angiotensin II.
   c. increased with increased delivered load of Na⁺.
   d. inhibited by K⁺-sparing diuretics.
   e. increased by ANP.

34. A reduction in dietary K⁺ intake would be expected to alter K⁺ transport in which segment of the nephron?
   a. Proximal convoluted tubule
   b. Descending limb of Henle
   c. Proximal straight tubule
   d. Collecting duct
   e. Thick ascending limb of Henle

35. Infusion of 1 L of which of the following solutions will lead to the largest increase in the volume of the ECF?
   a. Isotonic D_5W
   b. Isotonic NaCl
   c. Hypotonic NaCl
   d. Hypertonic NaCl

36. Which of the following structures is a barrier to the filtration of proteins across the glomerulus?
   a. Capillary endothelial cells
   b. Basement membrane
   c. Lacis cells
   d. Parietal epithelial cells
   e. Mesangial cells

37. Starling forces regulate sodium and water reabsorption by the proximal tubule. Which of the following changes in Starling forces would increase reabsorption?
   a. Increase in capillary hydrostatic pressure
   b. Increase in capillary oncotic pressure
   c. Decrease in capillary oncotic pressure
   d. Decrease in the permeability of the peritubular capillary to sodium and water

38. What will occur with a decrease in the extracellular fluid volume?
   a. Increase in glomerular filtration rate
   b. Increase in angiotensin II levels
   c. Increase in atrial natriuretic peptide (ANP) levels
   d. Increase in free water clearance
   e. Increase in fractional excretion of Na⁺

39. Which of the following increases the reabsorption of sodium and chloride in the distal tubule and collecting duct?
   a. Angiotensin II
   b. Peritubular Starling forces
   c. Atrial natriuretic peptide
   d. Aldosterone
   e. Urodilatin

40. Which of the following enhances urinary potassium excretion?
    a. An osmotic diuresis
    b. Acute metabolic acidosis
    c. Hypoaldosteronism
    d. Decreased tubular flow rate
    e. A water diuresis
41. Which of the following hormones plays an important role in keeping the plasma concentration of potassium within normal limits?
    a. Calcitriol
    b. Vasopressin
    c. Parathyroid hormone
    d. Insulin
    e. Glucagon
42. The use of a thiazide diuretic that inhibits NaCl reabsorption in the distal tubule does which of the following?
    a. Decreases the ability of the kidneys to excrete solute-free water
    b. Decreases the urinary excretion of NaCl
    c. Decreases the urinary excretion of K^+
    d. Increases the ability of the kidneys to excrete a concentrated urine
    e. Increases plasma K^+ concentration
43. Diuretics that inhibit NaCl reabsorption by the thick ascending limb of Henle's loop do which of the following?
    a. Stimulate calcium reabsorption by the thick ascending limb
    b. Decrease urine flow rate
    c. Stimulate urinary excretion of potassium
    d. Stimulate countercurrent multiplication
    e. Increase the osmolality of the medullary interstitial fluid

44. A 56-year-old woman has congestive heart failure with generalized edema. Which of the following plays an important role in the formation of edema in this woman?
    a. Increased interstitial hydrostatic pressure
    b. Decreased interstitial oncotic pressure
    c. Increased plasma oncotic pressure
    d. Decreased renal excretion of Na^+
    e. Decreased venous pressure
45. Vasopressin has which of the following actions?
    a. Increases the ability of water to cross the thick ascending limb of Henle's loop
    b. Increases the ability of urea to cross the cortical collecting duct
    c. Increases the ability of water to cross the cortical collecting duct
    d. Decreases glomerular filtration rate
    e. Increases the ability of water to cross the proximal tubule
46. An individual is on a hunger strike and ingests only water for a 3-week period. At the end of 3 weeks his maximum urine osmolality is 700 mOsm/kg H_2O. Before the hunger strike he was able to achieve a maximum urine osmolality of 1200 mOsm/kg H_2O. What is the most likely cause for the urine-concentrating defect in this individual?
    a. Failure to secrete ADH
    b. Impaired NaCl reabsorption by the thick ascending limb of Henle's loop
    c. Reduced GFR
    d. Decreased urea levels in the medullary interstitium
    e. Failure of collecting duct to respond to ADH

47. A healthy individual, weighing 60 kg, is infused with 1 L of isotonic saline to which 20 mEq of K^+ has been added. Following the infusion the plasma $[K^+]$ of this individual has increased from 3.5 mEq/L to 7.8 mEq/L. What is the most likely explanation for the development of hyperkalemia in this individual?
    a. Shift of K^+ from the ICF into the ECF
    b. Impaired renal excretion of K^+
    c. Addition of 20 mEq/L of K^+ to the ECF
    d. Contraction of the ECF volume
    e. Development of hyperosmolality

48. An individual with polyuria resulting from nephrogenic diabetes insipidus is treated with a thiazide diuretic. After several weeks of therapy, daily urine output has decreased. What is the most likely explanation for the ability of the thiazide diuretic to reduce urine output in this individual?
    a. Stimulation of ADH secretion
    b. Decrease in ECV
    c. Increase in the ability of water to cross the collecting duct
    d. Increase in the sensitivity of the collecting duct to ADH
    e. Stimulation of NaCl reabsorption by the thick ascending limb of Henle's loop

49. Two individuals ingest a diet containing 100 mEq/day of Na^+. One has normal renal function. The other has renal disease, and the GFR is half of the normal value. Assuming both individuals are in steady state Na^+ balance, what would be the expected Na^+ excretion of the individual with renal disease?
    a. 0 mEq/day
    b. 50 mEq/day
    c. 100 mEq/day
    d. 150 mEq/day
    e. 200 mEq/day

50. In response to a metabolic acidosis the kidneys increase the excretion of net acid. Which of the following is the most important component of this compensatory response?
    a. Increased filtered load of HCO_3^-
    b. Enhanced reabsorption of HCO_3^- by the proximal tubule
    c. Increased synthesis of NH_4^+
    d. Reduced H^+ secretion by the collecting duct
    e. Reduced secretion of HCO_3^- by the collecting duct

ANSWERS

1. c	26. c
2. b	27. b
3. a	28. a
4. b	29. c
5. b	30. a
6. a	31. e
7. b	32. b
8. a	33. c
9. d	34. d
10. b	35. d
11. c	36. b
12. b	37. b
13. c	38. b
14. d	39. d
15. a	40. a
16. e	41. d
17. b	42. a
18. c	43. c
19. b	44. d
20. a	45. c
21. a	46. d
22. a	47. a
23. d	48. b
24. e	49. c
25. a	50. c

Index

Page numbers followed by *t* indicate tables; followed by *i* indicate illustrations.

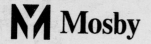 **Mosby**

Dedicated to Publishing Excellence

WE WANT TO HEAR
FROM YOU!

To help us publish the most useful materials for students, we would appreciate your comments on this book. Please take a few moments to complete the form below, and then tear it out and mail to us. Thank you for your input.

Koeppen: RENAL PHYSIOLOGY, 2e

1. For what courses are you using this book?
__medical school
__pharmacy school
__physician assistant program
__nursing school
__dental school
__osteopathic school
__undergrad
__other _____

__1st year
__2nd year
__3rd year
__4th year
__other

2. Was this book useful for your course? Why or why not?   _____Yes _____No

_____
_____
_____

3. What features of textbooks are important to you? (*check all that apply*)
__color figures
__summary tables and boxes
__price
__other _____

__summaries
__self-assessment questions

_____
_____

4. What influenced your decision to buy this text? (*check all that apply*)
__required/recommended by instructor
__recommendation by student
__bookstore display
__other _____

_____
_____

5. What other instructional materials did/would you find useful in this course?
__computer-assisted instruction
__lab time   __slides
__case studies book
__other _____

_____
_____

Are you interested in doing in-depth reviews of our medical textbooks? If so please fill out the information below.

NAME:_____

ADDRESS:_____

_____

TELEPHONE:_____

THANK YOU!

NO POSTAGE
NECESSARY
IF MAILED
IN THE
UNITED STATES

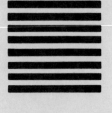

BUSINESS REPLY MAIL

FIRST CLASS MAIL   PERMIT No. 135   St. Louis, MO.

POSTAGE WILL BE PAID BY ADDRESSEE

**CHRIS REID
MEDICAL EDITORIAL
MOSBY–YEAR BOOK, INC.
11830 WESTLINE INDUSTRIAL DRIVE
ST. LOUIS, MO 63146-9987**

FOLD IN HALF AND TAPE HERE